Women's Health

Editor

JOYCE E. WIPF

MEDICAL CLINICS
OF NORTH AMERICA

www.medical.theclinics.com

Consulting Editors
DOUGLAS S. PAAUW
EDWARD R. BOLLARD

May 2015 • Volume 99 • Number 3

ELSEVIER

1600 John F. Kennedy Boulevard • Suite 1800 • Philadelphia, Pennsylvania, 19103-2899

http://www.theclinics.com

MEDICAL CLINICS OF NORTH AMERICA Volume 99, Number 3
May 2015 ISSN 0025-7125, ISBN-13: 978-0-323-37607-5

Editor: Jessica McCool
Developmental Editor: Susan Showalter

Medical Clinics of North America (ISSN 0025-7125) is published bimonthly by Elsevier Inc., 360 Park Avenue South, New York, NY 10010-1710. Months of publication are January, March, May, July, September, and November. Business and editorial offices: 1600 John F. Kennedy Boulevard, Suite 1800, Philadelphia, PA 19103-2899. Periodicals postage paid at New York, NY, and additional mailing offices. Subscription prices are USD $255.00 per year (US individuals), $471.00 per year (US institutions), $125.00 per year (US Students), $320.00 per year (Canadian individuals), $612.00 per year (Canadian institutions), $200.00 per year (Canadian and foreign students), $390.00 per year (foreign individuals), and $612.00 per year (foreign institutions). To receive student/resident rate, orders must be accompanied by name of affiliated institution, date of term, and the signature of program/residency coordinator on institution letterhead. Orders will be billed at individual rate until proof of status is received. Foreign air speed delivery is included in all Clinics' subscription prices. All prices are subject to change without notice. **POSTMASTER:** Send address changes to *Medical Clinics of North America*, Elsevier Health Sciences Division, Subscription Customer Service, 3251 Riverport Lane, Maryland Heights, MO 63043. **Customer Service: Telephone: 1-800-654-2452** (U.S. and Canada); **1-314-447-8871** (outside U.S. and Canada). **Fax: 314-447-8029. E-mail: journalscustomerserviceusa@elsevier.com** (for print support); **journalsonlinesupport-usa@elsevier.com** (for online support).

Reprints. For copies of 100 or more of articles in this publication, please contact the Commercial Reprints Department, Elsevier Inc., 360 Park Avenue South, New York, NY 10010-1710. Tel.: 212-633-3874; Fax: 212-633-3820; E-mail: reprints@elsevier.com.

Medical Clinics of North America is also published in Spanish by McGraw-Hill Interamericana Editores S. A., P.O. Box 5-237, 06500 Mexico, D.F., Mexico.

Medical Clinics of North America is covered in *MEDLINE/PubMed (Index Medicus), Current Contents, ASCA, Excerpta Medica, Science Citation Index, and ISI/BIOMED.*

PROGRAM OBJECTIVE

The goal of the *Medical Clinics of North America* is to keep practicing physicians up to date with current clinical practice by providing timely articles reviewing the state of the art in patient care.

TARGET AUDIENCE

All practicing physicians and other healthcare professionals.

LEARNING OBJECTIVES

Upon completion of this activity, participants will be able to:

1. Review methods of contraception and strategies in reproductive planning.
2. Discuss risk factors and screening methods for common infections, cancers, and diseases in women.
3. Describe the management of menopause, osteoporosis, and other age-related issues in women's health.

ACCREDITATION

The Elsevier Office of Continuing Medical Education (EOCME) is accredited by the Accreditation Council for Continuing Medical Education (ACCME) to provide continuing medical education for physicians.

The EOCME designates this enduring material for a maximum of 15 *AMA PRA Category 1 Credit*(s)™. Physicians should claim only the credit commensurate with the extent of their participation in the activity.

All other health care professionals requesting continuing education credit for this enduring material will be issued a certificate of participation.

DISCLOSURE OF CONFLICTS OF INTEREST

The EOCME assesses conflict of interest with its instructors, faculty, planners, and other individuals who are in a position to control the content of CME activities. All relevant conflicts of interest that are identified are thoroughly vetted by EOCME for fair balance, scientific objectivity, and patient care recommendations. EOCME is committed to providing its learners with CME activities that promote improvements or quality in healthcare and not a specific proprietary business or a commercial interest.

The planning committee, staff, authors and editors listed below have identified no financial relationships or relationships to products or devices they or their spouse/life partner have with commercial interest related to the content of this CME activity:
Caitlin Allen, MD; Lauren A. Beste, MD, MSc; Hollye C. Bondurant, PharmD; Lisa S. Callegari, MD, MPH; Ginger Evans, MD; Anjali Fortna, Mackenzie S. Fuller, BA; Carolyn Gardella, MD; Sharon K. Gill, MD; Anna L. Golob, MD; George N. Ioannou, BMBCh, MS; Kay M. Johnson, MD, MPH; Christine Kolehmainen, MD, MS; Mary B. Laya, MD, MPH; Ximena A. Levander, MD; Erica W. Ma, BA; Jessica McCool, Kim M. O'Connor, MD; Maryann K. Overland, MD; Andrea Prabhu, MD; Santha Priya; Eleanor Bimla Schwarz, MD, MS; Megan Suermann; Nancy Sugg, MD, MPH; Eliza L. Sutton, MD; Traci A. Takahashi, MD, MPH; Lauren Thaxton, MD, MBA; Alan G. Waxman, MD, MPH; Joyce E. Wipf, MD; Jennifer J. Wright, MD.

The planning committee, staff, authors and editors listed below have identified financial relationships or relationships to products or devices they or their spouse/life partner have with commercial interest related to the content of this CME activity:
Joann G. Elmore, MD, MPH is a consultant/advisor for the Informed Medical Decisions Foundation, a division of Healthwise, Incorporated.
Christoph I. Lee, MD, MSHS has a research grant from GE Healthcare, a division of the General Electric Company; is a consultant/advisor for Castlight Health; and receives royalties/patents from McGraw-Hill Education and UpToDate, Inc.

UNAPPROVED/OFF-LABEL USE DISCLOSURE

The EOCME requires CME faculty to disclose to the participants:

1. When products or procedures being discussed are off-label, unlabelled, experimental, and/or investigational (not US Food and Drug Administration [FDA] approved); and
2. Any limitations on the information presented, such as data that are preliminary or that represent ongoing research, interim analyses, and/or unsupported opinions. Faculty may discuss information about pharmaceutical agents that is outside of FDA-approved labelling. This information is intended solely for CME and is not intended to promote off-label use of these medications. If you have any questions, contact the medical affairs department of the manufacturer for the most recent prescribing information.

TO ENROLL

To enroll in the *Medical Clinics of North America* Continuing Medical Education program, call customer service at 1-800-654-2452 or sign up online at http://www.theclinics.com/home/cme. The CME program is available to subscribers for an additional annual fee of USD $295.

METHOD OF PARTICIPATION

In order to claim credit, participants must complete the following:

1. Complete enrolment as indicated above.
2. Read the activity.
3. Complete the CME Test and Evaluation. Participants must achieve a score of 70% on the test. All CME Tests and Evaluations must be completed online.

CME INQUIRIES/SPECIAL NEEDS

For all CME inquiries or special needs, please contact elsevierCME@elsevier.com.

MEDICAL CLINICS OF NORTH AMERICA

Contributors

CONSULTING EDITORS

DOUGLAS S. PAAUW, MD, MACP
Professor of Medicine, Division of General Internal Medicine, Rathmann Family Foundation Endowed Chair for Patient-Centered Clinical Education; Medicine Student Programs, Professor of Medicine, University of Washington School of Medicine, Seattle, Washington

EDWARD R. BOLLARD, MD, DDS, FACP
Professor of Medicine; Associate Dean of Graduate Medical Education, Designated Institutional Official (DIO), Department of Medicine, Penn State–Milton S. Hershey Medical Center, Penn State University College of Medicine, Hershey, Pennsylvania

EDITOR

JOYCE E. WIPF, MD, FACP
Section Chief of General Internal Medicine and Physician Director, Seattle VA Center of Excellence in Primary Care Education, Veterans Affairs Puget Sound Health Care System; Professor of Medicine, University of Washington, Seattle, Washington

AUTHORS

CAITLIN ALLEN, MD
Internal Medicine Resident, Department of Medicine, University of Wisconsin School of Medicine and Public Health, Madison, Wisconsin

LAUREN A. BESTE, MD, MSc
Primary Care Service, Health Services Research and Development, VA Puget Sound Health Care System; Division of General Internal Medicine, Department of Medicine, University of Washington, Seattle, Washington

HOLLYE C. BONDURANT, PharmD
Pharmacy Service, VA Puget Sound Health Care System, Seattle, Washington

LISA S. CALLEGARI, MD, MPH
Assistant Professor, Department of Obstetrics and Gynecology, University of Washington; Health Services Research and Development (HSR&D), Department of Veterans Affairs, VA Puget Sound Health Care System, Seattle, Washington

JOANN G. ELMORE, MD, MPH
Department of Medicine, University of Washington, Seattle, Washington

GINGER EVANS, MD
Acting Instructor, Department of Medicine, University of Washington; VA Puget Sound Health Care System, Seattle, Washington

MACKENZIE S. FULLER, BA
Department of Medicine, University of Washington, Seattle, Washington

CAROLYN GARDELLA, MD
Division of Women's Health, Department of Obstetrics and Gynecology, University of Washington; Department of Gynecology, VA Puget Sound Medical Center, Seattle, Washington

SHARON K. GILL, MD
Director, Women's Health Program, VA Puget Sound; Clinical Instructor, University of Washington, Seattle, Washington

ANNA L. GOLOB, MD
Acting Instructor, Division of General Internal Medicine, Department of Medicine, VAPSHCS, University of Washington, Seattle, Washington

GEORGE N. IOANNOU, BMBCh, MS
Hospital and Specialty Medicine Service, VA Puget Sound Health Care System; Division of Gastroenterology, Department of Medicine, University of Washington, Seattle, Washington

KAY M. JOHNSON, MD, MPH
Associate Professor, Department of Medicine, University of Washington School of Medicine and VA Puget Sound Health Care System, Seattle, Washington

CHRISTINE KOLEHMAINEN, MD, MS
Internal Medicine Physician and Associate Director of Women's Health; William S. Middleton Memorial Veteran's Hospital, Clinical Adjunct Assistant Professor, University of Wisconsin School of Medicine and Public Health, Madison, Wisconsin

MARY B. LAYA, MD, MPH
Associate Professor, Division of General Internal Medicine, Department of Medicine, General Internal Medicine Center, UWMC, University of Washington, Seattle, Washington

CHRISTOPH I. LEE, MD, MSHS
Departments of Health Services and Radiology, University of Washington, Seattle, Washington

XIMENA A. LEVANDER, MD
Department of Medicine, VA Puget Sound Health Care System, University of Washington, Seattle, Washington

ERICA W. MA, BA
Professor, Health Services Research and Development (HSR&D), Department of Veterans Affairs, VA Puget Sound Health Care System, Seattle Washington

KIM M. O'CONNOR, MD
Division of General Internal Medicine, Harborview Medical Center, The University of Washington; Associate Professor, Department of Medicine, General Internal Medicine Center, University of Washington General Internal Medicine Clinic, Seattle, Washington

MARYANN K. OVERLAND, MD
Department of Medicine, VA Puget Sound Health Care System, University of Washington, Seattle, Washington

ANDREA PRABHU, MD
Division of Women's Health, Department of Obstetrics and Gynecology, University of Washington, Seattle, Washington

ELEANOR BIMLA SCHWARZ, MD, MS
Research Assistant, Department of Medicine, University of California, Davis, Sacramento, California

NANCY SUGG, MD, MPH
Associate Professor, Department of Medicine, Harborview's Pioneer Square Clinic, University of Washington, Seattle, Washington

ELIZA L. SUTTON, MD
Associate Professor, Department of Medicine; Medical Director, Women's Health Care Center, University of Washington, Seattle, Washington

TRACI A. TAKAHASHI, MD, MPH
Associate Professor, Department of Medicine, VA Puget Sound Health Care System, University of Washington School of Medicine, Seattle, Washington

LAUREN THAXTON, MD, MBA
Department of Obstetrics and Gynecology, Albuquerque, New Mexico

ALAN G. WAXMAN, MD, MPH
Department of Obstetrics and Gynecology, Albuquerque, New Mexico

JENNIFER J. WRIGHT, MD
Division of General Internal Medicine, Harborview Medical Center, University of Washington; Assistant Professor, Department of Medicine, General Internal Medicine Center, University of Washington General Internal Medicine Clinic, Seattle, Washington

Contents

military experience. Health care providers need to be aware of the unique medical, psychiatric, and psychosocial needs of women veterans in order to best serve this patient population.

Preconception Care and Reproductive Planning in Primary Care **663**

Lisa S. Callegari, Erica W. Ma, and Eleanor Bimla Schwarz

Preconception care is designed to identify and reduce biomedical, behavioral, and social risks to the health of a woman or her baby before pregnancy occurs. Few women present requesting preconception care; however, 1 in 10 US women of childbearing age will become pregnant each year. As primary care physicians (PCPs) care for reproductive-aged women before, between, and after their pregnancies, they are ideally positioned to help women address health risks before conception, including optimizing chronic conditions, to prevent adverse pregnancy and longer-term health outcomes. PCPs can help women make informed decisions both about preparing for pregnancy and about using effective contraception when pregnancy is not desired.

Index **683**

Foreword

Women's Health

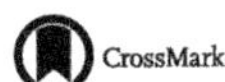

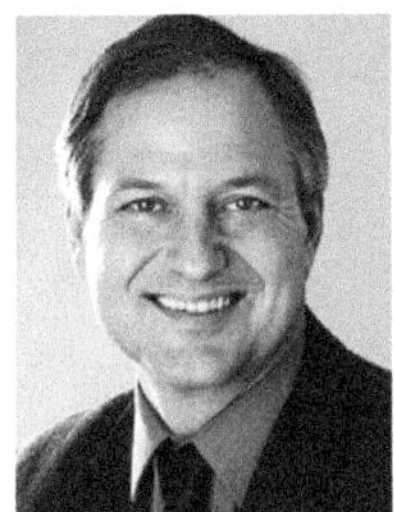

Douglas S. Paauw, MD, MACP
Consulting Editor

This issue of *Medical Clinics of North America* is dedicated to the important topic of Women's Health. Dr Joyce Wipf, an expert in women's health, has done an excellent job putting together a comprehensive issue, covering a number of key areas in women's health. Many traditional women's health issues are covered (breast cancer, cervical cancer screening, contraception, and menopause), but this issue covers areas that are becoming more understood as extremely important women's health topics (cardiovascular disease in women, intimate partner violence, and care of the Woman Veteran). I think the theme is extremely well covered, and this issue of *Medical Clinics of North America* will be very helpful in delivering outstanding clinical care.

Douglas S. Paauw, MD, MACP
Division of General Internal Medicine
Department of Medicine
University of Washington School of Medicine
Seattle, WA 98195, USA

E-mail address:
DPaauw@medicine.washington.edu

Med Clin N Am 99 (2015) xv
http://dx.doi.org/10.1016/j.mcna.2015.03.002
medical.theclinics.com

Preface
Women's Health

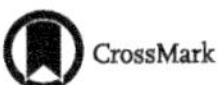

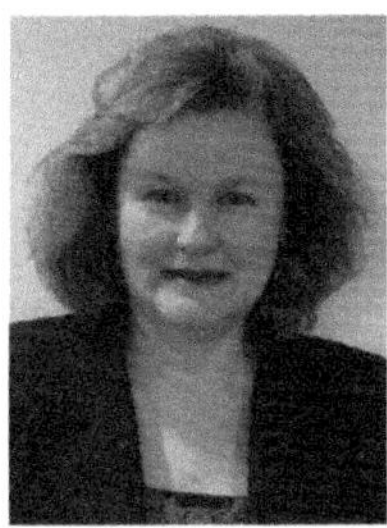

Joyce E. Wipf, MD, FACP
Editor

Women are complex. A woman's health care needs change dramatically with time and life events. It is inspiring and a joy to serve as a women's health care physician and provide guidance along this journey. Our work is challenging with continually evolving literature, data, and recommendations on clinical diagnosis, management, and screening, while taking into account essential factors of unique individual patient needs and preferences. What does "women's health" mean? Some may define it as obstetric and gynecologic conditions and gender-specific preventive health. Comprehensive women's health additionally includes primary care evaluation and management of acute and chronic medical conditions, risk assessment for screening all aspects of preventive health, and potential interprofessional collaboration.

While space constrains this issue from covering the myriad of classic topics in women's health, we focus on several important themes to provide thoughtful and in-depth reviews and the latest evidence-based practice. It is an exciting time to be a women's health provider! Even the time-honored annual health examination is changing—not going away, but focused on comprehensive preventive women's health. The articles describe recent information, sometimes reinterpretation of older data, and controversies that inform debates and support rationale for clinical approaches, guidelines, and constantly evolving recommended practice. Selected themes include the following:

- Reproductive health and contraception: Reproductive planning is an ongoing part of care of women of child-bearing age, as their personal life and needs may often change. Primary care providers need to be comfortable with prepregnancy planning, to optimize health status and conditions prior to pregnancy. Discussion includes a few selected medical conditions impacted by pregnancy.
- Common issues affecting a woman's quality of life: These include vulvar and vaginal conditions, sexual disorders, menopausal symptoms and changes, and osteoporosis.

Med Clin N Am 99 (2015) xvii–xviii
http://dx.doi.org/10.1016/j.mcna.2015.03.001

- Cancer screening: Critical review includes risk factors, evidence, and recommended approaches to cervical and breast cancer screening, benefits, and limitations of diagnostic testing and imaging.
- Emerging gender-specific data in medical conditions: Important examples discussed are cardiovascular risk assessment and liver disease in women.
- Intimate partner violence, sexual trauma, and posttraumatic stress: Personal traumas and their impact on well-being, mental health, and safety are essential issues to recognize and address in women's health care.

Special mention is warranted of the article on "Care of Women Veterans". Regardless of the setting and population of women we serve, increasingly, women's health providers will be caring for Women Veterans. Department of Veterans Affairs statistics report there are over 2.2 million Women Veterans in the United States. Comprehensive Women Veterans health care requires understanding of the impact of service and unique needs of the remarkable women who have served in our military. Each Veteran has a unique history and military experience, and medical interview will aid in determining if there are special health needs and conditions that may require consultant referral.

In summary, I am proud of this Women's Health issue and the expertise and dedication of contributing authors. Their articles help us to navigate complexities of women's health and to expand our knowledge and insights to foster excellence in clinical care.

Joyce E. Wipf, MD, FACP
Seattle VA Center of Excellence in Primary Care Education
VA Puget Sound Health Care System
University of Washington
1660 South Columbian Way (Mailstop S-123-COE)
Seattle, WA 98108, USA

E-mail address:
jwipf@uw.edu

Breast Cancer Screening

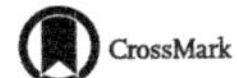

An Evidence-Based Update

Mackenzie S. Fuller, BA[a], Christoph I. Lee, MD, MSHS[b,c], Joann G. Elmore, MD, MPH[a,*]

KEYWORDS

- Breast cancer screening • Overdiagnosis • Mammography
- Clinical breast examination • Breast self-examination • MRI
- Informed decision making

KEY POINTS

- Mammography is the best-studied breast cancer screening modality and the only recommended imaging tool for screening the general population of women.
- Overall, there is a modest mortality benefit from routine breast cancer screening with mammography at the population level.
- Potential harms of routine screening include false-negative results, false-positive results with undue anxiety and benign biopsies, and overdiagnosis.
- Efforts should be made to help women make more informed decisions about participating in breast cancer screening.

INTRODUCTION

Breast cancer screening is used to identify women with asymptomatic cancer with the goal of enabling women to undergo less invasive treatments that lead to better outcomes, ideally at earlier stages and before the cancer progresses. There are important considerations for who should be screened, how often women should be screened, and with which imaging modality (or modalities). Ultimately, clinicians need to help women understand the benefits and risks of breast cancer screening to make informed decisions.

WHO SHOULD BE SCREENED?

Guidelines for who should undergo breast cancer screening vary within and among countries.[1] In the United States, the US Preventive Services Task Force recommends

---

This work was supported by the National Cancer Institute (K05 CA104699).
[a] Department of Medicine, University of Washington, 325 Ninth Avenue, Mailbox 359780, Seattle, WA 98104, USA; [b] Department of Health Services, University of Washington School of Public Health, Box 357660, Seattle, WA 98195, USA; [c] Department of Radiology, University of Washington, 825 Eastlake Avenue East, G3-200, Seattle, WA 98109, USA
* Corresponding author.
E-mail address: jelmore@u.washington.edu

Med Clin N Am 99 (2015) 451–468
http://dx.doi.org/10.1016/j.mcna.2015.01.002 **medical.theclinics.com**
0025-7125/15/$ – see front matter

that breast cancer screening with mammography be offered to women 50 to 74 years of age and that starting screening before age 50 years should be based on the individual woman's context, including her values regarding the benefits and risks.[2] The American Cancer Society recommends screening starting at age 40.[3] Screening women 40 to 49 years of age is more controversial than older ages, with less evidence available to determine the risk–benefit balance. Analyses using 6 different breast cancer simulation models of the National Cancer Institute–funded Cancer Intervention and Surveillance Modeling Network (CISNET) found that starting biennial (every 2 years) screening at age 40 years with mammography, in comparison to age 50 years, was associated with reduced breast cancer mortality by an additional 3%, but at the expense of more false-positive results and greater use of health care resources.[4]

There is little evidence to support screening women of average risk less than 40 years of age. These women have a lower incidence of breast cancer and were largely excluded from randomized controlled trials (RCTs) involving screening mammography. Similarly, there is little evidence regarding screening women more than 75 years of age because older women were also largely excluded from RCTs. Moreover, elderly women are more likely to have comorbid medical conditions and may experience less marginal benefit from screening. It is not recommended that people with limited life expectancy (<5 years) undergo routine screening, as early breast cancer detection and treatment could impair quality of life while not improving survival. However, women with limited life expectancy continue to be screened for breast cancer in the United States.[5]

HOW OFTEN SHOULD WOMEN BE SCREENED?

Countries vary in how often they recommend women undergo breast cancer screening. In a prospective cohort study of US women, it was found that after 10 years of screening with mammography, the cumulative probability of a woman receiving a false-positive recall (being called back for additional examination after abnormal screening but subsequently found to not have cancer) was lower with biennial screening than with annual screening.[6] In addition, analyses using 6 CISNET simulation models found that biennial screening mammography maintained most of the benefit of annual screening while reducing false-positive results by almost one-half.[4] The US Preventive Services Task Force, therefore, recommends currently that women without additional risk factors be offered screening mammography biennially starting at age 50.

METHODS OF BREAST CANCER SCREENING

Breast cancer screening modalities include both physical breast examinations as well as mammographic imaging. Additional supplemental screening with breast MRI may be considered for special high-risk populations.

Physical Examination

Breast self-examination

Many awareness campaigns encourage women to conduct monthly breast self-examinations. However, the evidence for mortality reduction from breast self-examination is limited. This topic has been investigated in RCTs, case-control studies, nonrandomized trials, and cohort studies.[7] Although breast self-examination may lead to detection of lesions at a smaller size, increased false-positive results and more testing have been noted with no reduction in mortality. Breast self-examination is no longer recommended by most guidelines.

Clinical breast examination

Clinical breast examination by a health care provider has been studied as a screening method used in conjunction with mammography. In the Canadian National Breast Screening Study of women age 50 to 59 years receiving either mammography and clinical breast examination or only clinical breast examination, the 25-year cumulative mortality from breast cancer diagnosed during the screening period was essentially equivalent between women who received mammography and clinical breast examination versus women who received only clinical breast examination.[8] Of note, the clinical breast examinations were performed by well-trained clinicians, the quality of the clinical breast examinations were evaluated periodically, and the clinicians spent 5 to 10 minutes examining each breast.[9] Community clinicians may not perform such high-quality clinical breast examinations, limiting the applicability of these results to general practice.

Imaging

Sample images of a screen-detected breast cancer noted in the right breast by full-field digital mammography and then seen on MRI and ultrasound are included in **Fig. 1**.

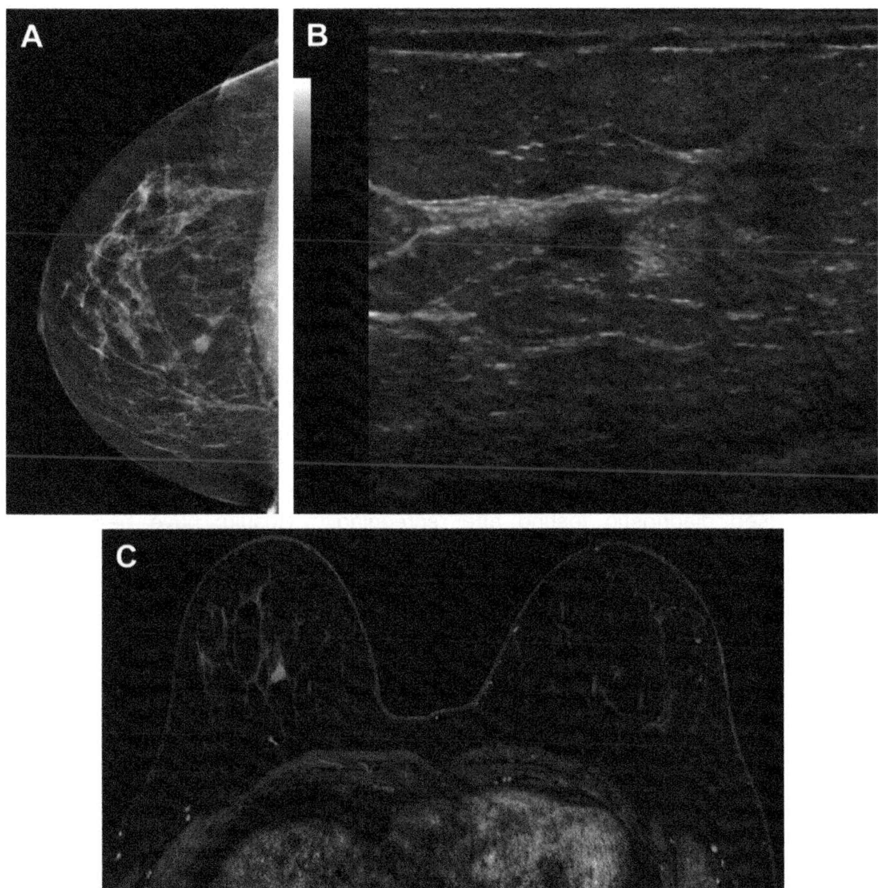

Fig. 1. Invasive cancer as seen by the following modalities: (*A*) screening mammogram, (*B*) ultrasound, and (*C*) MRI.

Screen-film mammography

Historically, screen-film mammography has been the standard method of breast cancer screening. In screen-film mammography, images were developed and fixed chemically, a process similar to film photography. Processing errors led to greater than 20% of images being rejected,[10] resulting in repeat imaging, which increased examination time, exposure to ionizing radiation, and costs. In the United States, screen-film mammography has now largely been replaced by full-field digital mammography.

Full-field digital mammography

In full-field digital mammography, images are displayed immediately on a computer monitor for interpretation, enabling more rapid interpretation than with screen-film mammography.[11] The digital display also enables the use of computer-aided detection (CAD) software, which recognizes suspicious image patterns to aid in cancer detection. Full-field digital mammography has been shown to have higher contrast, lower noise, and greater dynamic range than screen-film mammography.[12]

Several clinical trials have found full-field digital mammography to be of similar or greater accuracy than screen-film mammography.[13–15] The Digital Mammography Imaging Screening Trial (DMIST) found full-field digital mammography to be of similar accuracy to screen-film mammography overall and of greater accuracy than screen-film mammography for 3 subpopulations: women less than 50 years of age, premenopausal or perimenopausal women, and women with mammographically dense breast tissue.[16] Given this evidence and the other benefits of full-field digital mammography, including ease of storage and retrieval of images, full-field digital mammography has been progressively adopted as the modality of choice for breast cancer screening in the United States,[17] and now accounts for more than 95% of all functioning mammography units in the United States.[18]

Computer-aided detection

CAD software highlights potentially abnormal image features for radiologists. Early reports suggested that CAD was associated with improved detection of malignancies when used with either screen-film mammography or full-field digital mammography.[19,20] However, other reports suggest that CAD results in a significantly higher rate of false positives, as the programs usually add 2 to 5 marks per screening case on typical screening examinations.[19,21–23] In addition, the effect of CAD on patient outcomes (eg, mortality) is currently uncertain. CAD has been found to increase detection of ductal carcinoma in situ (DCIS) and, in women without breast cancer, is associated with increased diagnostic testing after screening.[24] Results have been mixed regarding the effect of CAD on the stage at which invasive breast cancer is detected.[24,25] Despite such uncertainty and lack of data on outcomes, CAD is widely used with screening mammography.[26]

Digital breast tomosynthesis

With digital breast tomosynthesis, a rotating gantry takes images of the breast from various angles to create a 3-dimensional view.[27] This technology, which has been approved by the US Food and Drug Administration, is now a standard feature in newer digital mammography units and rapidly diffusing into US community practice.[28] The radiation dose from digital breast tomosynthesis equals the dose from routine mammography; thus, combined full-field digital mammography and digital breast tomosynthesis currently doubles the radiation dose at screening.[29] In May 2013, however, the US Food and Drug Administration approved software allowing the reconstruction of a synthetic 2-dimensional mammography image from the 3-dimensional tomosynthesis acquisition, negating the doubling of radiation dose.

In 2-dimensional full-field digital mammography, fibroglandular tissue overlying tumors can mask them, reducing sensitivity. The 3-dimensional views that digital breast tomosynthesis provide enable radiologists to go through breast tissue slice by slice, reducing this masking effect. Two population-based screening studies in Europe and 1 large retrospective study in the United States have shown significantly increased cancer detection rates and decreased false-positive recall rates when digital breast tomosynthesis is added to full-field digital mammography.[30–32] Digital breast tomosynthesis may, therefore, reduce both patient morbidity and medical costs by reducing unnecessary diagnostic workups. In addition, digital breast tomosynthesis is less expensive and easier to incorporate into radiology workflow than other supplemental breast imaging tests, such as screening ultrasound and screening MRI.[28]

MRI and ultrasound

MRI and ultrasound are useful tools for evaluating abnormalities and diagnosing breast cancer, but they are not recommended as screening modalities for the general population. No studies have shown a mortality benefit for the general population from these imaging modalities. However, there may be mortality benefit for using MRI or ultrasound for supplemental screening in special very high-risk populations such as women with *BRCA1* and *BRCA2* mutations (see below).

Digital infrared thermal imaging

A number of emerging imaging technologies are being developed for breast cancer screening and diagnosis. One that is gaining popularity is digital infrared thermal imaging or breast thermography, which aims to detect malignancy by identifying higher local skin temperature owing to increased vascularization and inflammation caused by a developing malignancy.[33] Unfortunately, a recent systematic review concluded that there is currently insufficient evidence to recommend the use of this technology for breast cancer screening, with significant heterogeneity identified in published studies for both digital infrared thermal imaging's sensitivity (0.25–0.97) and specificity (0.12–0.85).[34]

Special Populations

Dense breasts

Dense breast tissue reduces screening mammography's sensitivity to detect breast cancer,[35] and women with dense breasts have 3 to 5 times greater lifetime risk of developing breast cancer than women with mostly fatty breasts,[36–38] regardless of other risk factors.[39] Breast density falls along a spectrum from almost entirely fat, to scattered fibroglandular densities, to heterogeneously dense, to extremely dense (**Fig. 2**). As of February 2015, 21 US states (AL, AZ, CA, CT, HI, OH, MA, MD, MI, MN, MO, NC, NJ, NV, NY, OR, PA, RI, TN, TX, VA) have enacted laws requiring that imaging centers notify patients with heterogeneously or extremely dense breasts that they may be at greater risk of developing breast cancer.[40] Some states also require, even though there are no supporting data, that women with dense breasts discuss potential benefits from additional screening (eg, ultrasound) beyond mammography with their physicians.[41]

ACRIN 6666, the largest trial comparing the addition of screening ultrasound to mammography in women with dense breasts and at least 1 other risk factor, demonstrated a detection rate of 4.3 additional cancers per 1000 women screened.[42] This increased detection was accompanied by an increase in biopsy rates from 2% to 5% of all women screened after adding ultrasound, with only 7.4% of the additional biopsies being positive for cancer, indicating a high false-positive rate.[42] Moreover, the ultrasound examinations in ACRIN 6666 were

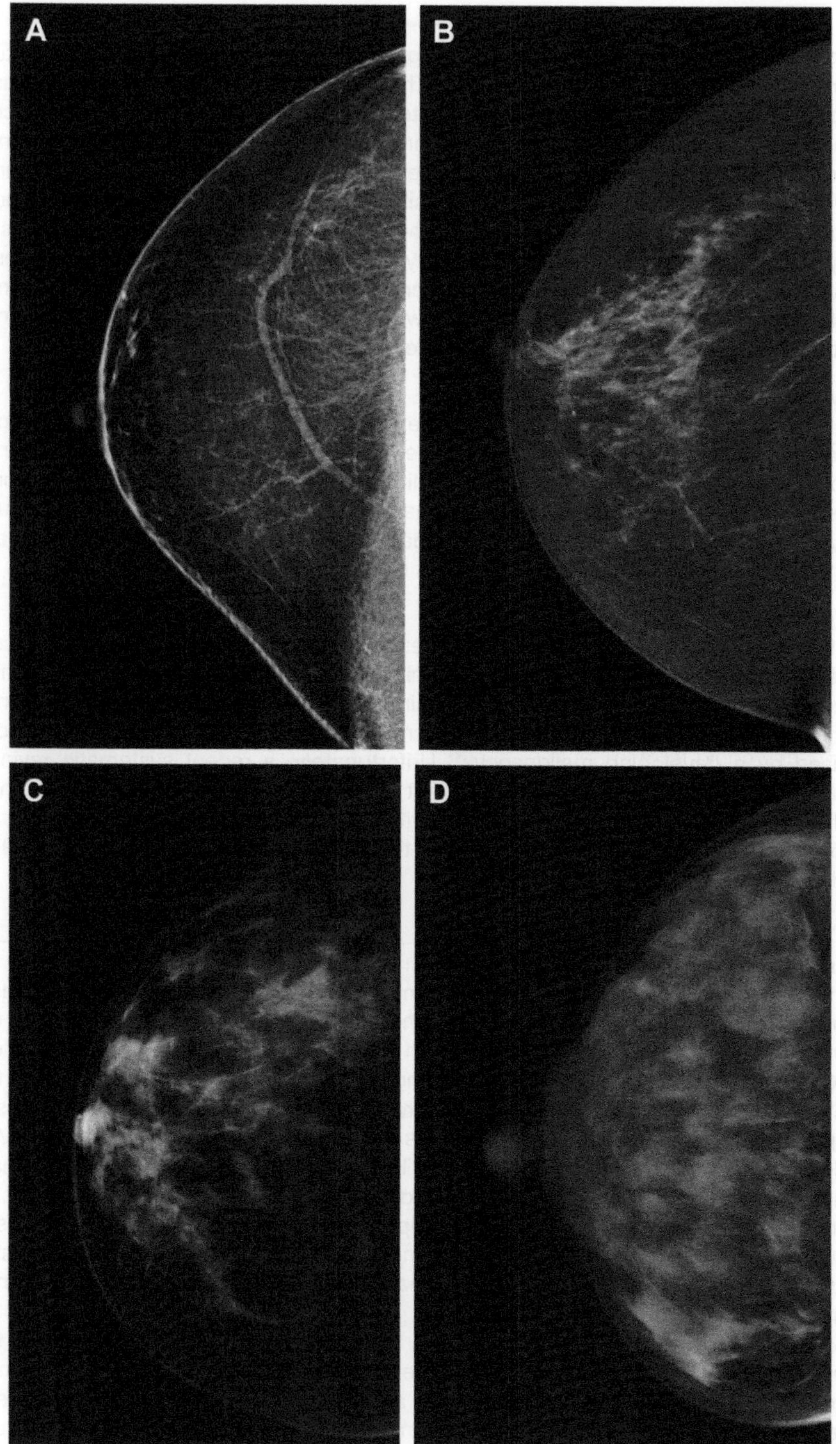

Fig. 2. Mammograms of varying breast densities from a craniocaudal view: (*A*) almost entirely fat, (*B*) scattered fibroglandular densities, (*C*) heterogeneously dense, and (*D*) extremely dense.

performed by subspecialty-trained breast imagers, raising uncertainty about what the results would be for screening ultrasound performed by general community radiologists and/or technologists.[41]

BRCA1 and BRCA2 mutations

Women with *BRCA1* and *BRCA2* gene mutations have a very high risk of developing breast and ovarian cancer during their lifetime. Two meta-analyses estimate cumulative risk of breast cancer by age 70 to be 55% to 65% for women with *BRCA1* and 45% to 47% for women with *BRCA2*.[43,44] Some carriers elect to undergo prophylactic mastectomy because of this increased risk. For women who do not choose this surgical option, there is debate about the best breast cancer screening strategy.

Generally, women with either of these mutations are advised to consider starting both screening mammography and screening MRI before the age of 40. In 1997, the Cancer Genetics Studies Consortium Task Force recommended that female carriers of *BRCA1* or *BRCA2* initiate annual mammograms between the ages of 25 and 35, using a consistent facility with prior films available for comparison.[45] Since then, the National Comprehensive Cancer Network has recommended both mammography and MRI screening starting at age 25,[46] the American College of Radiology recommends starting at age 30,[47] and the American Cancer Society recommends that individual preferences and circumstances guide the initiation of screening.[48]

Early evidence indicates, however, that mammography is less sensitive for women with *BRCA1* or *BRCA2* mutations than for women without these mutations.[49] In addition, tumors in women with these mutations grow rapidly, such that a detectable malignancy could form in between breast cancer screening examinations.[50]

There is mixed evidence concerning whether radiation, including from mammography, increases the risk of breast cancer in women with *BRCA1* and *BRCA2* mutations, with some studies showing that mutation carriers may be more prone to radiation-induced breast cancer than women without mutations[51] and other studies not showing an increased risk from radiation.[52,53] Although it is important to weigh the benefits of mammography against the risks, there is insufficient evidence to suggest that female carriers of *BRCA1* or *BRCA2* should avoid mammography owing to radiation exposure.

There have been several limitations on the studies describing outcomes of using MRI to screen women at high risk of breast cancer.[54–62] These limitations include limited numbers of screening rounds, lack of clarity regarding prevalent (first round of screening) and incident cancer detection rates, and varied underlying populations, equipment, protocols, and reporting of results. However, studies have demonstrated consistently that breast MRI is more sensitive than mammography or ultrasound in detecting hereditary breast cancer, although MRI has reduced specificity.[54–56,60,63,64] Some breast cancers are identified with mammography but missed with MRI. Annual MRI screening of women with the *BRCA1* mutation, in conjunction with annual screening mammography, has been shown in simulation modeling to be cost effective.[65,66] One approach to applying current guidelines to *BRCA1* gene mutation carriers is to alternate MRI and mammography screening in 6 month intervals beginning at age 30 years.[67]

Women with lifetime risk of breast cancer of greater than 20%

In addition to women with *BRCA* genes, annual MRI screening is recommended for women with a lifetime risk of breast cancer greater than 20%, which includes women with a strong family history of breast or ovarian cancer and women treated with radiation for Hodgkin lymphoma.[48] Unlike mammography, MRI does not use ionizing radiation, thus limiting a potential risk factor for developing breast cancer.

POTENTIAL BENEFITS AND RISKS

Potential Benefits

Mortality reduction

Screening mammography has been associated with reduced mortality from breast cancer in women 40 to 70 years of age, with absolute risk reduction increasing with age. **Fig. 3** shows the breast cancer mortality risk ratios found in RCTs of breast cancer screening. As shown in **Table 1**, adapted from a systematic review of the benefits and risks of screening mammography,[68] the number of breast cancer deaths averted with screening mammography in the next 15 years out of 10,000 women undergoing annual screening mammography for 10 years is 1 to 16 for women aged 40 years, 3 to 32 women aged 50 years, and 5 to 49 for women aged 60 years.

Decreased morbidity from therapies for cancers detected at earlier stages

When screening detects cancer at an earlier stage, a woman can undergo less invasive therapies than she would if the cancer were diagnosed at a later stage. Compared with cancers detected with physical examination (palpable tumors), breast cancers detected with screening mammography are usually smaller, less likely to have metastasized, more likely to be treated with breast conservation surgery (56% vs 32%), and less likely to require adjunct chemotherapy (28% vs 56%).[69,70] Thus, breast cancer screening is associated with increased treatment options and decreased morbidity from invasive therapies such as mastectomy and complete axillary node dissection.[71]

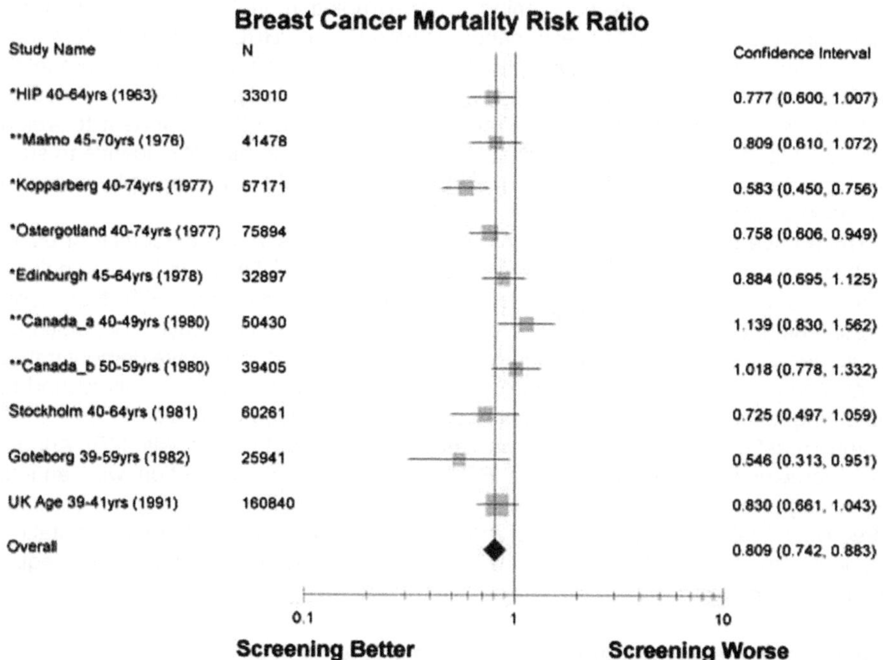

Breast Cancer Mortality Risk Ratio
Study Name
N
Confidence Interval
*HIP 40-64yrs (1963)
33010
0.777 (0.600, 1.007)
**Malmo 45-70yrs (1976)
41478
0.809 (0.610, 1.072)
*Kopparberg 40-74yrs (1977)
57171
0.583 (0.450, 0.756)
*Ostergotland 40-74yrs (1977)
75894
0.758 (0.606, 0.949)
*Edinburgh 45-64yrs (1978)
32897
0.884 (0.695, 1.125)
**Canada_a 40-49yrs (1980)
50430
1.139 (0.830, 1.562)
**Canada_b 50-59yrs (1980)
39405
1.018 (0.778, 1.332)
Stockholm 40-64yrs (1981)
60261
0.725 (0.497, 1.059)
Goteborg 39-59yrs (1982)
25941
0.546 (0.313, 0.951)
UK Age 39-41yrs (1991)
160840
0.830 (0.661, 1.043)
Overall
0.809 (0.742, 0.883)
0.1
1
10
Screening Better
Screening Worse

Fig. 3. Breast cancer screening randomized controlled trials. Results of a meta-analysis of randomized clinical trials of breast cancer screening. (*From* Glasziou P, Houssami N. The evidence base for breast cancer screening. Prev Med 2011;53(3):101; with permission.)

Table 1
Estimated benefits and risks of mammography screening for 10,000 women who undergo annual screening mammography over a 10-year period

Age of Women (y)	No. of Breast Cancer Deaths Averted with Mammography Screening Over Next 15 y[a]	No. of Women (95% CI) with ≥1 False-Positive Result During the 10 y[b]	No. (95% CI) with ≥1 False Positive Resulting in a Biopsy During the 10 y[b]	No. of Breast Cancers or DCIS Diagnosed During the 10 y that Would Never Become Clinically Important (Overdiagnosis)[c]
40	1–16	6130 (5940–6310)	700 (610–780)	?–104[d]
50	3–32	6130 (5800–6470)	940 (740–1150)	30–137
60	5–49	4970 (4780–5150)	980 (840–1130)	64–194

Abbreviation: DCIS, ductal carcinoma in situ.

[a] Number of deaths averted are from Welch and Passow[99]; the lower bound represents breast cancer mortality reduction if the breast cancer mortality RR were 0.95 (based on minimal benefit from the Canadian trials[100,101]), and the upper bound represents the breast cancer mortality reduction if the RR were 0.64 (based on the Swedish 2-County Trial[102]).

[b] False-positive and biopsy estimates and 95% CIs are 10-year cumulative risks reported in Hubbard et al[6] and Braithwaite et al.[103]

[c] Overdiagnosed cases are calculated by Welch and Passow[99]; the lower bound represents overdiagnosis based on results from the Malmö trial,[95] whereas the upper bound represents the estimate from Bleyer and Welch.[96]

[d] The lower bound estimate for overdiagnosis reported by Welch and Passow[99] came from the Malmö study.[95] The study did not enroll women younger than 50 years.

Adapted from Pace LE, Keating NL. A systematic assessment of benefits and risks to guide breast cancer screening decisions. JAMA 2014;311(13):1329.

Psychological benefit

Another benefit of screening mammography is the peace of mind some women receive from participating in screening and receiving a negative or "normal" mammogram. This benefit has not been well-documented or studied and is often ignored in risk–benefit discussions regarding population-based breast cancer screening.

Potential Risks

Pain and discomfort

During a mammogram, a woman's breasts are compressed to create uniform breast density, improve image resolution by reducing motion artifact, and reduce radiation dose. A systematic review of studies evaluating physical pain and discomfort from mammography found that reports of pain were associated with women's menstrual cycles and expectations, rather than with mammographic compression.[72] Although most women experienced some discomfort, few of these women considered compression a deterrent from undergoing screening.

Radiation exposure

Ionizing radiation can increase one's risk of developing breast cancer, as seen in women who have received therapeutic radiation to the chest (eg, for Hodgkin lymphoma).[73–75] The mean glandular dose from mammography in the United States is 1 to 2 mGy (100–200 mrad) per view, amounting to 2 to 4 mGy (200–400 mrad) per standard 2-view examination.[73,76] There is no way to know if and how many breast cancers are actually being caused by screening mammography. Still, the potential risk has prompted efforts to limit exposure by reducing the amount of radiation required for mammography screening, developing imaging modalities that do not use radiation (eg, ultrasound and MRI), and modifying screening strategies for subpopulations especially vulnerable to radiation.[77,78]

False positives

A false-positive result occurs when a screening mammogram is interpreted as abnormal in a woman who does not have cancer. In the United States, the false-positive rate is estimated to be 10% of women screened with mammography.[79,80] **Table 1** shows estimates that out of 10,000 women screened annually with mammography for 10 years, 4970 to 6130 women will receive at least 1 false-positive result in 10 years. It is estimated that 700 to 980 women who receive false positives undergo unnecessary biopsies. In a retrospective study that quantified the cumulative risk of receiving false-positive results by following women who were continually enrolled in a US health plan for a decade, the authors estimated the cumulative risk of a woman receiving at least 1 false-positive result as 49.1% (95% CI, 40.3–64.1) after 10 mammograms and 22.3% (95% CI, 19.2–27.5) after 10 clinical breast examinations.[81] The cumulative rates of breast biopsies for women without breast cancer were 18.6% (95% CI, 9.8–41.2) after 10 mammograms and 6.2% (95% CI, 3.7–11.2) after 10 clinical breast examinations.

The risk of false positives varies depending on the characteristics of women screened, the screening modality used, and the radiologist interpreting the examination.[82] Risk varies based on patient variables (eg, younger age, higher number of previous breast biopsies, family history of breast cancer, current estrogen use) and interpretive variables (eg, longer time between screening, failure to compare current with previous mammograms), and the radiologist's tendency to interpret mammograms as abnormal has the greatest effect on false-positive risk.

False-positive rates may vary by country as well.[83] One review of 32 breast cancer screening programs noted global variation in the percentage of mammograms interpreted as abnormal (ranging from 1.2% to 15%) and the number of biopsies performed (ranging from 5% to 85.5%).[84] A higher percentage of mammograms interpreted as abnormal in North America was noted, despite cancer rates being similar.[84] False-positive rates may be even higher with the use of additional screening modalities such as CAD and MRI. Studies suggest that 8% to 15% of women who undergo screening MRI are called back for additional evaluation and 3% to 15% will ultimately undergo breast biopsies.[55,56,85]

Anxiety

Emotional discomfort and anxiety can result from being called back for diagnostic workup after an abnormal mammogram. Several studies demonstrate that women who receive clear communication about negative screening results experience minimal anxiety about screening, whereas women who are recalled for additional diagnostic evaluation experience transient to persistent levels of anxiety.[86] In 1 study, women who initially received abnormal screening results but were subsequently found not to have cancer still experienced worry that affected their mood or functioning 3 months after screening.[87] A systematic review found that women who experience anxiety after a false-positive mammography result undergo more frequent future screening mammograms.[88]

False negatives

All breast cancer screening modalities can yield a false negative: a negative screening result when the patient does have breast cancer, as proven by biopsy but is clearly palpable on exam. For example, a lesion may not be viewable on imaging. Both women and their clinicians need to learn to not be falsely reassured by a normal imaging examination in the setting of a clinically detectable mass because this can lead to delays in diagnosis and treatment.

Cost

In the United States, mammography is estimated to account for almost $8 billion in annual health care expenditures.[89,90] Modeling estimates of screening mammography in the United States indicate that screening 85% of women would cost $10.1 billion with annual screening of women age 40 to 84 years (the American Cancer Society recommendation), $2.6 billion with biennial screening of women age 50 to 69 years (the European approach), and $3.5 billion with biennial screening for women age 50 to 74 years, personalized risk-based screening for women younger than age 50 years, and screening based on comorbid conditions for women age 75 years or older (US Preventive Services Task Force recommendations).[89] Other imaging modalities (eg, MRI) are more expensive than mammography, and they can result in greater recall for diagnostic evaluation.

Overdiagnosis

Overdiagnosis occurs when a woman is diagnosed with a breast cancer that would not have manifested with symptoms during a woman's lifetime; in other words, she would die of other causes before developing symptoms of breast cancer.[91] Once diagnosed, a woman might undergo treatments such as surgery, radiation, chemotherapy, and hormonal therapy, resulting in unnecessary costs and harms. Although it is difficult to determine the magnitude of overdiagnosis, the estimated range of breast cancer cases being overdiagnosed is between 7% and 50%.[92–96] As shown in **Table 1**, one estimate is that among 10,000 women undergoing screening mammography annually for 10 years, 30 to 194 women will be overdiagnosed with either DCIS or invasive breast cancer. Unfortunately, there is currently no way to determine at diagnosis of asymptomatic DCIS or invasive breast cancer whether or not the lesion will manifest symptomatically and ultimately cause harm to the woman; therefore, the current standard is to recommend treating all diagnosed DCIS and invasive breast cancer.

INTERPRETATION OF SCREENING MAMMOGRAPHY RESULTS

Clinicians receive screening mammography results for their patients in standardized lexicon using the American College of Radiology's Breast Imaging Reporting and Data System (BI-RADS).[97] Screening mammograms interpreted as normal or benign (BI-RADS assessment categories 1 and 2, respectively) correspond with a clinical management recommendation of continued routine screening, although the decision to continue screening should be based on the woman's preferences. Almost all abnormal screening mammograms are interpreted as BI-RADS assessment category 0, which indicates an incomplete assessment and request for additional diagnostic mammographic views and/or ultrasound. Some radiologists will provide a "probably benign" assessment at screening and recommend short-term follow-up mammography in 6 months. This designation corresponds with a radiologist's belief that the finding harbors less than 2% of malignancy. Rarely, radiologists will provide a BI-RADS 4 or 5 category assessment, deeming an imaging finding as suspicious for malignancy; these designations are usually reserved for after a complete diagnostic workup has been completed.

COMMUNICATION

Communication with Women Before Screening

Before women begin routine screening, clinicians should address patients' fears, concerns, and desires regarding screening, along with their underlying risk. Women may have an incorrect perception of their risk of dying of breast cancer. Although

1 in 8 women will be diagnosed with invasive breast cancer during their lifetime, the majority of women diagnosed will not die from their breast cancer. In addition, the majority of breast cancers are diagnosed in older women.

In terms of discussing breast cancer screening with women to facilitate informed decision making, physicians have traditionally been more likely to discuss the benefits than the harms of screening and frequently do not ask about women's preferences.[98] Therefore, physicians should make an effort to discuss both the benefits and the harms of screening with their patients (**Box 1**). In addition, once a woman has decided to undergo screening mammography, her physician should provide her with information to help her prepare for the examination and facilitate clear, useful test result interpretation.

Communication with Women After Screening

If a woman receives an abnormal screening result, she might be anxious about the possibility of having breast cancer. Clinicians should help women to navigate further testing and explain the likelihood that it could be a false positive based on the reported BI-RADS assessment. Women should understand that a positive screening result

Box 1
Topics to discuss with patients when deciding whether to participate in screening

Most Women Are at Lower Risk of Breast Cancer Death Than May Be Perceived

- Most women have a lower risk of breast cancer death than they might think. The "1 in 8" statistic refers to how many women will be diagnosed with breast cancer over their lifetime, with most women diagnosed in their 70s or 80s, not how many women will die of breast cancer over a certain period of time.

Mammography Is Not a Perfect Screening Test

- Although mammography will detect most cancers, some cancers will be missed, and some women will die of breast cancer regardless of whether they are screened.
- Often, women are called back for further testing because of an abnormality that is not cancer; this is called a "false-positive" result.
- Some women diagnosed with breast cancer will be cured regardless of whether the cancer was found by a mammogram.
- Some cancers that are found would have never caused problems (ie, symptoms). This is called "overdiagnosis."

Making a Decision about Mammography

- Some expert groups, including the United States Preventive Services Task Force, recommend that women aged 50 to 74 years undergo a screening mammogram every 2 years. Other expert groups recommend screening mammograms beginning at age 40 every 1 to 2 years.
- Whether a patient is likely to benefit from starting mammograms earlier or having them more frequently depends on her risks for breast cancer and her values and preferences.
- Each woman may feel differently about the possibility of having a false-positive result or being diagnosed with and treated for cancer that might not have caused problems. It is important to consider what these experiences might mean. It is also important to consider how women might feel if they decide not to undergo screening mammography and are later diagnosed with breast cancer, even if the likelihood that mammography would have made a difference is small.

Adapted from Pace LE, Keating NL. A systematic assessment of benefits and risks to guide breast cancer screening decisions. JAMA 2014;311(13):1332.

does not mean that they have cancer, only that they need additional examinations to rule out breast cancer. Similarly, women should understand that it is possible to receive a false-negative result, because no screening test is perfect.

SUMMARY

Mammography is the best-studied breast cancer screening modality and the only recommended imaging tool for screening the general population of women. Deciding when and how to participate in screening should involve a personalized discussion between a woman and her provider, weighing the individual breast cancer risk factors and competing comorbidities. In addition, a balanced discussion regarding both the benefits and risks of routine screening is warranted.

REFERENCES

1. International Cancer Screening Network. Breast cancer screening programs in 26 ICSN Countries, 2012: Organization, Policies, and Program Reach. 2013. Available at: http://appliedresearch.cancer.gov/icsn/breast/screening.html. Accessed September 4, 2014.
2. U.S. Preventive Services Task Force. Screening for breast cancer: U.S. preventive services task force recommendation statement. Ann Intern Med 2009;151(10):716–26.
3. Berg AO. Mammography screening: are women really giving informed consent? (Counterpoint). J Natl Cancer Inst 2003;95(20):1511–2 [discussion: 1512–3].
4. Mandelblatt JS, Cronin KA, Bailey S, et al. Effects of mammography screening under different screening schedules: model estimates of potential benefits and harms. Ann Intern Med 2009;151(10):738–47.
5. Royce TJ, Hendrix LH, Stokes WA, et al. Cancer screening rates in individuals with different life expectancies. JAMA Intern Med 2014;174:1558–65.
6. Hubbard RA, Kerlikowske K, Flowers CI, et al. Cumulative probability of false-positive recall or biopsy recommendation after 10 years of screening mammography: a cohort study. Ann Intern Med 2011;155(8):481–92.
7. Kosters JP, Gotzsche PC. Regular self-examination or clinical examination for early detection of breast cancer. Cochrane Database Syst Rev 2003;(2):CD003373.
8. Miller AB, Wall C, Baines CJ, et al. Twenty five year follow-up for breast cancer incidence and mortality of the Canadian National Breast Screening Study: randomised screening trial. BMJ 2014;348:g366.
9. Baines CJ, Miller AB, Bassett AA. Physical examination. Its role as a single screening modality in the Canadian National Breast Screening Study. Cancer 1989;63(9):1816–22.
10. Iared W, Shigueoka DC, Torloni MR, et al. Comparative evaluation of digital mammography and film mammography: systematic review and meta-analysis. Sao Paulo Med J 2011;129(4):250–60.
11. Pisano ED, Yaffe MJ. Digital mammography. Radiology 2005;234(2):353–62.
12. Shtern F. Digital mammography and related technologies: a perspective from the National Cancer Institute. Radiology 1992;183(3):629–30.
13. Skaane P. Studies comparing screen-film mammography and full-field digital mammography in breast cancer screening: updated review. Acta Radiol 2009;50(1):3–14.
14. Skaane P, Hofvind S, Skjennald A. Randomized trial of screen-film versus full-field digital mammography with soft-copy reading in population-based

screening program: follow-up and final results of Oslo II study. Radiology 2007;244(3):708–17.
15. Skaane P, Skjennald A, Young K, et al. Follow-up and final results of the Oslo I Study comparing screen-film mammography and full-field digital mammography with soft-copy reading. Acta Radiol 2005;46(7):679–89.
16. Pisano ED, Gatsonis CA, Yaffe MJ, et al. American College of Radiology Imaging Network digital mammographic imaging screening trial: objectives and methodology. Radiology 2005;236(2):404–12.
17. Houssami N, Ciatto S. The evolving role of new imaging methods in breast screening. Prev Med 2011;53(3):123–6.
18. US Food and Drug Administration. Mammography Quality Standards Act and Program (MQSA) National Statistics. 2014. Available at: http://www.fda.gov/Radiation-EmittingProducts/MammographyQualityStandardsActandProgram/FacilityScorecard/ucm113858.htm. Accessed September 26, 2014.
19. Warren Burhenne LJ, Wood SA, D'Orsi CJ, et al. Potential contribution of computer-aided detection to the sensitivity of screening mammography. Radiology 2000;215(2):554–62.
20. Brem RF, Baum J, Lechner M, et al. Improvement in sensitivity of screening mammography with computer-aided detection: a multiinstitutional trial. AJR Am J Roentgenol 2003;181(3):687–93.
21. The JS, Schilling KJ, Hoffmeister JW, et al. Detection of breast cancer with full-field digital mammography and computer-aided detection. AJR Am J Roentgenol 2009;192(2):337–40.
22. Yang SK, Moon WK, Cho N, et al. Screening mammography-detected cancers: sensitivity of a computer-aided detection system applied to full-field digital mammograms. Radiology 2007;244(1):104–11.
23. Freer TW, Ulissey MJ. Screening mammography with computer-aided detection: prospective study of 12,860 patients in a community breast center. Radiology 2001;220(3):781–6.
24. Fenton JJ, Xing G, Elmore JG, et al. Short-term outcomes of screening mammography using computer-aided detection: a population-based study of Medicare enrollees. Ann Intern Med 2013;158(8):580–7.
25. Fenton JJ, Abraham L, Taplin SH, et al. Effectiveness of computer-aided detection in community mammography practice. J Natl Cancer Inst 2011;103(15):1152–61.
26. Rao VM, Levin DC, Parker L, et al. How widely is computer-aided detection used in screening and diagnostic mammography? J Am Coll Radiol 2010;7(10):802–5.
27. Diekmann F, Bick U. Breast tomosynthesis. Semin Ultrasound CT MR 2011;32(4):281–7.
28. Gur D. Tomosynthesis: potential clinical role in breast imaging. AJR Am J Roentgenol 2007;189(3):614–5.
29. Lee CI, Lehman CD. Digital breast tomosynthesis and the challenges of implementing an emerging breast cancer screening technology into clinical practice. J Am Coll Radiol 2013;10(12):913–7.
30. Ciatto S, Houssami N, Bernardi D, et al. Integration of 3D digital mammography with tomosynthesis for population breast-cancer screening (STORM): a prospective comparison study. Lancet Oncol 2013;14(7):583–9.
31. Skaane P, Bandos AI, Gullien R, et al. Comparison of digital mammography alone and digital mammography plus tomosynthesis in a population-based screening program. Radiology 2013;267(1):47–56.

32. Friedewald SM, Rafferty EA, Rose SL, et al. Breast cancer screening using tomosynthesis in combination with digital mammography. JAMA 2014;311(24):2499–507.
33. Anbar M. Clinical thermal imaging today. IEEE Eng Med Biol Mag 1998;17(4):25–33.
34. Vreugdenburg TD, Willis CD, Mundy L, et al. A systematic review of elastography, electrical impedance scanning, and digital infrared thermography for breast cancer screening and diagnosis. Breast Cancer Res Treat 2013;137(3):665–76.
35. Ciatto S, Visioli C, Paci E, et al. Breast density as a determinant of interval cancer at mammographic screening. Br J Cancer 2004;90(2):393–6.
36. McCormack VA, dos Santos Silva I. Breast density and parenchymal patterns as markers of breast cancer risk: a meta-analysis. Cancer Epidemiol Biomarkers Prev 2006;15(6):1159–69.
37. Byrne C, Schairer C, Wolfe J, et al. Mammographic features and breast cancer risk: effects with time, age, and menopause status. J Natl Cancer Inst 1995;87(21):1622–9.
38. Boyd NF, Guo H, Martin LJ, et al. Mammographic density and the risk and detection of breast cancer. N Engl J Med 2007;356(3):227–36.
39. Vachon CM, van Gils CH, Sellers TA, et al. Mammographic density, breast cancer risk and risk prediction. Breast Cancer Res 2007;9(6):217.
40. Are you dense advocacy Inc. D.E.N.S.E. state efforts. Available at: http://www.areyoudenseadvocacy.org/dense/. Accessed September 8, 2014.
41. Lee CI, Bassett LW, Lehman CD. Breast density legislation and opportunities for patient-centered outcomes research. Radiology 2012;264(3):632–6.
42. Berg WA, Zhang Z, Lehrer D, et al. Detection of breast cancer with addition of annual screening ultrasound or a single screening MRI to mammography in women with elevated breast cancer risk. JAMA 2012;307(13):1394–404.
43. Antoniou A, Pharoah PD, Narod S, et al. Average risks of breast and ovarian cancer associated with BRCA1 or BRCA2 mutations detected in case Series unselected for family history: a combined analysis of 22 studies. Am J Hum Genet 2003;72(5):1117–30.
44. Chen S, Parmigiani G. Meta-analysis of BRCA1 and BRCA2 penetrance. J Clin Oncol 2007;25(11):1329–33.
45. Burke W, Daly M, Garber J, et al. Recommendations for follow-up care of individuals with an inherited predisposition to cancer. II. BRCA1 and BRCA2. Cancer Genetics Studies Consortium. JAMA 1997;277(12):997–1003.
46. National Comprehensive Cancer Network (NCCN). NCCN clinical practice guidelines in oncology: breast cancer. 2nd edition. Jenkintown (PA): National Comprehensive Cancer Network; 2011.
47. Lee CH, Dershaw DD, Kopans D, et al. Breast cancer screening with imaging: recommendations from the Society of Breast Imaging and the ACR on the use of mammography, breast MRI, breast ultrasound, and other technologies for the detection of clinically occult breast cancer. J Am Coll Radiol 2010;7(1):18–27.
48. Saslow D, Boetes C, Burke W, et al. American Cancer Society guidelines for breast screening with MRI as an adjunct to mammography. CA Cancer J Clin 2007;57(2):75–89.
49. Tilanus-Linthorst M, Verhoog L, Obdeijn IM, et al. A BRCA1/2 mutation, high breast density and prominent pushing margins of a tumor independently contribute to a frequent false-negative mammography. Int J Cancer 2002;102(1):91–5.

50. Tilanus-Linthorst MM, Kriege M, Boetes C, et al. Hereditary breast cancer growth rates and its impact on screening policy. Eur J Cancer 2005;41(11): 1610–7.
51. Andrieu N, Easton DF, Chang-Claude J, et al. Effect of chest X-rays on the risk of breast cancer among BRCA1/2 mutation carriers in the international BRCA1/2 carrier cohort study: a report from the EMBRACE, GENEPSO, GEO-HEBON, and IBCCS Collaborators' Group. J Clin Oncol 2006;24(21):3361–6.
52. Narod SA, Lubinski J, Ghadirian P, et al. Screening mammography and risk of breast cancer in BRCA1 and BRCA2 mutation carriers: a case-control study. Lancet Oncol 2006;7(5):402–6.
53. Goldfrank D, Chuai S, Bernstein JL, et al. Effect of mammography on breast cancer risk in women with mutations in BRCA1 or BRCA2. Cancer Epidemiol Biomarkers Prev 2006;15(11):2311–3.
54. Warner E, Plewes DB, Hill KA, et al. Surveillance of BRCA1 and BRCA2 mutation carriers with magnetic resonance imaging, ultrasound, mammography, and clinical breast examination. JAMA 2004;292(11):1317–25.
55. Kriege M, Brekelmans CT, Boetes C, et al. Efficacy of MRI and mammography for breast-cancer screening in women with a familial or genetic predisposition. N Engl J Med 2004;351(5):427–37.
56. Leach MO, Boggis CR, Dixon AK, et al. Screening with magnetic resonance imaging and mammography of a UK population at high familial risk of breast cancer: a prospective multicentre cohort study (MARIBS). Lancet 2005;365(9473): 1769–78.
57. Lehman CD, Blume JD, Weatherall P, et al. Screening women at high risk for breast cancer with mammography and magnetic resonance imaging. Cancer 2005;103(9):1898–905.
58. Lehman CD, Isaacs C, Schnall MD, et al. Cancer yield of mammography, MR, and US in high-risk women: prospective multi-institution breast cancer screening study. Radiology 2007;244(2):381–8.
59. Sardanelli F, Podo F, D'Agnolo G, et al. Multicenter comparative multimodality surveillance of women at genetic-familial high risk for breast cancer (HIBCRIT study): interim results. Radiology 2007;242(3):698–715.
60. Kuhl C, Weigel S, Schrading S, et al. Prospective multicenter cohort study to refine management recommendations for women at elevated familial risk of breast cancer: the EVA trial. J Clin Oncol 2010;28(9):1450–7.
61. Shah P, Rosen M, Stopfer J, et al. Prospective study of breast MRI in BRCA1 and BRCA2 mutation carriers: effect of mutation status on cancer incidence. Breast Cancer Res Treat 2009;118(3):539–46.
62. Rijnsburger AJ, Obdeijn IM, Kaas R, et al. BRCA1-associated breast cancers present differently from BRCA2-associated and familial cases: long-term follow-up of the Dutch MRISC Screening Study. J Clin Oncol 2010;28(36): 5265–73.
63. Weinstein SP, Localio AR, Conant EF, et al. Multimodality screening of high-risk women: a prospective cohort study. J Clin Oncol 2009;27(36):6124–8.
64. Sardanelli F, Podo F, Santoro F, et al. Multicenter surveillance of women at high genetic breast cancer risk using mammography, ultrasonography, and contrast-enhanced magnetic resonance imaging (The High Breast Cancer Risk Italian 1 Study): final results. Invest Radiol 2011;46(2):94–105.
65. Plevritis SK, Kurian AW, Sigal BM, et al. Cost-effectiveness of screening BRCA1/2 mutation carriers with breast magnetic resonance imaging. JAMA 2006; 295(20):2374–84.

66. Lee JM, McMahon PM, Kong CY, et al. Cost-effectiveness of breast MR imaging and screen-film mammography for screening BRCA1 gene mutation carriers. Radiology 2010;254(3):793–800.
67. Cott Chubiz JE, Lee JM, Gilmore ME, et al. Cost-effectiveness of alternating magnetic resonance imaging and digital mammography screening in BRCA1 and BRCA2 gene mutation carriers. Cancer 2012;119:1266–76.
68. Pace LE, Keating NL. A systematic assessment of benefits and risks to guide breast cancer screening decisions. JAMA 2014;311(13):1327–35.
69. Barth RJ Jr, Gibson GR, Carney PA, et al. Detection of breast cancer on screening mammography allows patients to be treated with less-toxic therapy. AJR Am J Roentgenol 2005;184(1):324–9.
70. Leung JW. Screening mammography reduces morbidity of breast cancer treatment. AJR Am J Roentgenol 2005;184(5):1508–9.
71. Freedman GM, Anderson PR, Goldstein LJ, et al. Routine mammography is associated with earlier stage disease and greater eligibility for breast conservation in breast carcinoma patients age 40 years and older. Cancer 2003;98(5): 918–25.
72. Armstrong K, Moye E, Williams S, et al. Screening mammography in women 40 to 49 years of age: a systematic review for the American College of Physicians. Ann Intern Med 2007;146(7):516–26.
73. Elmore JG, Lee CI. Radiation-related risks of imaging studies. UpToDate 2012. Available at: http://www.uptodate.com/contents/radiation-related-risks-of-imaging-studies. Accessed November 21, 2012.
74. Olsson H, Baldetorp B, Ferno M, et al. Relation between the rate of tumour cell proliferation and latency time in radiation associated breast cancer. BMC Cancer 2003;3:11.
75. Janjan NA, Zellmer DL. Calculated risk of breast cancer following mantle irradiation determined by measured dose. Cancer Detect Prev 1992;16(5–6):273–82.
76. Suleiman OH, Spelic DC, McCrohan JL, et al. Mammography in the 1990s: the United States and Canada. Radiology 1999;210(2):345–51.
77. Helzlsouer KJ, Harris EL, Parshad R, et al. Familial clustering of breast cancer: possible interaction between DNA repair proficiency and radiation exposure in the development of breast cancer. Int J Cancer 1995;64(1):14–7.
78. Swift M, Morrell D, Massey RB, et al. Incidence of cancer in 161 families affected by ataxia-telangiectasia. N Engl J Med 1991;325(26):1831–6.
79. Johns LE, Moss SM, Age Trial Management Group. False-positive results in the randomized controlled trial of mammographic screening from age 40 ("Age" trial). Cancer Epidemiol Biomarkers Prev 2010;19(11):2758–64.
80. Breast Cancer Surveillance Consortium (NCI). 2012. Available at: http://breastscreening.cancer.gov/. Accessed November 20, 2012.
81. Elmore JG, Barton MB, Moceri VM, et al. Ten-year risk of false positive screening mammograms and clinical breast examinations. N Engl J Med 1998;338(16): 1089–96.
82. Christiansen CL, Wang F, Barton MB, et al. Predicting the cumulative risk of false-positive mammograms. J Natl Cancer Inst 2000;92(20):1657–66.
83. Smith-Bindman R, Chu PW, Miglioretti DL, et al. Comparison of screening mammography in the United States and the United Kingdom. JAMA 2003; 290(16):2129–37.
84. Elmore JG, Nakano CY, Koepsell TD, et al. International variation in screening mammography interpretations in community-based programs. J Natl Cancer Inst 2003;95(18):1384–93.

85. Kuhl CK, Schrading S, Leutner CC, et al. Mammography, breast ultrasound, and magnetic resonance imaging for surveillance of women at high familial risk for breast cancer. J Clin Oncol 2005;23(33):8469–76.
86. Brett J, Bankhead C, Henderson B, et al. The psychological impact of mammographic screening. A systematic review. Psychooncology 2005;14(11):917–38.
87. Lerman C, Trock B, Rimer BK, et al. Psychological side effects of breast cancer screening. Health Psychol 1991;10(4):259–67.
88. Brewer NT, Salz T, Lillie SE. Systematic review: the long-term effects of false-positive mammograms. Ann Intern Med 2007;146(7):502–10.
89. O'Donoghue C, Eklund M, Ozanne EM, et al. Aggregate cost of mammography screening in the United States: comparison of current practice and advocated guidelines. Ann Intern Med 2014;160(3):145–53.
90. Elmore JG, Gross CP. The cost of breast cancer screening in the United States: a picture is worth... a billion dollars? Ann Intern Med 2014;160(3):203.
91. Welch HG, Black WC. Overdiagnosis in cancer. J Natl Cancer Inst 2010;102(9):605–13.
92. Gotzsche PC, Jorgensen KJ, Maehlen J, et al. Estimation of lead time and overdiagnosis in breast cancer screening. Br J Cancer 2009;100(1):219 [author reply: 220].
93. Duffy SW, Lynge E, Jonsson H, et al. Complexities in the estimation of overdiagnosis in breast cancer screening. Br J Cancer 2008;99(7):1176–8.
94. Gotzsche PC, Nielsen M. Screening for breast cancer with mammography. Cochrane Database Syst Rev 2006;(4):CD001877.
95. Zackrisson S, Andersson I, Janzon L, et al. Rate of over-diagnosis of breast cancer 15 years after end of Malmo mammographic screening trial: follow-up study. BMJ 2006;332(7543):689–92.
96. Bleyer A, Welch HG. Effect of three decades of screening mammography on breast-cancer incidence. N Engl J Med 2012;367(21):1998–2005.
97. American College of Radiology. ACR breast imaging reporting and data system (BI-RADS). Breast imaging atlas. 5th edition. Renton (VA): American College of Radiology; 2013.
98. Hoffman RM, Lewis CL, Pignone MP, et al. Decision-making processes for breast, colorectal, and prostate cancer screening: the DECISIONS survey. Med Decis Making 2010;30(Suppl 5):53S–64S.
99. Welch H, Passow HJ. Quantifying the benefits and harms of screening mammography. JAMA Intern Med 2014;174(3):448–54.
100. Miller AB, To T, Baines CJ, et al. The Canadian National Breast Screening Study-1: breast cancer mortality after 11 to 16 years of follow-up. A randomized screening trial of mammography in women age 40 to 49 years. Ann Intern Med 2002;137(5 Pt 1):305–12.
101. Miller AB, To T, Baines CJ, et al. Canadian National Breast Screening Study-2: 13-year results of a randomized trial in women aged 50-59 years. J Natl Cancer Inst 2000;92(18):1490–9.
102. Tabar L, Vitak B, Chen TH, et al. Swedish two-county trial: impact of mammographic screening on breast cancer mortality during 3 decades. Radiology 2011;260(3):658–63.
103. Braithwaite D, Zhu W, Hubbard RA, et al. Screening outcomes in older US women undergoing multiple mammograms in community practice: does interval, age, or comorbidity score affect tumor characteristics or false positive rates? J Natl Cancer Inst 2013;105(5):334–41.

Cervical Cancer Prevention

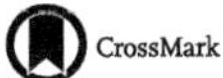

Immunization and Screening 2015

Lauren Thaxton, MD, MBA, Alan G. Waxman, MD, MPH*

KEYWORDS

• Cervical cancer screening • Human papillomavirus • Cytology • HPV vaccine

KEY POINTS

- Immunization against 4 types of human papillomavirus (HPV) is now recommended for girls and boys aged 11 to 12, with catch-up vaccination up to age 26.
- The 2012 screening guidelines recommend either cytology or cotesting with cytology plus a high-risk HPV test.
- The negative predictive value of cotesting is high enough to extend the interval between screening tests to 5 years.

INTRODUCTION

Worldwide, approximately half a million new cases of cervical cancer are diagnosed per year, almost half of which are fatal. The burden of disease is highest in developing countries where cervical screening and immunization are not readily available. In the United States, where screening for cervical cancer has been routine for more than 50 years, cervical cancer is uncommon, with only 12,360 new cases and 4,020 deaths estimated for 2014.[1] Approximately half of newly diagnosed cases of invasive cervical cancer are in women who have never been screened.[2] It is now well established that human papillomavirus (HPV) is the necessary agent in the pathogenesis of cervical cancer. This virus is present in 99.7% of all cervical neoplasms,[3] including essentially all squamous cell cancers and adenocarcinomas. Worldwide, HPV has also been associated with a significant proportion of cancer in sites beyond the cervix, including the anus (88%), vulva (43%), penis (50%), vagina (70%), and oropharynx (13%–56%).[4]

HPV is a double-stranded, encapsulated DNA virus. There are more than 100 types of HPV, at least 40 of which are known to infect the human genital tract and 15 are potentially oncogenic.[5] Ninety percent of cervical cancers worldwide are caused by just 9 types with types 16 and 18 responsible for two-thirds to three-quarters of cases.[6]

Department of Obstetrics and Gynecology, 1 University of New Mexico, MSC 10 5580, Albuquerque, NM 87131, USA
* Corresponding author.
E-mail address: awaxman@salud.unm.edu

Med Clin N Am 99 (2015) 469–477
http://dx.doi.org/10.1016/j.mcna.2015.01.003 medical.theclinics.com
0025-7125/15/$ – see front matter

PRIMARY PREVENTION: THE HUMAN PAPILLOMAVIRUS VACCINES

In 2006, the Food and Drug Administration (FDA) approved the first vaccine against HPV, Gardasil. In premarketing studies, Gardasil showed a high level of protection against cervical, vulvar, and vaginal lesions caused by 4 HPV types: 6, 11, 16, and 18.[7,8] In 2009, a bivalent vaccine, Cervarix, was approved by the FDA to target cervical intraepithelial neoplasia caused by HPV types 16 and 18.[9] The efficacy of both these vaccines is very high if given before initial exposure to the virus.[8,9] Gardasil has subsequently been approved for prevention of anal intraepithelial lesions in both male and female patients. The Advisory Committee on Immunization Practices (ACIP) and major professional organizations, including The American College of Obstetricians and Gynecologists (ACOG) and the American Academy of Pediatrics, recommend routine 3-dose vaccination at ages 11 to 12 (ie, before the onset of intercourse). Gardasil is approved for use in male and female patients, Cervarix for female patients only. Immunization may given to children as young as age 9 and those who have not completed the full 3 doses may be vaccinated up to age 26.[10,11] In December 2014, the FDA approved Gardasil 9, a vaccine that protects against the four HPV types in Gardasil, plus types 31, 33, 45, 52, and 58. These five HPV types in addition to HPV types 16 and 18, are responsible for 90% of cervical cancers.[6] At the time of this writing, the ACIP has not yet issued recommendations regarding this new vaccine.

SCREENING FOR CERVICAL CANCER

In 1941, George Papanicolaou and Herbert Traut[12] published a clinical trial demonstrating the value of the cytology test for cervical cancer.[12] Over the next 2 decades, clinic-based and community-based demonstration projects of the Papanicolaou (Pap) test showed both a decline in invasive cancer and general acceptability of the test to the women to be screened.[13] Since that time, screening recommendations regarding onset and frequency of screening have changed many times as our understanding of the pathogenesis of cervical cancer and the performance characteristics of available screening tests has expanded. Additionally, novel technologies, such as liquid-based cytology and HPV testing, have been developed.

Why Add Human Papillomavirus Testing to the Papanicolaou Test?

Although the widespread use of cervical cytology in the United States has been accompanied by a marked decline in cervical cancer incidence, the sensitivity of a single Pap test to identify cervical intraepithelial neoplasia (CIN) grade 2 or worse is limited, and estimated in several studies between 51% and 55%.[14–16] Moreover, the interreviewer reliability of the Pap test is low, on the order of 50% to 78%.[17] In addition, cytology is poor at detecting adenocarcinoma.[18] The Pap test has worked as well as it has despite the poor sensitivity of a single test because it is repeated periodically during the span of a woman's lifetime. Studies have shown a cumulative risk of CIN3 or worse of 0.17% to 0.50% 3 years after a negative cytology without reference to previous screening.[18–20]

Testing for HPV is now readily available, and studies have consistently shown that testing for HPV has a higher sensitivity and a higher negative predictive value compared with cytology alone.[21] Increased sensitivity, however, comes at a cost of lower specificity.

Katki and colleagues[18] analyzed the course of more than 300,000 women in the Kaiser Permanente Northern California (KPNC) system who were screened with cytology plus an HPV DNA test. In this study, abnormal cytology alone identified a cumulative incidence of CIN3 or worse of 4.7% over 5 years. The cumulative incidence among those testing positive for HPV regardless of cytology, on the other hand, was 7.6%. Of those whose cytology was negative at baseline but HPV test was positive for high-risk types, 5.9% developed CIN3 or worse by 5 years.

Ronco and colleagues[22] combined data from 4 European studies (Swedescreen, Population Based Screening Study Amsterdam [POBASCAM], A Randomised Trial of HPV Testing in Primary Cervical Screening [ARTISTIC], New Technologies for Cervical Cancer Screening [NTCC]) that included over 176,000 women randomized to cytology-based or HPV-based screening. The HPV group included both cotesting and screening with HPV alone. Although the rates of cervical cancer were comparable between the 2 groups over the first 2.5 years, there was 60% less cancer over the next 5.5 years in the group screened with HPV tests. Early diagnosis of precancer in the HPV-based test group allowed early treatment and prevention of invasion.

Although the rates of squamous cell carcinoma of the cervix have declined in the United States, adenocarcinoma seems to be on the rise.[23] Like squamous cell carcinoma, adenocarcinoma is an HPV-mediated disease. The offending type of HPV in squamous cancer is HPV 16 in 50% to 60% of cases and HPV 18 in only 10% to 20% of cases. In adenocarcinoma, this ratio is reversed with 30% attributable to HPV-16 and 40% to 60% to HPV-18.[24] In an analysis of KPNC patients, HPV testing was found to be significantly more efficient at detecting adenocarcinoma in situ (AIS) and adenocarcinoma than was cytology. Whereas 60% of AIS lesions and 85% of adenocarcinomas were cytology negative, only 20% and 22%, respectively, tested negative for high-risk HPV.[18]

The increase in sensitivity provided by addition of HPV testing to cytology allows a longer interval to be safely permitted between screens. A joint European study comparing cytology with HPV testing alone in 24,000 women in 6 countries showed a risk of CIN3 or worse of 0.51% 3 years after a negative Pap test and 0.27% 6 years after a negative HPV test.[20] The KPNC database showed a cumulative risk of CIN3 or worse of 0.26% and 0.08% 5 years after negative cytology alone and negative cotesting respectively.[25] Hence, testing with both cytology and HPV at 5 year intervals gives greater protection than testing with cytology alone at 3 year intervals. In addition, it is more likely to diagnose adenocarcinoma and adenocarcinoma in situ.

An important caveat is to use FDA-approved and clinically validated tests for high-risk HPV. The performance characteristics of these tests have been established based on large randomized clinical trials against defined endpoints such as CIN2, CIN3, and cancer. Other, laboratory-developed, tests may be analytically validated to insure internal validity for diagnosing HPV; however, management guidelines are based on established HPV load and established clinical endpoints. In addition, laboratory-developed tests are exempt from FDA oversight. Currently, there are 4 FDA-approved high-risk HPV assays: Hybrid Capture 2, Cervista, Cobas, and Aptima. Each tests for 13 or 14 high-risk HPV types at established clinically validated thresholds.

These 4 HPV tests are all approved for clinical use in the United States for 2 indications: reflex testing with atypical squamous cells of undetermined significance (ASC-US) cytology and cotesting in women aged 30 and older. In April of 2014, the FDA approved extended indications for use of the Cobas HPV test, to include primary screening in women age 25 and older. The ATHENA trial showed a 12% risk of CIN3 or worse in women who were cytology negative but positive for HPV type 16 and 10% risk in women who were positive for 16 or 18.[26] The FDA approval allows for direct referral to colposcopy if the Cobas test reveals a positive HPV-16 or positive HPV-18. Cytology triage is recommended for patients testing positive for 1 or more of 12 other high-risk HPV types. Use of this algorithm in women over the age of 25 compared favorably compared with the current recommendations for detecting CIN2 or worse and CIN3 or worse.

The guidelines that follow are recommended by the US Preventive Services Task Force, American Cancer Society, ACOG, and other professional organizations.[27–29]

CURRENT SCREENING GUIDELINES

When to Enter Screening

Cervical cancer screening should begin at age 21, regardless of age of sexual debut (**Table 1**). This recommendation is based on the natural history of HPV infection and dysplasia in adolescents and young women. In a study of female university students, the cumulative incidence of HPV infection over 24 months was 32.3%.[30] Despite this exposure, the incidence of cervical cancer before age 20 is exceedingly low at 0.1 per 100,000,[31] because most HPV infection in this age group spontaneously regresses. In a similar study of female university students, the cumulative incidence of HPV infection over 36 months was 43% and the median duration of infection was 8 months. By 12 months following diagnosis of infection, 70% of women were no longer infected and by 24 months only 9% continued to be infected.[32]

This is not to say that the female adolescent does not require well-woman care. ACOG continues to recommend regular visits in this age group to discuss safe sex practices, HPV vaccination, and contraception.[29] This does not require invasive pelvic examination, and providers are encouraged to test for gonorrhea and chlamydia by urine samples rather than traditional cervical swabs.

Screening Intervals

For women 21 to 29 years old, screening should be completed using cytology (Pap testing) alone every 3 years. This recommendation for triennial cytologic screenings is based on modeling studies showing that annual screening provides minimal benefit in cancer risk reduction while doubling the number of colposcopies

Table 1
2012 Cervical cancer screening recommendations

When to start screening	Age 21 regardless of age at coitarche	—
Screening interval	Ages 21–29	Cytology alone every 3 y (HPV testing for ASC-US triage age 25–29)
	Ages 30–64	Cotesting every 5 y or cytology alone every 3 y[a]
When to stop screening	Age 65 with 3 consecutive negative Paps or 2 consecutive negative HPV tests in prior 10 y and no history of CIN2+ in the last 20 y or posthysterectomy with removal of the cervix with no history of CIN2+ in 20 y	

Screening recommendations by American Cancer Society, American Society for Colposcopy and Cervical Pathology, and American Society for Clinical Pathology, and the US Preventive Services Task Force.

[a] Both options acceptable. ACS/ASCCP/ASCP preferred option is cotesting every 5 years. USPSTF preferred option is every 3 years.

Adapted from Moyer VA. U.S. Preventive Services Task Force. Screening for cervical cancer: U.S. Preventive Services Task Force recommendation statement. Ann Intern Med 2012;156(12):880–91; and Saslow D, Solomon D, Lawson HW, et al. American Cancer Society, American Society for Colposcopy and Cervical Pathology, and American Society for Clinical Pathology screening guidelines for the prevention and early detection of cervical cancer. J Low Genit Tract Dis 2012;16(3):175–204.

performed.[33] Cotesting with cytology and HPV testing is not recommended in this age group because of the high prevalence of high-risk HPV infection and rarity of progression of those infections to invasive cancer.[34] As discussed above, the Cobas HPV test is FDA-approved after age 25 for primary screening.

For women 30 to 64 years old, screening options include cytology every 3 years or cotesting with cytology plus HPV testing at 5-year intervals. The screening guidelines recommended by the American Cancer Society, American Society for Colposcopy and Cervical Pathology, and American Society for Clinical Pathology recommend cotesting at 5-year intervals with triennial cytology as a fallback method if HPV testing is not available.[28] Conversely, the US Preventive Services Task Force recommends cytology every 3 years as the default screening method with cotesting every 5 years reserved for those women wanting to extend the interval.[27]

When to Exit Screening

Women with adequate prior screening and no history if CIN2 or greater in the prior 20 years should exit screening at age 65. Adequate prior screening is defined as 3 consecutive negative Pap tests or 2 consecutive negative HPV tests within the 10 years before exiting, with most recent test within the last 5 years. Screening should not be resumed after it has been stopped even if the patient reports a new sexual partner.[28]

Women in this group are recommended to exit screening for many reasons. The prevalence of HPV declines with age leaving postmenopausal women less than half as likely as young women to acquire the infection.[35,36] Additionally, natural history studies have shown that the progression from HPV to CIN3 to invasive disease occurs over a similarly long timeline regardless of age of viral infection.[34,37] Therefore, even if exposed to HPV, older women are less likely to develop invasive cancer during the remainder of their lives. Low-grade cytologic abnormalities reported in this age group are more likely to be false-positive because of the decreased incidence of disease as well as atrophic changes that can be mistaken for atypia. Postmenopausal women with false-positive test results will, in turn, require expensive, potentially painful, and anxiety-provoking downstream workups with little risk reduction benefit.[38]

Special Considerations

Total hysterectomy with no history of dysplasia

Women with a prior history of removal of the cervix for benign indications without a history of CIN2 or worse, do not merit further cervical cancer screening and should not resume screening at any point, even in the event of a new sexual partner. Hysterectomy is the second most common surgical procedure performed on women in the United States. It is important for the primary care physician to note that in some instances the cervix is left in situ, known as a supracervical hysterectomy. For this reason, discussion with the patient about the details of her surgical history, as well as examination, is important before discontinuation of screening. Cytology in this group is no longer a screening test for cervical cancer. Instead, it screens for primary vaginal cancer, a very rare disease with an estimated incidence of 0.7 per 100,000 women.[39] In a retrospective cohort study of cytology from the vaginal cuff, the positive predictive value of cuff cytology for identification of vaginal cancer was zero.[40]

Continued screening after treatment of cervical intraepithelial neoplasia grade 2 or worse

The risk of cervical cancer after treatment of a precancerous lesion, although very low, remains elevated above the baseline population for 20 years after treatment.[41]

Therefore, screening should continue for 20 years even if this requires screening past the age of 65.

Screening of human immunodeficiency virus–positive women

Although screening guidelines for the general population have been revised, as outlined above, recommendations for human immunodeficiency virus (HIV)–positive women have not changed in the past decade. HIV-positive and other significantly immunocompromised women, such as solid organ transplant patients, should be screened twice in the year of diagnosis, then annually thereafter.

Screening vaccinated women

Recommendations for screening should not be modified by history of HPV vaccination. This recommendation is based on relatively low vaccination rates among young women aged 13 to 17 years old; only 37.6% have completed the 3-shot series as of 2014.[42] A large proportion of the screened population has not yet reached the age of recommended screening. Because the vaccines are approved for women up to 26 years old, many women have been vaccinated after exposure to the virus. The vaccines are prophylactic only. Therefore, women vaccinated after exposure can expect significantly less protection than those immunized before exposure; in most cases this means before the onset of sexual activity.

FUTURE CONSIDERATIONS

In 2007, Australia instituted a free school-based HPV immunization program. Since then, 70% to 72% of girls aged 15 to 17 years have received all 3 doses of the vaccine. In 2013, the program was extended to boys. In the period after initiation of the immunization program, they have seen a 61% decrease in new cases of genital warts, caused by HPV types 6 and 11, covered by the Gardasil vaccine.[43] They have seen an early decline in CIN2 and CIN3 as well.[44] Vaccine coverage in the United States is opportunistic and is roughly half that of Australia. Reasons parents give for not vaccinating their daughters include safety concerns even though the HPV vaccines compare favorably with other vaccines in terms of rarity of severe adverse events.[42] They also cite lack of knowledge about HPV, that their daughters do not need the vaccine, that they are not sexually active, and (most telling) that their health care providers did not recommend the vaccine.[42] It is not known what level of coverage will provide the degree of herd immunity needed to change the screening guidelines to reflect an immunized population. Ongoing vaccine-related research, such as the efficacy of fewer than 3 doses and the effect of implementing the new vaccine for 9 high-risk HPV types,[6] will undoubtedly contribute to the discussion of screening protocols in the postvaccine era. All that can be certainly predicted is that, just as screening recommendations have changed multiple times since the 1950s, they will surely be revised again in the near future.

REFERENCES

1. American Cancer Society. Cancer facts and figures 2014. Atlanta (GA): American Cancer Society; 2014.
2. Sawaya GF, Grimes DA. New technologies in cervical cytology screening: a word of caution. Obstet Gynecol 1999;94(2):307–10.
3. Walboomers JM, Jacobs MV, Manos MM, et al. Human papillomavirus is a necessary cause of invasive cervical cancer worldwide. J Pathol 1999;189: 12–9.

4. Forman D, de Martel C, Lacey C, et al. Global burden of human papillomavirus and related diseases. Vaccine 2012;30S:F12–23.
5. Munoz N, Bosch FX, de Sanjosé S, et al. Epidemiologic classification of human papillomavirus types associated with cervical cancer. N Engl J Med 2003;348: 518–27.
6. Serrano B, Alemany L, Tous S, et al. Potential impact of a nine-valent vaccine in human papillomavirus related cervical disease. Infect Agent Cancer 2012;7(1): 38.
7. Garland SM, Hernandez-Avila M, Wheeler CM, et al. Quadrivalent vaccine against human papillomavirus to prevent anogenital diseases. N Engl J Med 2007;356:1928–43.
8. The FUTURE II Study Group. Quadrivalent vaccine against human papillomavirus to prevent high-grade cervical lesions. N Engl J Med 2007;356:1915–27.
9. Paavonen J, Naud P, Salmerón J, et al. Efficacy of human papillomavirus (HPV)-16/18 AS04-adjuvanted vaccine against cervical infection and precancer caused by oncogenic HPV types (PATRICIA): final analysis of a double-blind, randomised study in young women. Lancet 2009;374(9686):301–14.
10. Centers for Disease Control and Prevention (CDC). FDA licensure of bivalent human papillomavirus vaccine (HPV2, Cervarix) for use in females and updated HPV vaccination recommendations from the Advisory Committee on Immunization Practices (ACIP). MMWR Morb Mortal Wkly Rep 2010;59(20):626–9 [Erratum in MMWR Morb Mortal Wkly Rep 2010;59:1184].
11. Centers for Disease Control and Prevention (CDC). Recommendations on the use of quadrivalent human papillomavirus vaccine in males—Advisory Committee on Immunization Practices (ACIP), 2011. MMWR Morb Mortal Wkly Rep 2011;60(50): 1705–8.
12. Papanicolaou GN, Traut HF. The diagnostic value of vaginal smears in carcinoma of the uterus. Am J Obstet Gynecol 1941;42:193–206.
13. Waxman AG. Guidelines for cervical cancer screening: history and rationale. Clin Obstet Gynecol 2005;48(1):77–97.
14. Cuzick J, Clavel C, Petry KU, et al. Overview of the European and North American studies on HPV testing in primary cervical screening. Int J Cancer 2006;119: 1095–101.
15. McRory DC, Batcher DB, Bastian L, et al. Evaluation of cervical cytology: evidence report/technology assessment no.5. Rockville (MD): Agency for Healthcare Policy and Research; 1999. AHCPR Publication no. 99–E010.1115.
16. Mayrand MH, Duarte-Franco E, Mansour N, et al. Human papillomavirus DNA versus Papanicolaou screening tests for cervical cancer. N Engl J Med 2007; 357:1579–88.
17. Stoler MH, Schiffman M, Atypical Squamous Cells of Undetermined Significance-Low-grade Squamous Intraepithelial Lesion Triage Study (ALTS) Group. Interobserver reproducibility of cervical cytologic and histologic interpretations: realistic estimates from the ASCUS-LSIL Triage Study. JAMA 2001; 285:1500–5.
18. Katki HA, Kinney WK, Fetterman B, et al. Cervical cancer risk for women undergoing concurrent testing for human papillomavirus and cervical cytology: a population-based study in routine clinical practice. Lancet Oncol 2011;12: 663–72.
19. Sherman ME, Lorincz AT, Scott DR, et al. Baseline cytology, human papillomavirus testing, and risk for cervical neoplasia: a 10-year cohort analysis. J Natl Cancer Inst 2003;95(1):46–52.

20. Dillner J, Rebolj M, Birembaut P, et al. Long term predictive values of cytology and human papillomavirus testing in cervical cancer screening: joint European cohort study. BMJ 2008;337:a1754.
21. Castle PE, Cremer M. Human papillomavirus testing in cervical cancer screening. Obstet Gynecol Clin North Am 2013;40:377–90.
22. Ronco G, Dillner J, Elfstrom KM, et al. Efficacy of HPV-based screening for prevention of invasive cervical cancer: follow-up of four European randomized controlled trials. Lancet 2014;383:524–32.
23. Smith HO, Tiffany MF, Qualls CR, et al. The rising incidence of adenocarcinoma relative to squamous cell carcinoma of the uterine cervix in the United States—a 24-year population-based study. Gynecol Oncol 2000;78(2):97–105.
24. Herzog TJ, Monk BJ. Reducing the burden of glandular carcinomas of the uterine cervix. Am J Obstet Gynecol 2007;197(6):566–71.
25. Katki HA, Schiffman M, Castle PE, et al. Benchmarking CIN 3+ risk as the basis for incorporating HPV and Pap cotesting into cervical screening and management guidelines. J Low Genit Tract Dis 2013;17(5):S28–35.
26. Wright TC Jr, Stoler MH, Sharma A, et al. Evaluation of HPV-16 and HPV-18 genotyping for the triage women with high-risk HPV+ cytology negative results. Am J Clin Pathol 2011;136:578–86.
27. Moyer VA, U.S. Preventive Services Task Force. Screening for cervical cancer: U.S. preventive services task force recommendation statement. Ann Intern Med 2012;156(12):880–91.
28. Saslow D, Solomon D, Lawson HW, et al. American Cancer Society, American Society for Colposcopy and Cervical Pathology, and American Society for Clinical Pathology screening guidelines for the prevention and early detection of cervical cancer. J Low Genit Tract Dis 2012;16(3):175–204.
29. Committee on Practice Bulletins—Gynecology. Screening for cervical cancer. Practice Bulletin 131. American College of Obstetricians and Gynecologists. Obstet Gynecol 2012;120:1222–38.
30. Winer RL, Lee S, Hughes JP, et al. Genital human papillomavirus infection: incidence and risk factors in a cohort of female university students. Am J Epidemiol 2003;157:218–26.
31. Howlader N, Noone AM, Krapcho M, et al. SEER cancer statistics review, 1975–2011. Bethesda (MD): National Cancer Institute; 2014. Available at: http://seer.cancer.gov/csr/1975_2011/. based on November 2013 SEER data submission, posted to the SEER web site.
32. Ho GY, Bierman R, Beardsley L, et al. The natural history of cervical papillomavirus infection in young women. N Engl J Med 1998;338:423–8.
33. Kulasingam S, Havrilesky L, Ghebre R, et al. Screening for cervical cancer: a decision analysis for the US Preventive Services Task Force. Rockville (MD): Agency for Healthcare Research and Quality; 2011. AHRQ Pub. No. 11-05157-EF1.
34. Schiffman M, Wentzensen N. From human papillomavirus to cervical cancer. Obstet Gynecol 2010;116(1):177–85.
35. Dunne EF, Unger ER, Sternberg M, et al. Prevalence of HPV infection among females in the United States. JAMA 2007;297:813–9.
36. Gyllensten U, Gustavsson I, Lindell M, et al. Primary high-risk HPV screening for cervical cancer in post-menopausal women. Gynecol Oncol 2012;125:343–5.
37. Rodriguez AC, Schiffman M, Herrero R, et al. Rapid clearance of human papillomavirus and implications for clinical focus on persistent infections. J Natl Cancer Inst 2008;100:513–7.

38. Sawaya GF, Grady D, Kerlikowske K, et al. The positive predictive value of cervical smears in previously screened postmenopausal women: the Heart and Estrogen/progestin Replacement Study (HERS). Ann Intern Med 2000;133:942–50.
39. Wu X, Matanoski G, Chen VW, et al. Descriptive epidemiology of vaginal cancer incidence and survival by race, ethnicity, and age in the United States. Cancer 2008;113(Suppl 10):2873–82.
40. Pearce KF, Haefner HK, Sarwar SF, et al. Cytopathological findings on vaginal Papanicolaou smears after hysterectomy for benign gynecologic disease. N Engl J Med 1996;335:1559–62.
41. Melnikow J, McGahan C, Sawaya GF, et al. Cervical intraepithelial neoplasia outcomes after treatment: long-term follow-up from the British Columbia Cohort Study. J Natl Cancer Inst 2009;101(10):721–8.
42. Stokley S, Jeyarajah J, Yankey D, et al. Human papillomavirus vaccination coverage among adolescents, 2007–2013 and postlicensure vaccine safety monitoring, 2006–2014—United States. MMWR Morb Mortal Wkly Rep 2014;63:620–4.
43. Harrison C, Britt H, Garland S. Decreased management of genital warts in young women in Australian general practice post introduction of National HPV Vaccination Program: results from a nationally representative cross-sectional general practice study. PLoS One 2014;9(9):e105967.
44. Brotherton JM, Fridman M, May CL, et al. Early effect of the HPV vaccination programme on cervical abnormalities in Victoria, Australia: an ecological study. Lancet 2011;377(9783):2085–92.

Oral Contraception

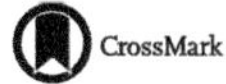

Ginger Evans, MD[a,*], Eliza L. Sutton, MD[b]

KEYWORDS

- Oral contraception • Ethinyl estradiol • Levonorgestrel • Venous thromboembolism
- Medical eligibility criteria

KEY POINTS

- Oral contraceptives (OC) offer noncontraceptive benefits, including improvement of acne, hirsutism, and dysmenorrhea.
- Many OC formulations exist; ethinyl estradiol at 20 to 30 mcg with levonorgestrel seems to confer a lower risk of venous thromboembolism than OCs with other progestins.
- Medical eligibility criteria, developed by the World Health Organization and adapted by individual countries, provide a resource to assess patients' medical situations for contraindications to OCs.
- Blood pressure measurement is the only physical examination or testing needed before OC prescription.
- Continuous daily use of OCs and extended (3 month) cycles are reasonable alternatives to cyclic monthly use and can further improve menstrual-associated symptoms.

INTRODUCTION

The development of hormonal contraception marked a breakthrough in the technology of pregnancy prevention and planning. Hormonal contraception relies on a progestin to

- Thicken cervical mucus, forming a mechanical barrier
- Suppress ovulation by suppressing the midcycle surge of follicle-stimulating hormone (FSH) and luteinizing hormone (LH)
- Keep the endometrium thin and thus inhospitable for implantation

Estrogen contributes to ovulation suppression and also prevents sloughing of the endometrium, thus reducing irregular bleeding, which can be a limiting side effect of progestin-only methods.

Disclosure: No financial relationships to disclose.
[a] VA Puget Sound Health Care System, 1660 South Columbian Way, S-123-PCC, Seattle, WA 98108, USA; [b] Women's Health Care Center, University of Washington, 4245 Roosevelt Way Northeast, Box 354765, Seattle, WA 98105, USA
* Corresponding author.
E-mail address: gingere@u.washington.edu

Med Clin N Am 99 (2015) 479–503
http://dx.doi.org/10.1016/j.mcna.2015.01.004
0025-7125/15/$ – see front matter Published by Elsevier Inc.

HISTORY AND SAFETY OF THE PILL

In 1960, the Food and Drug Administration (FDA) approved the first oral contraceptive (OC), a pill containing mestranol 150 mcg and norethynodrel, 3 years after its approval for the treatment of menstrual disorders.[1] The pill has been popular, but the early high-dose formulation was associated with increased mortality from venous thromboembolism (VTE) and arterial vascular events.[2,3] With the development of other formulations, the effect of the estrogen dose and the specific progestin on thromboembolism risk were recognized,[4] leading to the development of lower-dose, lower-risk formulations. Current formulations of combination OCs (COCs) contain one-third to one-fifth of the amount of estrogen in the first COC, plus any of 8 synthetic progestins in a dizzying array of patterns (**Table 1**).

In 1973, a progestin-only pill (POP), popularly called the *mini pill*, became available. The sole active ingredient in the only POP available in the United States and Canada is norethindrone. The POP is less effective than other hormonal methods of contraception and commonly causes irregular bleeding, but it is safer than combined hormonal contraceptives (CHCs) for women in whom exogenous estrogen is contraindicated.

In 1996, the World Health Organization (WHO) developed and began a periodic review called *Medical Eligibility Criteria for Contraceptive Use* (hereafter referred to as *MEC*); the fourth edition of MEC was released in 2009[6] with subsequent updates. The MEC suggests a weighing of risks and benefits ranging from level 1 to level 4 (**Box 1**) for each form of contraception with regard to specific patient factors and medical conditions and has been adopted and adapted by individual countries for their own use. Free resources to assist in the clinical use of the MEC are available for download at the Centers for Disease Control and Prevention's Web site.[7]

PREGNANCY PREVENTION

Modern CHCs are effective for contraception, with perfect use theoretically resulting in only 0.3 pregnancies per 100 women in the first year. Actual effectiveness depends significantly on adherence. Typical use of COCs results in about 9 pregnancies per 100 women in the first year, performing significantly better than barrier methods, spermicides, withdrawal, and fertility awareness (rhythm) methods but not as well as intrauterine devices (IUDs), progestin implants or injections, or sterilization.[8] For comparison, 85% of sexually active heterosexual women conceive in 1 year without contraception.[8]

NONCONTRACEPTIVE HEALTH BENEFITS

Since the original introduction of COCs, many noncontraceptive benefits have been discovered and used; in addition, benefits have been attributed to COCs that are not currently substantiated by research (**Box 2**). Because patients are frequently unaware of the noncontraceptive benefits, health care providers have an important opportunity to debunk myths and educate patients on the real and relevant benefits.[9–11]

Acne is an important consideration to many young adult patients. All COCs are effective for relief of acne in clinical trials.[12,22] In general, about half (50%–90%) of patients will experience improvement in acne after 6 to 9 months, with an average of 30% to 60% reduction in inflammatory lesions.[29,30] The estrogen component of a COC decreases circulating free androgen via 2 mechanisms: (1) suppression of LH-driven androgen production by ovaries and (2) induction of hepatic synthesis of sex hormone binding globulin (SHBG), which leads to lower levels of free testosterone.

The comparative effectiveness against acne between formulations of COCs is unclear.[12,22] The ring and patch may not be as effective against acne as OCs because

Table 1
Ingredients and formulations of hormonal contraceptives available in the United States

Estrogen Forms and Doses	Progestin Forms	Phasing Number of Days at Each Dose of Active Medication	Cycle Number of Active Pills Per Pill Pack
EE	First-generation	**Monophasic** (estrogen and progestin dose stable over ≥21 d)	21-d Pack
10 mcg[a]	Ethynodiol diacetate	Multiphasic (progestin dose changes over 21 d)	21
20 mcg	Norethindrone	Biphasic (10 + 11)	28-d Pack
25 mcg	Norethindrone acetate	Triphasic (7 + 7 + 7)	21
30 mcg	Second-generation	Estrophasic (estrogen dose changes over ≥21 d)	24[c]
35 mcg	**Levonorgestrel**	20/30/35 mcg EE[c] (5 + 7 + 9; monophasic in progestin)	28
40 mcg[a]	Norgestrel	30/40/30 mcg EE (6 + 5 + 10; also triphasic in progestin)	91-d Pack
50 mcg	Third-generation	3/2/1 mg EV[c] (2 + 5 + 17 + 2 + 2; also multiphasic in progestin)	84
EV[a,b]	Desogestrel	Estrophasic (estrogen dose changes over ≥84 d)	84 + 7 of 10 mcg EE
3 mg	*Etonorgestrel*[c] (ring, implant)	20/25/30/10 mcg EE (42 + 21 + 21 + 7; monophasic in progestin)[5]	
2 mg	*Norelgestromin*[c] (patch)		
1 mg	Norgestimate		
Mestranol	Fourth-generation		
(EE prodrug)	Dienogest[b]		
50 mcg	Drospirenone		

This information is current as of September 2014. New brands with new synthetic hormones and formulations, and generics of previously approved brands, become available frequently.

Bold indicates recommended first-line COC.

Italics indicate progestins available only in nonoral contraceptives.

Abbreviations: EE, ethinyl estradiol; EV, estradiol valerate.

[a] Available only within an estrophasic formulation (as of September 2014).

[b] As a component of OC, available only as brand name (as of September 2014).

[c] Available only as brand name (as of September 2014).

Box 1
Key: MEC for contraceptive use

Level	Definition/Meaning
1	Level 1 medical conditions present no contraindication to the contraceptive method; the method may be used without restriction
2	Advantages of method generally outweigh proven and/or theoretic risks for women with level 2 medical conditions.
3	Proven and/or theoretic risks usually outweigh advantages for women with level 3 medical conditions.
4	Health risk from the method is considered unacceptable for women with level 4 medical conditions; the method is contraindicated.

Adapted from Centers for Disease Control and Prevention. U S. medical eligibility criteria for contraceptive use, 2010. MMWR Recomm Rep 2010;59(RR-4):2.

they bypass first-pass hepatic metabolism, so do not induce SHBG synthesis.[22,30] POPs are not effective against acne because they lack the therapeutic estrogen component. The progestin component of COCs binds androgen receptors, which could worsen acne. However, in a COC, the androgen-reducing effect of the estrogen component outweighs the proandrogenic effect of the progestin component resulting in an overall decrease in acne. Multiple different progestin formulations are available

Box 2
Proven benefits and unproven/disproven noncontraceptive effects of COCs

Proven Benefits

Acne

- All COCs are effective.[12]
- New antiandrogenic progestins (eg, drospirenone) are superior in some trials.[12–14]

PCOS

- COCs are effective for associated menstrual disorders, acne, and hirsutism.[15]

Primary dysmenorrhea[16–18]

Secondary dysmenorrhea from endometriosis[15,19,20]

PMDD[21]

- Only drospirenone-containing COCs have demonstrated a benefit
- Trials of other COCs have not shown a benefit over placebo

Menorrhagia[22,23]

Reduction in risk of endometrial, ovarian, and colon cancer[24]

Unproven or disproven effects of COCs

PMS[25,26]

Leiomyoma growth[22]

Functional ovarian cysts (treatment)[27]

Bone mineral density[28]

Abbreviations: PCOS, polycystic ovary syndrome; PMDD, premenstrual dysphoric disorder; PMS, premenstrual syndrome.

(see **Table 1**). Later-generation progestins are less androgenic, including drospirenone, which was derived from spironolactone and, therefore, has antiandrogenic and antimineralocorticoid properties. Drospirenone was superior for the treatment of acne to triphasic norgestimate/ethinyl estradiol (EE) and nomegestrol acetate/17β-estradiol in comparative trials[12–14] but also can cause hyperkalemia (because of its antimineralocorticoid effect), necessitating laboratory monitoring in some women.[22] It is not known how COCs compare with other acne therapy.[12]

For primary dysmenorrhea, nonsteroidal antiinflammatory drugs are generally the first-line treatment; but COCs are also effective.[16] Based on small trials, the response could be as high as 80%,[17] and the magnitude of benefit was significant (with a pain score decrease in one trial from 60 out of 100 to 20 out of 100 on a visual analogue scale) after only one cycle of therapy.[18] There is no evidence for the benefit of one COC over another.[16] COCs may also be used for menorrhagia, with an anticipated decrease in blood flow of about 40% to 50%.[22,23] Continuous administration could theoretically decrease this further given the fewer number of scheduled bleeding episodes. Secondary dysmenorrhea associated with endometriosis is also an indication for COCs.[15,20]

COCs address the effects of anovulation and androgenic excess in women with polycystic ovary syndrome (PCOS), reducing acne and hirsutism associated with this condition.[15] COCs are associated with higher high-density lipoprotein and triglyceride levels in women with PCOS without affecting metabolic measures, including glucose and insulin, in a clinically significant manner.[31]

Premenstrual dysphoric disorder (PMDD) is a severe form of premenstrual syndrome (PMS). Only OCs containing drospirenone are FDA approved for the treatment of PMDD based on clinical trials.[21,22] The benefit is uncertain for milder symptoms (PMS).[25] PMS symptoms not severe enough to meet the definition of PMDD may be treated with nonhormonal measures, such as exercise, relaxation, and selective serotonin reuptake inhibitors.[26]

OCs are not effective for the treatment of functional ovarian cysts.[27] COCs can prevent formation of functional ovarian cysts,[32] particularly corpus luteum cysts; however, multiphasic COCs and the lower-dose COCs currently in use (EE ≤35 mcg) may be less effective than higher-dose monophasic COCs.[33]

OCs may improve bleeding symptoms associated with leiomyomas, but they do not positively or negatively affect their growth.[22]

Lastly, the use of OCs for prophylaxis against menstrual migraine (without aura) has mixed evidence.[34] Continuous/extended use of COCs, or tetraphasic preparations that gradually step down estrogen doses, may prevent the premenstrual decrease in estrogen levels that may precipitate headaches.[34–37]

RISKS AND CONTRAINDICATIONS

Pregnancy is associated with a higher risk of morbidity and mortality than contraception; however, women in modern times are typically exposed to contraception for more of their lives than to pregnancy. The risks of CHC are essentially a subset of the risks of pregnancy via the estrogenic effect on (1) the coagulation system, increasing the risks of venous and arterial thrombosis and thromboembolism, and (2) estrogen-dependent tissues, particularly breast and liver. For clinical decision making, the risk comparison should include the risks and efficacy of different methods of contraception.

Relative and absolute contraindications to CHCs are listed in **Table 2**, including several conditions in which the US MEC and UK MEC assign different levels of risk.

Table 2
Conditions in which the risks of COCs outweigh the benefits

Condition			Risk Level 4	Risk Level 3
VTE (DVT and/or PE)	Current VTE		X	—
	Higher risk of VTE	History of VTE with higher risk recurrence	X	—
		Known thrombogenic mutation	X	—
		Major surgery with prolonged immobilization	X	—
		Postpartum <21 d	X	—
		Systemic lupus erythematosus with positive or unknown antiphospholipid antibody status	X	—
		Budd-Chiari syndrome: should not use COCs[40] but not listed by MEC level	X	—
	Lower risk of VTE	History of VTE with lower risk recurrence	—	X
		Post partum 21–42 d with other risk for VTE (including age $\geq$35 y, smoking, BMI $\geq$30, preeclampsia, cesarean section, postpartum hemorrhage)[39]	—	X
		Inflammatory bowel disease with increased risk VTE	—	X
		Obesity (BMI $\geq$35 kg/m^2 is level 3 in UK) MEC based on VTE risk and cardiovascular risk[38] but level 2 in US MEC[40]	—	Level 3 in UK MEC, level 2 in US MEC
		Family history of VTE in a first-degree relative before 45 y of age is level 3 in UK MEC[38] but family history of VTE in first-degree relatives is level 2 in US MEC[40]	—	Level 3 in UK MEC, Level 2 in US MEC

Arterial thrombosis (particularly cardiovascular)	Diabetes	Duration >20 y[a]	X	X
		Known vascular disease[a]	X	X
		Nephropathy, neuropathy, retinopathy[a]	X	X
	Hypertension	Controlled hypertension (systolic blood pressure <140 and diastolic blood pressure <90)	—	X
		Systolic blood pressure 140–150 or diastolic blood pressure 90–99	—	X
		Systolic blood pressure ≥160 or diastolic blood pressure ≥100	X	—
	Cardiovascular risks, including age, diabetes, hypertension, hyperlipidemia	Lower risk based on number & severity of factors	—	X
		Higher risk based on number & severity of factors	X	—
	Current or past ischemic heart disease		X	—
	History of stroke		X	—
	Migraine	With aura, any age	X	—
		Without aura, ≥35 y	(For COC continuation)	(For COC initiation)
	Smoking, age ≥35 y	≥15 Cigs/d	X	—
		<15 Cigs/d	—	X
	Vascular disease		X	—
	Complicated valvular heart disease		X	—
	Complicated congenital heart disease[38]		X	—
	Peripartum cardiomyopathy	Moderate to severely impaired cardiac function, <6 or ≥6 mo post partum	X	—
		<6 mo Post partum and normal to mildly reduced cardiac function	X	—
		≥6 mo Post partum and normal to mildly reduced cardiac function	—	X

(*continued on next page*)

Table 2
(*continued*)

Condition			Risk Level 4	Risk Level 3
Liver or biliary disease	Hepatic adenoma or hepatocellular carcinoma		X	—
	Severe (decompensated) cirrhosis		X	—
	Viral hepatitis[a] (acute or flare)		X	X
	Current or medically treated gallbladder disease		—	X
	History of cholestasis caused by COC use		—	X
Breast neoplasm	Current breast cancer		X	—
	History of breast cancer, clinically disease-free for ≥5 y		—	X
	Undiagnosed breast mass[38]		—	For COC initiation, in UK MEC
Other or combined risks	Complicated organ transplant		X	—
Lactation[39] (see also **Table 3** and VTE risk section of this table)		<21 d Post partum	X	—
		21 to <30 d Post partum	—	X
Lack of efficacy because of malabsorption	History of bariatric surgery with intestinal bypass		—	X

Pregnancy poses risk in the disease conditions listed earlier.
Information is from US MEC[40] except where otherwise noted.
UK MEC determination is given where condition is not mentioned in US MEC or listing differs significantly.
Abbreviations: BMI, body mass index; Cigs, cigarettes; DVT, deep vein thrombosis; PE, pulmonary embolism.
[a] Level 3 or 4 based on severity and other risk factors.

Table 3
Initiating OC in the postpartum period

Days Post Partum	CHC Breastfeeding	CHC Not Breastfeeding	POP Breastfeeding	POP Not Breastfeeding
<21	4	4	2	1
21–29	3	3 If other VTE risk[a] 2 If no other VTE risk	2	1
30–42	3 If other VTE risk[a] 2 If no other VTE risk[a]	3 If other VTE risk[a] 2 If no other VTE risk[a]	1	1
>42	2	1	1	1

[a] VTE risk here also includes smoking, obesity, and complications of recent pregnancy, including preeclampsia, caesarian delivery, or postpartum hemorrhage.

Adapted from Centers for Disease Control and Prevention. Update to CDC's U.S. medical eligibility criteria for contraceptive use, 2010: revised recommendations for the use of contraceptive methods during the postpartum period. MMWR Morb Mortal Wkly Rep 2011;60(26):882.

Misconceptions about the risks of hormonal contraception and lack of knowledge about the benefits are common among women who are potential candidates for OC use.[9,41] In addition, CHCs are sometimes prescribed for women with level 3 and 4 contraindications. Analysis of data from a national health survey in the United States found that 23.7% of nearly 3000 women aged 18 to 44 years who took CHCs had level 3 or 4 conditions (see **Box 1**, **Table 2**), including 9% who had level 4 conditions in which CHCs are contraindicated; the most common conditions were (1) migraine and an age of 35 years or older or migraine with aura, (2) hypertension, and (3) multiple risk factors for cardiovascular disease.[42]

VTE remains the major risk of COCs, occurring at 3.5 times more than the baseline risk of approximately 0.37 per 1000 user-years for nonpregnant women[5] but still a significantly lower risk than during pregnancy and the postpartum period. VTEs attributable to OCs occur at about 0.63 per 1000 user-years, with excess deaths from VTE attributable to OCs occurring in about 5 women per 1 million user-years.[43]

Cancer may be a concern for some women considering CHCs. In fact, OC use is associated with lifetime reduction in 3 types of cancer:

- Endometrial cancer incidence: OR 0.57 (95% CI 0.43 – 0.77)[24]
- Ovarian cancer incidence: OR 0.73 (95% CI 0.66 – 0.81), related to duration of use (OR 0.91 for use ≤12 months and OR 0.42 for use >10 years)[44]
- Colorectal cancer incidence: OR 0.86 (95% CI 0.79 – 0.95)[24]

On the other hand, OC use is associated with increased likelihood of 2 or 3 types of cancer:

- Breast cancer incidence overall: OR 1.08 (95% CI 1.00–1.17)[24]
  - Longer use and current use are associated with higher risk in women 20–44, with OR 1.5 (95% CI 1.1-2.2) for current use ≥5 years and OR 1.6 (95% CI 1.1-2.5) for lifetime use ≥15 years.[45]
  - OC initiation before age 20–25 is associated with higher risk of diagnosis by age 40 for women with BRCA1, for OC initiation before age 20 (OR 1.40, 95% CI 1.14-1.70) and possibly from age 20–25 (OR 1.19, 95% CI 0.99-1.42), compared with older ages.[46]
- Cervical cancer and precancer incidence is increased in setting of persistent human papillomavirus infection and OC use, however risk estimation is limited by the heterogeneity of studies[24]

- The increased risk of cervical cancer is observed with current or recent OC use and may either persist[24] or decline to baseline[47] after cessation of OCs.
- Benign liver tumors (focal nodular hyperplasia and hepatic adenoma) are associated with OC use, and incidence of hepatocellular carcinoma may be increased (OR 1.57, 95% CI 0.96 – 2.54, from heterogeneous studies).[48] For comparison, in men hepatic adenomas occur less often, but the risk of transformation to hepatocellular carcinoma is about 10-fold higher[49]

PRESCRIBING ORAL CONTRACEPTIVES

Prescribers may find the number of different formulations challenging to navigate and may incorrectly think breast and pelvic examinations are necessary before initial prescription and subsequent refills.

A basic medical history should be obtained before CHC prescription. Relative and absolute contraindications to CHCs are listed in **Table 2** and include hypertension, vasculopathy, advanced liver disease, and breast cancer, with the last 2 also contraindications to POP.[40] In pulmonary hypertension, pregnancy is contraindicated because of the 30% to 50% maternal mortality risk; however, CHCs are generally not advised[50]: Acute or chronic VTEs can cause or exacerbate pulmonary hypertension; drug-drug interactions may reduce the efficacy of systemic hormonal approaches,[51,52] and estrogen might play an etiologic role in the condition.[50]

Venous Thromboembolism Risk Factors by History

Risk factors for VTE should be reviewed before prescription of a CHC, including family medical history. However, family history of VTE is a poor means of screening for thrombophilia in women who are candidates for CHCs. The *sensitivity* of a positive family history of VTE for detecting thrombophilic laboratory findings in patients is 11% for affected first-degree relatives and 16% for affected first- *and* second-degree relatives; the *positive predictive value* for finding such a thrombophilic defect is 8% and 9%, respectively.[53] A negative family history, thus, fails to accurately assess patients' risk of thrombophilia and may be falsely reassuring. A positive family history (especially of late-life or provoked VTE in single or distant relatives) could unduly limit the prescription of effective contraception.

Despite limitations in predicting known thrombophilic mutations, a positive family history does modestly predict a woman's overall risk of future VTE. In an observational study of young women, a positive family history for VTE was associated with 2.4-fold increased risk of VTE even in the absence of a prothrombin gene mutation or factor V Leiden.[54] In a case-control study of people with a first episode of VTE, family history of a first-degree relative affected before 45 to 50 years of age or a family history of several affected relatives was associated with 2- to 4-fold increased risk of VTE.[55]

Family history of VTE is considered level 2 for use of CHCs in the WHO MEC[6] and the US MEC[40] because the absolute risk of VTE is low and because of the poor performance of family history as a screening tool. However, in the UK MEC, family history of VTE in a first-degree relative before 45 years of age is level 3.[56]

Given the uncertainties and the discrepant guidelines discussed earlier, the low absolute risk for VTE even for women on CHCs, and the availability of other effective methods of contraception, the authors concur with the recommendations that a family history of young or multiple relatives with VTE warrants discussion with patients of their potentially heightened relative risk of VTE on a CHC, plus consideration of other contraceptive options and/or testing for thrombophilic conditions.[57,58]

Testing for thrombophilic conditions is not cost-effective for the general population of women starting CHCs.[57,59]

Physical Examination

Physical examination[60] and testing[60,61] other than blood pressure measurement is not required before prescription. Blood pressure should be measured before initiation of CHC; hypertension is a contraindication to CHCs though not to POPs (see **Table 2**).[40,60] Given the lack of need for a physical examination and testing, in September 2014, Planned Parenthood began offering to women in Minnesota and Washington online video visits for prescription of hormonal contraception, with patients required to obtain a blood pressure reading in the community.[62]

Body mass index (BMI) may be taken into consideration. In the WHO[6] and US MEC,[40] a BMI of 30 kg/m^2 or greater is level 2, whereas in the UK MEC, a BMI of 30 to 35 kg/m^2 is level 2 and a BMI of 35 kg/m^2 or greater is level 3 because of the risk of cardiovascular disease and VTE (see **Table 2**).[38]

Generic Versus Brand Name Drugs

To gain FDA approval, generic formulations of brand medications must be therapeutically equivalent to the brand (same active ingredients at same doses) and must demonstrate bioequivalence (mean area under the drug concentration-time curve within 90% confidence level of brand in crossover studies). In one study, initiation of generic or insurance-preferred brand medications (including OCs) was associated with 62% and 30% greater odds, respectively, of patients having adequate adherence (>80% of medication doses taken) than patients started on higher-tier medications.[63] On the other hand, concerns about side effects and the perceived possibility of lower efficacy of medications may affect the acceptability of a generic OC for some women. The American Congress of Obstetricians and Gynecologists (ACOG)[64] supports a low threshold for use of whichever oral contraceptive patients and clinicians think will be most effective based on various considerations, including cost and patient preference.

Medication Interactions

OCs can interact with medications of several classes, reducing the efficacy either of the contraceptive or of the other medications. The interactions significant enough to warrant consideration of either a different approach to contraception or a different medication for the underlying condition are listed next, all level 3 for CHCs and for POP except where noted:

- Rifamycin-class antibiotics (rifampin, rifabutin, and rifapentine)[40]
- Some antiepileptic medications: barbiturates, carbamazepine, phenytoin, primidone, oxcarbazepine, and topiramate[40]
- Lamotrigine (level 3 for CHCs; level 1 for POP)[40]
- Ritonavir-boosted antiretroviral therapy (highly active antiretroviral therapy including ritonavir to inhibit CYP3A4)[40]
- St John's wort[65] (not listed in MEC)
- Armodafinil and modafinil[66] (not listed in MEC)
- Dual endothelin receptor antagonist bosentan[51,52] (not listed in MEC)

Other highly active antiretroviral therapy medications affect the serum levels of hormones in CHCs; however, the clinical relevance of these effects remains murky.[67]

Thinking regarding the effect of antibiotics on efficacy of OCs has changed over time, except for antibiotics in the rifamycin class. Some studies show no overall effect on nonrifamycin antibiotics on blood levels of steroid hormones,[68] and the MEC classifies all nonrifamycin antibiotics as level 1.[40] However, the interaction may be clinically significant in some individuals, particularly with the use of tetracyclines and penicillins[69]; a 2011 population study in the Netherlands found that OC users who conceived had an odds ratio of 2.21 (95% confidence interval: 1.03–4.75) of having taken antibiotics around the time of conception.[70]

CHOOSING BETWEEN MANY COMBINATION ORAL CONTRACEPTIVE OPTIONS

See **Box 3** for tips on selecting from among COCs. Because the side effect profile and noncontraceptive benefits are largely similar between different formulations of COCs, patient preference can strongly influence the choice. The cost difference between generic and brand name formulations can be marked, which may be a consideration for some patients.

Monophasic COC preparations should be first-line agents, as there is insufficient evidence to demonstrate that triphasic preparations are better in terms of effectiveness, bleeding patterns, or discontinuation rates.[72]

In a 2014 Cochrane Review,[5] researchers recommended 30 μg of EE with levonorgestrel (LNG) as the first-line COC. This recommendation was based on a meta-analysis of 26 studies examining the differential VTE risk between various formulations of COCs, with the VTE risk found to depend on both the dose of EE and the type of progestin. The lowest COC dose of EE (20 μg) has the lowest VTE risk but may also increase unscheduled bleeding that can adversely affect compliance. Of the progestins, LNG (20 μg or 30 μg) had the lowest VTE risk (other types carried a 50%–80% higher risk).

CYCLIC VERSUS CONTINUOUS USE OF COMBINATION ORAL CONTRACEPTIVES

When the COC was first introduced in 1960, it was formulated with 21 active pills, followed by a 7 days of placebo. The withdrawal bleed on placebo pills was meant to mimic a woman's natural cycle and, thus, increase acceptability among users.[73–75]

Continuous or extended use of COCs was recommended by some practitioners long before the FDA approval in 2003 of Seasonale®, the first brand formulated for withdrawal bleeding every 3 months (once per season). Since that formulation was approved, the method has become more widely used, both for the treatment of menstrual-related symptoms (eg, menstrual migraine and endometriosis) and for convenience. Several COCs packaged for extended-cycle use and for continuous use are

Box 3
Tips for selecting a COC

- Patient preference should be strongly considered.[64]
- Generic formulations cost less than brand name formulations and are bioequivalent.[71]
- Monophasic preparations are preferred.[72]
- Of the available progestins, LNG (with 20 μg or 30 μg EE) increases the VTE risk the least.[5]
- 20 μg EE may increase the VTE risk less than higher dosages of estrogen.[5]
- 30 μg EE results in less unscheduled bleeding and lower discontinuation rates.[12]
- Even relatively androgenic progestins, like LNG, tend to improve acne.[12]

Abbreviation: LNG, levonorgestrel.

currently on the market, but any monophasic COC can be used continuously by having patients take only the active pills from each pack and beginning the next pack directly, without 7 days of no pill or placebo every 28 days. However, third-party payers may not cover the additional pack required every 12 weeks to use cyclic COCs in this manner.

Multiple researchers have demonstrated that most women prefer to have less or no bleeding if given the opportunity,[76,77] which can be achieved in several ways:

- Continuous use of active monophasic COCs indefinitely
- Continuous use of active monophasic COCs for periods of time longer than 28 days (for example, 84 days) followed by a scheduled withdrawal bleed
- Continuous use of active monophasic COCs until persistent unscheduled bleeding begins, at which time patients initiate a hormone-free interval of 7 days or less and, thus, a withdrawal bleed

Advocates of continuous use argue that the hormone-free interval serves no biological purpose and could theoretically lead to decreased effectiveness because of the rare possibility of escape ovulation, decreased compliance, and more missed pills; worsened quality of life; and more menstrual-related symptoms and work absenteeism.

Critics of continuous use articulate 2 main concerns: (1) a lack of long-term data supporting its safety and (2) overmedicalization of normal menstruation. In other words, they voice concern that continuous-use COCs might recruit more users that are looking for lifestyle benefits (amenorrhea) without necessarily needing/desiring the contraceptive benefits and, therefore, exposing themselves to risks of COCs without a strong indication.[78]

Efficacy

Studies monitoring signs of ovulation have demonstrated follicular development occurring in the hormone-free interval of cyclic COCs.[79] Delay in initiation of the next cycle of active pills after a placebo week can lead to contraceptive failure. Some researchers have postulated that continuous use of COCs may be more effective than cyclic use,[80] but the authors of a recent Cochrane review concluded that contraceptive efficacy of extended-cycle COC use was similar to cyclic COC use in 8 randomized controlled trials (RCTs).[81]

Bleeding and Endometrial Effect

Extended-cycle COC use results in less scheduled bleeding with variable reports on the frequency of spotting or unscheduled bleeding. Most studies show a similar number of days with bleeding between cyclic COCs and extended-cycle COCs and similar discontinuation rates,[81] with the unscheduled bleeding of extended use declining over the first several months of use[81,82] and fewer menstrual symptoms with extended-cycle use.[81]

Sonographic studies of the endometrial lining in continuous and extended-cycle COC users have demonstrated normal endometrial stripes, and biopsies have confirmed a lack of hyperplasia.[73,80,81,83]

Return to Fertility

Median time to return of menses is 32 days after stopping continuous COCs,[73,84,85] and 99% of women return to spontaneous menses or pregnancy within 90 days of stopping COCs.[84] Furthermore, within the confines of a 1-year study, the duration of use was not related to time to return to menses.[84]

PATIENT COUNSELING

Initiation

There are 3 methods for initiation of CHCs and POP:

- Start on same day the CHC is prescribed (called *quick start*, *same day start*, or *immediate start*)
- Start on first day of next menses
- Start on the first Sunday on or after the start of next menses (*Sunday start*)

The quick-start method is acceptable if patients are unlikely to be pregnant. Ovulation is inhibited after 7 days of use. Compared with the other approaches, the quick-start method may result in higher initial continuation rates[86]; but that difference is lost over time for COCs.[86,87] Bleeding rates and pregnancy rates are similar.[86,87] The quick-start method is used when OCs are begun in amenorrheic patients in the postpartum period.

Common Minor Side Effects, Including Management

Breast tenderness and nausea with or without vomiting are commonly reported with initiation of CHCs, are attributed to the estrogen component, and are less problematic with 20 mcg EE COCs than with higher EE doses.[88] Nausea can be managed by taking the pill at bedtime or switching to a 20-mcg EE formulation.

On the other hand, breakthrough bleeding (BTB) is more common with 20-mcg EE COCs than with higher EE doses and leads to more frequent discontinuation of the lower-dose pills.[88] BTB is also common on POP. For low-dose EE COCs and for POP, taking the pill at the same time every day can reduce the chance of BTB.

All of these side effects tend to improve over several months with continued use; counseling patients to expect them and that they should resolve within a few months can improve OC continuation rates.

If BTB on COC does not resolve with time (and another cause is not found) or if patients do not find waiting 3 months acceptable, BTB can be managed by increasing the EE dose from 20 mcg EE to 30 to 35 mcg EE or switching to a COC with a different progestin. If patients have been taking the COC as an extended cycle, stopping the active hormone for 4 to 7 days to allow a withdrawal bleed, then resuming extended use, may be effective for several months, at which time it can be repeated.

Potential for weight gain on COC may be a concern for some women; however, studies show no significant effect and no difference in discontinuation rates for weight gain between COC and placebo.[89]

Potential Major Side Effects

Any symptom suggestive of VTE or arterial thrombosis should be evaluated promptly.

Headaches can occur with initiation of CHCs. New or worsened migraines, severe headaches, or headaches associated with neurologic signs or symptoms should prompt discontinuation of the CHC and initiation of appropriate medical evaluation.

Methods to Improve Adherence

For OCs, the quick-start method (also called *immediate start* or *same-day start*) is associated with better *initial* adherence[86] as discussed earlier. Daily text messages improve OC continuation rates,[90] and special counseling can help patients identify cues to daily dosing.[91] Several dozen smartphone applications are available, varying in reminder methods (light, sound, vibration, and/or pop-up reminders) and also in technical reliability.[92] Dispensing a larger quantity of pill packs at once is associated with fewer pregnancies but more “pill wastage.”[93]

Although not the focus of this article, the contraceptive patch and ring are relevant to a discussion of adherence to hormonal contraception. Adherence is better with the CHC patch than the COC pill in weeks in which it is used,[94,95] but side effects may result in a greater chance of discontinuation of the patch.[95] The CHC ring has been associated with better adherence compared with the patch and ring in some studies.[96]

Advice for Missed Pills

Ovulation is most likely to occur when pills are missed in the first or last week of active hormone in cyclic use or any other lapse that results in a hormone-free stretch of more than 7 days. Estrogen dose matters; missing 1 to 4 doses of COC results in more follicular activity in women who have been on 20-mcg EE formulations than in women who have been on 30-mcg EE pills.[97] Patients should be given advice on aids to adherence as well as clear instructions on what to do if 1 or more doses is missed (**Fig. 1**).

Follow-up

No routine follow-up is needed after the initiation of POP or CHC; however, women should be encourage to return for follow-up should side effects or any other issues

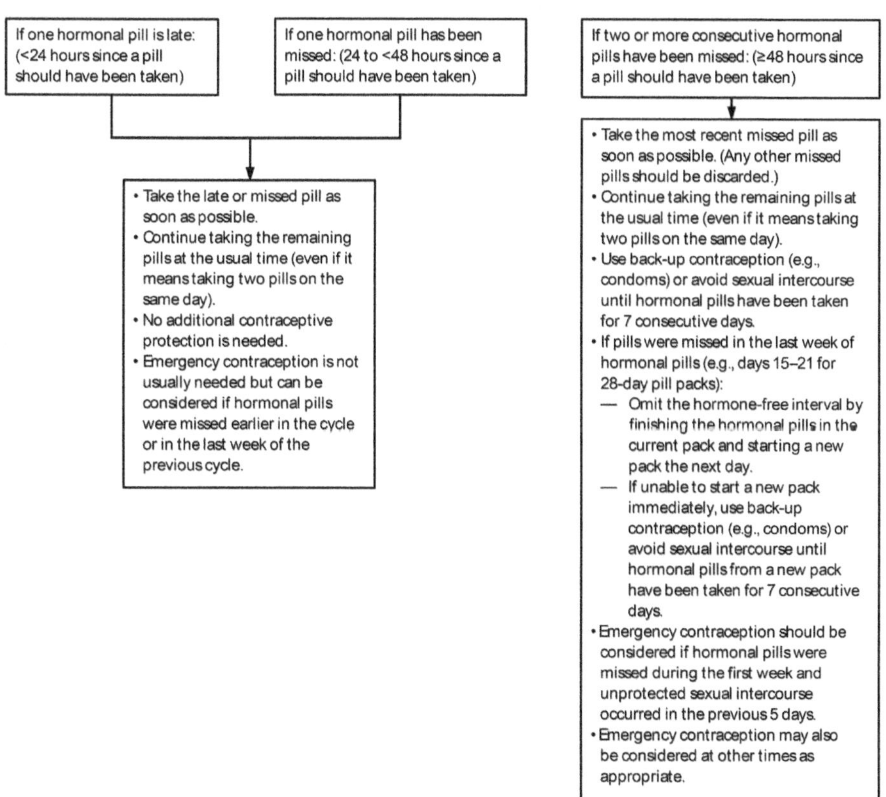

Fig. 1. Recommended actions after late or missed COC doses. (*From* Centers for Disease Control and Prevention. U.S. Selected Practice Recommendations for Contraceptive Use, 2013: adapted from the World Health Organization selected practice recommendations for contraceptive use, 2nd edition. MMWR Recomm Rep 2013;62(RR-05):1–60.)

or concerns arise.[60] Significant changes in health status that may increase the risk or reduce the efficacy of the contraceptive method should prompt a reevaluation of its use.[60] As is advised for all adults, women on CHC[60] should have blood pressure measured periodically.

CONSIDERATIONS FOR SPECIAL POPULATIONS

A woman's fertility may span 30 or more years of her life, during which adjustments in the best choice of contraception should be expected. She will likely experience changes in her own menstrual cycle, menstrual-associated symptoms, comorbidities, parity, desire for future fertility, timing or frequency of sexual activity, other coprescribed medications, and so forth. All of these may influence the balance of benefit and risk for a woman choosing a contraceptive method. The following are a few subgroups for which questions commonly arise.

Teenage Years

Compared with the 1990s, adolescents in the United States are less likely to report being sexually active and more likely to report using effective forms of contraception; but the teen pregnancy rate remains higher than in other developed countries,[98] and about 78% of teen pregnancies are unintended.[99] In 2009, teens aged 15 to 19 years in the United States had 705,000 pregnancies and 410,000 live births.[98]

During 2006 to 2010, 43% of teens aged 15 to 19 years reported having had sex, which represents a 16% decline from a prior finding of 51% in 1995.[100] Almost 80% of female teenagers who had sex reported having used contraception for the first intercourse, with 68% of those using condoms, 16% using OC, and 6% using injection, patch, ring, or emergency contraception.[101] Among female teenagers who had sex in the prior month but were not pregnant, postpartum, or seeking pregnancy, overall 48% used a hormonal method or IUD without a condom; 12% used a hormonal method or IUD with a condom; 16% used condoms alone or a method of similar efficacy; 6% used a less effective method, such as withdrawal; and 18% did not use any contraception.[100] Compared with 1995, this reflects a 26% increase in the use of more effective methods and a 7% decrease in the use of no contraceptive method.[100]

Age, itself, is not a contraindication to any reversible form of contraception. Teens should be counseled that condoms are needed to protect against sexually transmitted infections; but given their high contraceptive failure rate with typical use, an additional contraceptive method should also be strongly considered. Although outside the scope of this article, Long-acting reversible contraceptives (LARCs) are highly efficacious and safe in this population but are underused, with about 2.5% of teens using IUDs[102] and about 0.5% using progestin implant.[103] The ACOG recommends that adolescents be encouraged to consider LARC methods.[103] CHCs also remain a reasonable choice for contraception for teens and offer control of irregular and/or heavy periods. COCs have the additional noncontraceptive benefit of improving acne.

Adolescents face some unique barriers to obtaining and optimally using contraception that should be considered by health care practitioners.[104]

Confidentiality can be a significant concern. Policies need to be in place to maintain confidentiality of medical records, reimbursements, and so forth; patients should be repeatedly reassured about efforts to maintain confidentiality.

Misinformation can be prevalent and should be corrected. Providing accurate information on sex and contraceptive choices to adolescents does not lead to increased rates of sexual activity, earlier onset of intercourse, or a greater number of partners.[104,105] Patients may have exaggerated concern or inaccurate information about risks of COCs; practitioners can help by dispelling myths about weight gain, mood swings, or acne. Teens should also be reassured that a pelvic examination is typically not needed before prescribing OCs.[60]

Adherence to user-dependent hormonal contraceptive methods is a significant challenge in this population. Typical-use failure rates for COCs are about 8% in the general population but 15% to 26% in teenagers,[104] hence, the recommendation to consider LARC or injection. When OCs are chosen, the clinician should counsel patients on the importance of not missing pills, emphasize the noncontraceptive benefits of OCs, offer (but not require) frequent follow-up, and troubleshoot ways to keep use confidential from a parent or other adult if that is important to patients. Alternatively, if patients are open to involving their mother, this can increase compliance.[104] Lastly, emergency contraception should also be proactively discussed and prescribed so it is readily available if the need should arise.

Postpartum

Effective contraception in the postpartum period is important. Unintended pregnancies can have long-lasting detrimental effects on the mother-child relationship.[106] Interpregnancy intervals less than 6 months adversely affect fetal health by increasing preterm birth and neonatal death.[106,107] Cross-culturally, about half (ranging about 32%–60%) of mothers have resumed sexual activity by 6 weeks post partum.[1–4,6,7,40,108] Contraceptive counseling by practitioners before and after delivery significantly increases the percentage of women who choose a highly effective method of contraception.[109]

When considering OC options in the postpartum period, the main consideration for nonbreastfeeding mothers is the risk of VTE, which is 11-fold[110] to 50-fold[111] higher in the first 3 months post partum than in nonpregnant women and as much as 84-fold higher[111] in the first 6 weeks post partum compared with the nonpregnant state. Coagulation and fibrinolysis variables are altered post partum, potentially as a mechanism for reducing the risk of postpartum hemorrhage.[40] MEC recommendations for the postpartum period are given in **Table 3**.

Additional considerations with breastfeeding include (1) hormone uptake into breast milk and its effect on the infant and (2) effect of hormones on breast milk production. Although the estrogen component of COCs may decrease milk production, POPs do not have a demonstrable effect on milk production. Exogenous progestin is transferred to breast milk[112]; however, no long-term effects have been detected with observation of breastfed children whose mothers took POPs up to 8 years.[113] COCs have not been shown to have adverse effects on infants.[40,114]

Perimenopause

Perimenopause includes several years of decreasing fertility during the menopausal transition and ends 12 months after the final menstrual period.[115,116] There is a wide range of experiences and symptoms related to perimenopause; but physiologic changes, cycle changes, and perimenopausal symptoms can last more than 6 years[117] and commonly intensify over the 4 years preceding the final menstrual period.[118]

Contraception is indicated for pregnancy prevention during perimenopause. Fecundity is variable from woman to woman and affected by genetics, comorbidities, smoking, coital frequency, and male fertility. Although fertility rates decrease starting in a woman's late 20s, the annual chance of pregnancy in heterosexual cohabitating women in their mid 40s, not using any contraception, can still be estimated around 10%[119]; pregnancy can occur into the sixth decade of life. It is estimated that only about half of couples are truly sterile at 45 years of age.[120] Furthermore, when pregnancies do occur in this period, there is a higher risk of miscarriage (about 33% by 45 years of age),[120,121] pregnancy complications, and perinatal mortality (about 1.0%–1.4% to women 40 years and older).[122]

The full spectrum of options for contraception is available to women in perimenopause; age, itself, is not a contraindication to any of the options. The US MEC categorizes 40 years of age and older as level 2 with the comment that cardiovascular risk factors increase with age and advises that "[i]n the absence of other adverse clinical conditions, CHCs can be used until menopause."[40]

The estrogen component of COCs can have noncontraceptive benefits for perimenopause-related symptoms commonly experienced at this time,[118] including irregular cycles, heavy menstrual bleeding, and vasomotor symptoms.

The most concerning potential complications of COCs are detailed in prior sections but are generally VTE and cardiovascular disease (heart attack and stroke). The presence of comorbidities that contribute to these diseases increases with age (eg, diabetes, hypertension); age is an independent risk factor for VTE. COCs should generally not be prescribed to women aged 35 years and older who smoke or to women with multiple risk factors for cardiovascular disease, of which age is one.[40]

Although outside the scope of this article, LARC options (IUDs and progestin implant) should also be considered for women in this age group, especially those who have relative or absolute contraindications to exogenous estrogen.

Deciding when to stop hormonal contraception should be an individualized decision. In a healthy, nonsmoking woman who has continued COCs throughout perimenopause, it would be ideal to stop COCs shortly after menopause has begun (after her final natural menstrual period would have occurred). This timing is, of course, difficult to identify prospectively and complicated by the suppression of her natural menses by the COCs. Continued withdrawal bleeds do not mean menopause has not developed; likewise, amenorrhea while on cyclic COCs does not necessarily predict menopause.[119] The most common method of stopping is to have a woman who is approaching 50 years old stop her COC while using a nonhormonal backup method. If this trial period is not feasible for a particular woman, practitioners can check an FSH level at the end of each hormone-free interval and presume menopause has developed if FSH is 30 IU/L or greater. However, this approach can be misleading, failing to identify menopause even though it has developed.[119]

REFERENCES

1. Colton FB. Steroids and "the pill": early steroid research at Searle. Steroids 1992;57(12):624–30.
2. Risk of thromboembolic disease in women taking oral contraceptives. A preliminary communication to the Medical Research Council by a Subcommittee. Br Med J 1967;2(5548):355–9.
3. Markush RE, Seigel DG. Oral contraceptives and mortality trends from thromboembolism in the United States. Am J Public Health Nations Health 1969;59(3): 418–34.
4. Inman WH, Vessey MP, Westerholm B, et al. Thromboembolic disease and the steroidal content of oral contraceptives. A report to the Committee on Safety of Drugs. Br Med J 1970;2(5703):203–9.
5. de Bastos M, Stegeman BH, Rosendaal FR, et al. Combined oral contraceptives: venous thrombosis. Cochrane Database Syst Rev 2014;(3):CD010813.
6. World Health Organization. Medical eligibility criteria for contraceptive use, 4th edition. 2010. Available at: http://whqlibdoc.who.int/publications/2010/9789241563888_eng.pdf?ua=1. Accessed September 21, 2014.

7. United States medical eligibility criteria (US MEC) for contraceptive use, 2010. Centers for Disease Control and Prevention Web site. Available at: http://www.cdc.gov/reproductivehealth/unintendedpregnancy/usmec.htm. Accessed January 20, 2014.
8. Trussell J. Contraceptive failure in the United States. Contraception 2011;83(5):397–404.
9. Kaunitz AM. Oral contraceptive health benefits: perception versus reality. Contraception 1999;59(Suppl 1):29S–33S.
10. Peipert JF, Gutmann J. Oral contraceptive risk assessment: a survey of 247 educated women. Obstet Gynecol 1993;82(1):112–7.
11. Tessler SL, Peipert JF. Perceptions of contraceptive effectiveness and health effects of oral contraception. Womens Health Issues 1997;7(6):400–6.
12. Arowojolu AO, Gallo MF, Lopez LM, et al. Combined oral contraceptive pills for treatment of acne. Cochrane Database Syst Rev 2012;(7):CD004425.
13. Thorneycroft IH, Gollnick H, Schellschmidt I. Superiority of a combined contraceptive containing drospirenone to a triphasic preparation containing norgestimate in acne treatment. Cutis 2004;74(2):123–30.
14. Mansour D, Verhoeven C, Sommer W, et al. Efficacy and tolerability of a monophasic combined oral contraceptive containing nomegestrol acetate and 17β-oestradiol in a 24/4 regimen, in comparison to an oral contraceptive containing ethinylestradiol and drospirenone in a 21/7 regimen. Eur J Contracept Reprod Health Care 2011;16(6):430–43.
15. Bozdag G, Yildiz BO. Combined oral contraceptives in polycystic ovary syndrome - indications and cautions. Front Horm Res 2013;40:115–27.
16. Wong CL, Farquhar C, Roberts H, et al. Oral contraceptive pill as treatment for primary dysmenorrhoea. Cochrane Database Syst Rev 2009;(2):CD002120.
17. Osayande AS, Mehulic S. Diagnosis and initial management of dysmenorrhea. Am Fam Physician 2014;89(5):341–6.
18. Harada T, Momoeda M, Terakawa N, et al. Evaluation of a low-dose oral contraceptive pill for primary dysmenorrhea: a placebo-controlled, double-blind, randomized trial. Fertil Steril 2011;95(6):1928–31.
19. ACOG Committee on Practice Bulletins–Gynecology. ACOG practice bulletin No. 108: polycystic ovary syndrome. Obstet Gynecol 2009;114(4):936–49.
20. Harada T, Momoeda M, Taketani Y, et al. Low-dose oral contraceptive pill for dysmenorrhea associated with endometriosis: a placebo-controlled, double-blind, randomized trial. Fertil Steril 2008;90(5):1583–8.
21. Yonkers KA, Brown C, Pearlstein TB, et al. Efficacy of a new low-dose oral contraceptive with drospirenone in premenstrual dysphoric disorder. Obstet Gynecol 2005;106(3):492–501.
22. ACOG practice bulletin No. 110: noncontraceptive uses of hormonal contraceptives. Obstet Gynecol 2010;115(1):206–18.
23. Larsson G, Milsom I, Lindstedt G, et al. The influence of a low-dose combined oral contraceptive on menstrual blood loss and iron status. Contraception 1992;46(4):327–34.
24. Gierisch JM, Coeytaux RR, Urrutia RP, et al. Oral contraceptive use and risk of breast, cervical, colorectal, and endometrial cancers: a systematic review. Cancer Epidemiol Biomarkers Prev 2013;22(11):1931–43.
25. Lopez LM, Kaptein AA, Helmerhorst FM. Oral contraceptives containing drospirenone for premenstrual syndrome. Cochrane Database Syst Rev 2012;(2):CD006586.
26. Marjoribanks J, Brown J, O'Brien PM, et al. Selective serotonin reuptake inhibitors for premenstrual syndrome. Cochrane Database Syst Rev 2013;(6):CD001396.

27. Grimes DA, Jones LB, Lopez LM, et al. Oral contraceptives for functional ovarian cysts. Cochrane Database Syst Rev 2014;(4):CD006134.
28. Lopez LM, Chen M, Mullins S, et al. Steroidal contraceptives and bone fractures in women: evidence from observational studies. Cochrane Database Syst Rev 2012;(8):CD009849.
29. George R, Clarke S, Thiboutot D. Hormonal therapy for acne. Semin Cutan Med Surg 2008;27(3):188–96.
30. Katsambas AD, Dessinioti C. Hormonal therapy for acne: why not as first line therapy? Facts and controversies. Clin Dermatol 2010;28(1):17–23.
31. Halperin IJ, Kumar SS, Stroup DF, et al. The association between the combined oral contraceptive pill and insulin resistance, dysglycemia and dyslipidemia in women with polycystic ovary syndrome: a systematic review and meta-analysis of observational studies. Hum Reprod 2011;26(1):191–201.
32. Vessey M, Metcalfe A, Wells C, et al. Ovarian neoplasms, functional ovarian cysts, and oral contraceptives. Br Med J (Clin Res Ed) 1987;294(6586): 1518–20.
33. Lanes SF, Birmann B, Walker AM, et al. Oral contraceptive type and functional ovarian cysts. Am J Obstet Gynecol 1992;166(3):956–61.
34. Newman LC, Yugrakh MS. Menstrual migraine: treatment options. Neurol Sci 2014;35(Suppl 1):57–60.
35. Chai NC, Peterlin BL, Calhoun AH. Migraine and estrogen. Curr Opin Neurol 2014;27(3):315–24.
36. Sulak P, Willis S, Kuehl T, et al. Headaches and oral contraceptives: impact of eliminating the standard 7-day placebo interval. Headache 2007;47(1): 27–37.
37. Macìas G, Merki-Feld GS, Parke S, et al. Effects of a combined oral contraceptive containing oestradiol valerate/dienogest on hormone withdrawal-associated symptoms: results from the multicentre, randomised, double-blind, active-controlled HARMONY II study. J Obstet Gynaecol 2013;33(6):591–6.
38. Faculty of Sexual and Reproductive Healthcare. UK medical eligibility criteria for contraceptive use (UKMEC 2009). Royal College of Obstetricians and Gynaecologists. Available at: http://www.fsrh.org/pdfs/UKMEC2009.pdf. Accessed September 20, 2014. November 2009 (revised May 2010).
39. Centers for Disease Control and Prevention. Update to CDC's U.S. medical eligibility criteria for contraceptive use, 2010: revised recommendations for the use of contraceptive methods during the postpartum period. MMWR Morb Mortal Wkly Rep 2011;60(26):878–83.
40. Centers for Disease Control and Prevention. U S. medical eligibility criteria for contraceptive use, 2010. MMWR Recomm Rep 2010;59(RR-4):1–86.
41. Lee J, Jezewski MA. Attitudes toward oral contraceptive use among women of reproductive age: a systematic review. ANS Adv Nurs Sci 2007;30(1): E85–103.
42. Yu J, Hu XH. Inappropriate use of combined hormonal contraceptives for birth control among women of reproductive age in the United States. J Womens Health (Larchmt) 2013;22(7):595–603.
43. Tricotel A, Raguideau F, Collin C, et al. Estimate of venous thromboembolism and related-deaths attributable to the use of combined oral contraceptives in France. PLoS One 2014;9(4):e93792.
44. Havrilesky LJ, Gierisch JM, Moorman PG, et al. Oral contraceptive use for the primary prevention of ovarian cancer. Evid Rep Technol Assess (Full Rep) 2013;(212):1–514.

45. Beaber EF, Malone KE, Tang MT, et al. Oral contraceptives and breast cancer risk overall and by molecular subtype among young women. Cancer Epidemiol Biomarkers Prev 2014;23(5):755–64.
46. Kotsopoulos J, Lubinski J, Moller P, et al. Timing of oral contraceptive use and the risk of breast cancer in BRCA1 mutation carriers. Breast Cancer Res Treat 2014;143(3):579–86.
47. Vessey M, Yeates D. Oral contraceptive use and cancer: final report from the Oxford-Family Planning Association contraceptive study. Contraception 2013; 88(6):678–83.
48. Maheshwari S, Sarraj A, Kramer J, et al. Oral contraception and the risk of hepatocellular carcinoma. J Hepatol 2007;47(4):506–13.
49. Farges O, Ferreira N, Dokmak S, et al. Changing trends in malignant transformation of hepatocellular adenoma. Gut 2011;60(1):85–9.
50. Pugh ME, Hemnes AR. Development of pulmonary arterial hypertension in women: interplay of sex hormones and pulmonary vascular disease. Womens Health (Lond Engl) 2010;6(2):285–96.
51. van Giersbergen PL, Halabi A, Dingemanse J. Pharmacokinetic interaction between bosentan and the oral contraceptives norethisterone and ethinyl estradiol. Int J Clin Pharmacol Ther 2006;44(3):113–8.
52. Galiè N, Hoeper MM, Humbert M, et al. Guidelines for the diagnosis and treatment of pulmonary hypertension: the Task Force for the Diagnosis and Treatment of Pulmonary Hypertension of the European Society of Cardiology (ESC) and the European Respiratory Society (ERS), endorsed by the International Society of Heart and Lung Transplantation (ISHLT). Eur Heart J 2009;30(20): 2493–537.
53. Cosmi B, Legnani C, Bernardi F, et al. Value of family history in identifying women at risk of venous thromboembolism during oral contraception: observational study. BMJ 2001;322(7293):1024–5.
54. Spannagl M, Heinemann LA, Dominh T, et al. Comparison of incidence/risk of venous thromboembolism (VTE) among selected clinical and hereditary risk markers: a community-based cohort study. Thromb J 2005;3:8.
55. Bezemer ID, van der Meer FJ, Eikenboom JC, et al. The value of family history as a risk indicator for venous thrombosis. Arch Intern Med 2009;169(6):610–5.
56. Venous thromboembolism and hormonal contraception (green-top guideline No. 40). Royal College of Obstetricians and Gynaecologists. London. Available at: https://www.rcog.org.uk/globalassets/documents/guidelines/gtg40venousthromboembolism0910.pdf. Accessed September 19, 2014. Published September 27, 2010.
57. National Clinical Guideline Centre (UK). Venous thromboembolic diseases: the management of venous thromboembolic diseases and the role of thrombophilia testing [Internet]. London: Royal College of Physicians (UK); 2012.
58. De Stefano V, Rossi E. Testing for inherited thrombophilia and consequences for antithrombotic prophylaxis in patients with venous thromboembolism and their relatives. A review of the Guidelines from Scientific Societies and Working Groups. Thromb Haemost 2013;110(4):697–705.
59. Wu O, Robertson L, Twaddle S, et al. Screening for thrombophilia in high-risk situations: a meta-analysis and cost-effectiveness analysis. Br J Haematol 2005;131(1):80–90.
60. Division of Reproductive Health, National Center for Chronic Disease Prevention and Health Promotion, Centers for Disease Control and Prevention. U.S. selected practice recommendations for contraceptive use, 2013: adapted

from the World Health Organization selected practice recommendations for contraceptive use, 2nd edition. MMWR Recomm Rep 2013;62(RR-05):1–60.
61. Tepper NK, Steenland MW, Marchbanks PA, et al. Laboratory screening prior to initiating contraception: a systematic review. Contraception 2013;87(5):645–9.
62. Planned Parenthood. Available at: http://www.plannedparenthood.org/get-care/online/video-visit. Accessed September 19, 2014.
63. Shrank WH, Hoang T, Ettner SL, et al. The implications of choice: prescribing generic or preferred pharmaceuticals improves medication adherence for chronic conditions. Arch Intern Med 2006;166(3):332–7.
64. Committee on Gynecologic Practice American College of Obstetricians and Gynecologists. ACOG committee opinion No. 375: brand versus generic oral contraceptives. Obstet Gynecol 2007;110(2 Pt 1):447–8.
65. Rahimi R, Abdollahi M. An update on the ability of St. John's wort to affect the metabolism of other drugs. Expert Opin Drug Metab Toxicol 2012;8(6):691–708.
66. Robertson P, Hellriegel ET, Arora S, et al. Effect of modafinil on the pharmacokinetics of ethinyl estradiol and triazolam in healthy volunteers. Clin Pharmacol Ther 2002;71(1):46–56.
67. Robinson JA, Jamshidi R, Burke AE. Contraception for the HIV-positive woman: a review of interactions between hormonal contraception and antiretroviral therapy. Infect Dis Obstet Gynecol 2012;2012:890160.
68. Archer JS, Archer DF. Oral contraceptive efficacy and antibiotic interaction: a myth debunked. J Am Acad Dermatol 2002;46(6):917–23.
69. Dickinson BD, Altman RD, Nielsen NH, et al, Council on Scientific Affairs, American Medical Assocation. Drug interactions between oral contraceptives and antibiotics. Obstet Gynecol 2001;98(5 Pt 1):853–60.
70. Koopmans PC, Bos JH, de Jong-van den Berg LT. Are antibiotics related to oral combination contraceptive failures in the Netherlands? A case-crossover study. Pharmacoepidemiol Drug Saf 2012;21(8):865–71.
71. Sober SP, Schreiber CA. Controversies in family planning: are all oral contraceptive formulations created equal? Contraception 2011;83(5):394–6.
72. Van Vliet HA, Grimes DA, Lopez LM, et al. Triphasic versus monophasic oral contraceptives for contraception. Cochrane Database Syst Rev 2011;(11):CD003553.
73. Panicker S, Mann S, Shawe J, et al. Evolution of extended use of the combined oral contraceptive pill. J Fam Plann Reprod Health Care 2014;40(2):133–41.
74. Tyrer L. Introduction of the pill and its impact. Contraception 1999;59(Suppl 1):11S–6S.
75. Coutinho EM. To bleed or not to bleed, that is the question. Contraception 2007;76(4):263–6.
76. den Tonkelaar I, Oddens BJ. Preferred frequency and characteristics of menstrual bleeding in relation to reproductive status, oral contraceptive use, and hormone replacement therapy use. Contraception 1999;59(6):357–62.
77. Wright KP, Johnson JV. Evaluation of extended and continuous use oral contraceptives. Ther Clin Risk Manag 2008;4(5):905–11.
78. Hitchcock CL, Prior JC. Evidence about extending the duration of oral contraceptive use to suppress menstruation. Womens Health Issues 2004;14(6):201–11.
79. Baerwald AR, Olatunbosun OA, Pierson RA. Ovarian follicular development is initiated during the hormone-free interval of oral contraceptive use. Contraception 2004;70(5):371–7.
80. Steinauer J, Autry AM. Extended cycle combined hormonal contraception. Obstet Gynecol Clin North Am 2007;34(1):43–55, viii.

81. Edelman AB, Gallo MF, Jensen JT, et al. Continuous or extended cycle vs. cyclic use of combined oral contraceptives for contraception. Cochrane Database Syst Rev 2005;(3):CD004695.
82. Miller L, Notter KM. Menstrual reduction with extended use of combination oral contraceptive pills: randomized controlled trial. Obstet Gynecol 2001;98(5 Pt 1): 771–8.
83. Foidart JM, Sulak PJ, Schellschmidt I, et al. The use of an oral contraceptive containing ethinylestradiol and drospirenone in an extended regimen over 126 days. Contraception 2006;73(1):34–40.
84. Davis AR, Kroll R, Soltes B, et al. Occurrence of menses or pregnancy after cessation of a continuous oral contraceptive. Fertil Steril 2008;89(5):1059–63.
85. Barnhart KT, Schreiber CA. Return to fertility following discontinuation of oral contraceptives. Fertil Steril 2009;91(3):659–63.
86. Brahmi D, Curtis KM. When can a woman start combined hormonal contraceptives (CHCs)? A systematic review. Contraception 2013;87(5):524–38.
87. Lopez LM, Newmann SJ, Grimes DA, et al. Immediate start of hormonal contraceptives for contraception. Cochrane Database Syst Rev 2012;(12):CD006260.
88. Gallo MF, Nanda K, Grimes DA, et al. 20 μg versus >20 μg estrogen combined oral contraceptives for contraception. Cochrane Database Syst Rev 2013;(8): CD003989.
89. Gallo MF, Lopez LM, Grimes DA, et al. Combination contraceptives: effects on weight. Cochrane Database Syst Rev 2014;(1):CD003987.
90. Castaño PM, Bynum JY, Andrés R, et al. Effect of daily text messages on oral contraceptive continuation: a randomized controlled trial. Obstet Gynecol 2012;119(1):14–20.
91. Halpern V, Lopez LM, Grimes DA, et al. Strategies to improve adherence and acceptability of hormonal methods of contraception. Cochrane Database Syst Rev 2013;(10):CD004317.
92. Gal N, Zite N, Wallace L. A systematic review of smartphone oral contraceptive reminder applications. Obstet Gynecol 2014;123(Suppl 1):9S.
93. Steenland MW, Rodriguez MI, Marchbanks PA, et al. How does the number of oral contraceptive pill packs dispensed or prescribed affect continuation and other measures of consistent and correct use? A systematic review. Contraception 2013;87(5):605–10.
94. Archer DF, Cullins V, Creasy GW, et al. The impact of improved compliance with a weekly contraceptive transdermal system (Ortho Evra) on contraceptive efficacy. Contraception 2004;69(3):189–95.
95. Lopez LM, Grimes DA, Gallo MF, et al. Skin patch and vaginal ring versus combined oral contraceptives for contraception. Cochrane Database Syst Rev 2013;(4):CD003552.
96. Martínez-Astorquiza-Ortiz de Zarate T, Díaz-Martín T, Martínez-Astorquiza-Corral T, MIA Study Investigators. Evaluation of factors associated with noncompliance in users of combined hormonal contraceptive methods: a cross-sectional study: results from the MIA study. BMC Womens Health 2013;13:38.
97. Zapata LB, Steenland MW, Brahmi D, et al. Effect of missed combined hormonal contraceptives on contraceptive effectiveness: a systematic review. Contraception 2013;87(5):685–700.
98. Curtin SC, Abma JC, Ventura SJ, et al. Pregnancy rates for U.S. women continue to drop. NCHS Data Brief 2013;(136):1–8.
99. Mosher WD, Jones J, Abma JC. Intended and unintended births in the United States: 1982-2010. Natl Health Stat Report 2012;(55):1–28.

100. Centers for Disease Control and Prevention. Sexual experience and contraceptive use among female teens - United States, 1995, 2002, and 2006-2010. MMWR Morb Mortal Wkly Rep 2012;61(17):297–301.
101. Martinez G, Copen CE, Abma JC. Teenagers in the United States: sexual activity, contraceptive use, and childbearing, 2006-2010 national survey of family growth. Vital Health Stat 23 2011;(31):1–35.
102. Whitaker AK, Sisco KM, Tomlinson AN, et al. Use of the intrauterine device among adolescent and young adult women in the United States from 2002 to 2010. J Adolesc Health 2013;53(3):401–6.
103. Committee on Adolescent Health Care Long-Acting Reversible Contraception Working Group The American College of Obstetricians and Gynecologists. Committee opinion no. 539: adolescents and long-acting reversible contraception: implants and intrauterine devices. Obstet Gynecol 2012;120(4):983–8.
104. American Academy of Pediatrics Committee on Adolescence, Blythe MJ, Diaz A. Contraception and adolescents. Pediatrics 2007;120(5):1135–48.
105. Kirby DB, Laris BA, Rolleri LA. Sex and HIV education programs: their impact on sexual behaviors of young people throughout the world. J Adolesc Health 2007; 40(3):206–17.
106. Cameron S. Postabortal and postpartum contraception. Best Pract Res Clin Obstet Gynaecol 2014;28(6):871–80.
107. Smith GC, Pell JP, Dobbie R. Interpregnancy interval and risk of preterm birth and neonatal death: retrospective cohort study. BMJ 2003;327(7410):313.
108. Teal SB. Postpartum contraception: optimizing interpregnancy intervals. Contraception 2014;89(6):487–8.
109. Zapata LB, Murtaza S, Whiteman MK, et al. Contraceptive counseling and postpartum contraceptive use. Am J Obstet Gynecol 2015;212(2):171.e1–8.
110. Heit JA, Kobbervig CE, James AH, et al. Trends in the incidence of venous thromboembolism during pregnancy or postpartum: a 30-year population-based study. Ann Intern Med 2005;143(10):697–706.
111. Pomp ER, Lenselink AM, Rosendaal FR, et al. Pregnancy, the postpartum period and prothrombotic defects: risk of venous thrombosis in the MEGA study. J Thromb Haemost 2008;6(4):632–7.
112. Shikary ZK, Betrabet SS, Patel ZM, et al. ICMR task force study on hormonal contraception. Transfer of levonorgestrel (LNG) administered through different drug delivery systems from the maternal circulation into the newborn infant's circulation via breast milk. Contraception 1987;35(5):477–86.
113. Speroff L, Mishell DR. The postpartum visit: it's time for a change in order to optimally initiate contraception. Contraception 2008;78(2):90–8.
114. Nilsson S, Mellbin T, Hofvander Y, et al. Long-term follow-up of children breastfed by mothers using oral contraceptives. Contraception 1986;34(5):443–57.
115. McKinlay SM. The normal menopause transition: an overview. Maturitas 1996; 23(2):137–45.
116. Soules MR, Sherman S, Parrott E, et al. Executive summary: Stages of Reproductive Aging Workshop (STRAW). Climacteric 2001;4(4):267–72.
117. Long ME, Faubion SS, Maclaughlin KL, et al. Contraception and hormonal management in the perimenopause. J Womens Health (Larchmt) 2015;24(1):3–10.
118. Ferrell RJ, Simon JA, Pincus SM, et al. The length of perimenopausal menstrual cycles increases later and to a greater degree than previously reported. Fertil Steril 2006;86(3):619–24.
119. Baldwin MK, Jensen JT. Contraception during the perimenopause. Maturitas 2013;76(3):235–42.

120. Leridon H. A new estimate of permanent sterility by age: sterility defined as the inability to conceive. Popul Stud (Camb) 2008;62(1):15–24.
121. Hansen JP. Older maternal age and pregnancy outcome: a review of the literature. Obstet Gynecol Surv 1986;41(11):726–42.
122. Jacobsson B, Ladfors L, Milsom I. Advanced maternal age and adverse perinatal outcome. Obstet Gynecol 2004;104(4):727–33.

Intrauterine Devices and Other Forms of Contraception: Thinking Outside the Pack

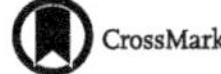

Caitlin Allen, MD[a,*], Christine Kolehmainen, MD, MS[b]

KEYWORDS

- Contraception • Intrauterine devices • Subcutaneous implants • Barrier methods
- Emergency contraception

KEY POINTS

- Intrauterine, subdermal, injectable, patch, and ring contraceptive methods are as effective or more effective than combined oral contraceptive pills.
- Intrauterine devices and subdermal implants are highly effective, long-acting, reversible contraception options that are preferred for women of all ages, including adolescents, nulliparous women, and women with multiple sexual partners.
- Explaining pregnancy rates for typical use versus perfect use is important when discussing contraception with patients.
- Patients should be advised of all side effects, including impacts on sexual desire and the risk of acquiring a sexually transmitted infection, for all hormonal and nonhormonal contraceptive methods.
- Emergency contraception is available, safe, and effective for up to 120 hours after an unprotected sexual encounter in nonpregnant women.

INTRODUCTION

At present about half of all pregnancies are unplanned or ill timed.[1] Half of unintended pregnancies are caused by contraceptive failure because of incorrect or inconsistent use.[2] Highly effective contraception is important for reducing the unintended pregnancy rate in the United States and has been listed as a top priority by the Centers for Disease Control (CDC) as a winnable battle to reduce the teen pregnancy rate.[3]

Disclosures: None.
[a] Department of Medicine, University of Wisconsin School of Medicine and Public Health, 5120 MFCB, 1685 Highland Avenue, Madison, WI 53705, USA; [b] William S. Middleton Memorial Veteran's Hospital, University of Wisconsin School of Medicine and Public Health, 11G, 2500 Overlook Terrace, Madison, WI 53703, USA
* Corresponding author.
E-mail address: callen@uwhealth.org

Med Clin N Am 99 (2015) 505–520
http://dx.doi.org/10.1016/j.mcna.2015.01.005 **medical.theclinics.com**
0025-7125/15/$ – see front matter

Most women discuss contraception with their primary care provider and inquire about the convenience of the contraceptive method, the amount of time or effort needed to use the method, side effects, return to fertility after cessation, potential noncontraceptive benefits, and the impact on sexual function.

This article discusses options for contraception other than oral contraceptive pills, including new recommendations that expand the use of the highly effective intrauterine devices (IUDs). **Table 1** and **Fig. 1** summarize the methods grouped into 5 categories: long-acting, reversible contraception (LARC; IUD, implant), sterilization, other nonoral hormonal contraception (injection, ring, patch), barrier methods (condoms, diaphragm, cervical cap), and other methods (withdrawal and fertility-based awareness). It provides details on their efficacy, time to efficacy, and return to fertility. After a brief discussion of the impact of contraception on sexuality, it closes with information on emergency contraceptive options for women who have unprotected intercourse and do not desire a pregnancy.

LONG-ACTING REVERSIBLE CONTRACEPTIVE: INTRAUTERINE DEVICES AND SUBDERMAL IMPLANTS

Women who use combined oral contraceptives (COCs), the patch, and the ring have a 20-fold increased risk of method failure compared with women who use long-acting reversible contraceptives (LARCs).[4] Moreover, in one study, women less than 21 years of age who used COCs had almost twice the rate of unintended pregnancy of older women using the same method.[4] Despite these high failure rates with COCs and low failure rates with IUDs, less than 10% of women in the United States use an IUD or implant.[4,5] The Contraceptive Choice project showed that, in the absence of knowledge, financial, or logistical barriers, women chose LARC methods more than any other contraceptive method.[6] Addressing these barriers could increase rates of use for these highly effective methods.

Two IUDs and 1 subdermal implant are available: the copper T280A IUD (Paragard), the levonorgestrel (LNG) IUD (Mirena), and the etonogestrel subdermal implant (Nexplanon, formerly Implanon) (**Table 2**). An additional low-dose LNG IUD (Skyla) was US Food and Drug Administration (FDA) approved in 2013 for prevention of pregnancy for 3 years, but because of limited data and clinical evaluations it is not discussed in this article.[7]

- The T-shaped copper IUD is made of polyethylene and has 380 copper coils wrapped around the stem and arms.[8] This method is useful for women who cannot or do not want hormonal methods.
- The LNG-IUD, also T shaped, releases a small amount of progesterone locally to the intrauterine tissue, causing atrophy.[9]
- The etonogestrel subdermal implant is about the size of a matchstick. Inserted in the groove between the biceps and the triceps muscle on the underside of the upper arm, the implant provides a controlled release of progestin, inhibiting ovulation.[8]

Table 2 lists the duration of efficacy, mechanism of action, approximate cost, timing to initiate, contraindications, and common adverse side effects for each of these long-acting reversible methods.

The American Congress of Obstetricians and Gynecologists (ACOG) recommends encouraging LARC use for most women, including nulliparous women; those with a history of sexually transmitted infections, pelvic inflammatory disease (PID), or ectopic pregnancy; and adolescents to reduce unplanned pregnancies.[8] Typical use pregnancy rates for the implant are the lowest of the LARCs, at 0.05 per 100 women in

Table 1
Contraceptive options beyond combined oral contraceptive (COC) pills

Type of Contraception		Efficacy Perfect (%)[a,1,14]	Efficacy Typical (%)[b,1,14]	Continuation at 1 y (%)[c,d,1,14]	Onset of Efficacy	Resumption of Fertility	Sexual Satisfaction Grade[e]
LARC	IUDs						
	Copper IUD (Paragard)	0.6	0.8	78	Copper: immediate[9]	Ovulation within 10 d to 2 wk[9]; Copper: 2–3.7 mo	****[65]
	LNG-IUD (Mirena)	0.2	0.2	80	LNG: backup for 7 d[9]	LNG: 4 mo[13]	****[65]
	Subdermal etonogestrel implant (Implanon)	0.05	0.05	84	Backup 7 d; unless during menses[9]	Ovulation 10 d to 2 wk[9]; 2.9–7 mo[13]	***
Permanent contraception	Sterilization: female	0.5	0.5	100	See **Table 3**; varies	NA	****[30]
	Sterilization: male	0.15	0.15	100	3 mo[26]	NA	****
Nonoral hormonal methods	Injectable Progestin (Depo-Provera)	0.2	6	56	Backup 7 d; unless during menses[34]	4.5–5 mo[13]	***
	Vaginal ring (NuvaRing)	0.3	9	67	Backup 7 d, unless during menses[58]	Assuming similar to COC, 2.5–3 mo[13]	***[59]
	Transdermal patch (OrthaEvra)	0.3	9	67	Backup 7 d, unless during menses[58]	Assuming similar to COC, 2.5–3 mo[13]	***
	COCs (for comparison)	0.3	9	67	See above	See above	NA
Barrier methods	Male condom	2	15–18	43	Immediate	Immediate	*[50]
	Female condom	5	15–18	41	Immediate	Immediate	*
	Diaphragm and cervical cap	6	15–18	21	Immediate	Immediate	**[60]
Other	Withdrawal	4	22	46	Immediate	Immediate	*
	Fertility awareness methods	3–5	24	47	Immediate	Immediate	*

Abbreviations: COC, combined oral contraceptive; LARC, long-acting reversible contraception; LNG, levonorgestrel; NA, not available.

[a] Percentage of couples with unintended pregnancies during the first year of use who use the method perfectly (ie, correctly and consistently).

[b] Typical couples who initiate the use of a method (not necessarily for the first time) with the percentage of unintended pregnancy at 1 year.

[c] Among couples attempting to avoid pregnancy, the percentage who continue to use the method for 1 year.

[d] Resumption of fertility includes median time to ovulation and median cycles/time to pregnancy.

[e] Sexual satisfaction grade: *, have to interrupt intercourse to use method; **, minimal interruption to intercourse to use method (prepare 3–48 hours before intercourse); ***, no interruption to intercourse but may influence sexual drive/desire; ****, no preparation or interruption to intercourse, and minimal impact on sexual desire.

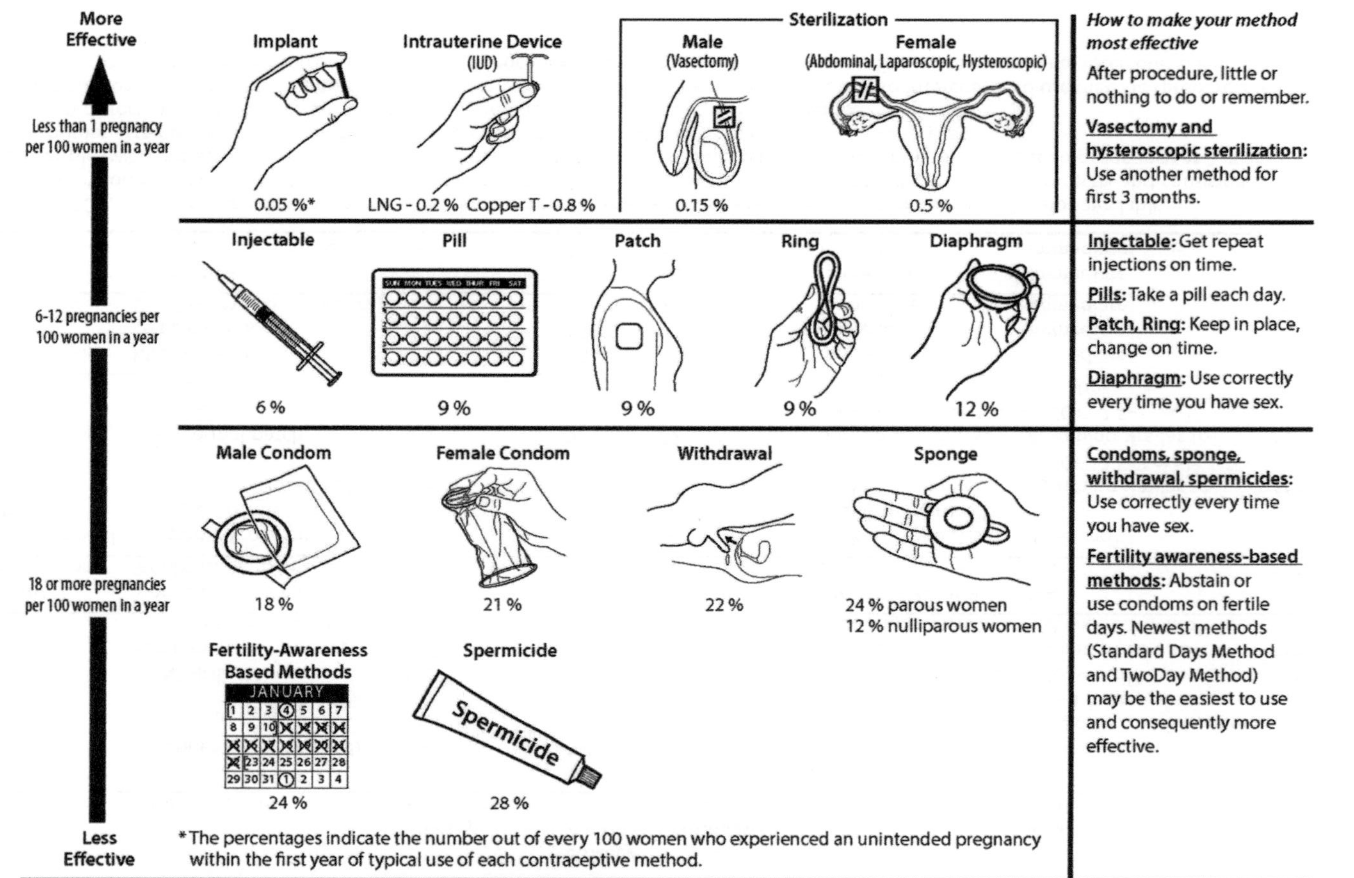

Fig. 1. Effectiveness of contraceptive methods. (*From* Centers for Disease Control. Available at: http://www.cdc.gov/reproductivehealth/UnintendedPregnancy/PDF/effectiveness_of_contraceptive_methods.pdf. Accessed January 6, 2015.)

Table 2
LARCs (IUDs and subdermal implant)

	Copper IUD	LNG-IUD	Subdermal Implant: Etonogestrel
FDA-approved Effectiveness (y)	Up to 10 y (but may be effective up to 12 y[61])	Up to 5 y (but may be effective up to 7 y[61])	Up to 3 y
Mechanism of Action	Inflammatory response of uterine lining Copper ions toxic to sperm: inhibit transport; before/after fertilization before implantation[8]	Thickening of cervical mucus Inflammatory response of uterine lining: endometrial suppression Sperm dysmotility; ovum dysmotlity[8]	Inhibition of ovulation, decrease in menstrual lining, and increase in cervical mucus
Approximate Retail Cost ($)	440[9]	700[9]	625[9]
When to Place	At any point in the cycle[8]	At any point in the menstrual cycle, but backup method should be used for 7 d if not during menses[8]	At any point in the menstrual cycle, but backup method should be used for 7 d if not during menses[8]
Contraindications to Use[a]	Distorted uterine cavity Gestational trophoblastic disease AIDS (see drug interaction) Insertion while awaiting cervical cancer treatment	Distorted uterine cavity Current or previous breast cancer Insertion while awaiting cervical cancer treatment Severe decompensated liver failure Gestational trophoblastic disease AIDS (see drug interaction)	Current or previous breast cancer Severe decompensated liver failure
Most Common Adverse Effect	Abnormal bleeding and pain	Headache, nausea, breast tenderness, cyst formation, depression	Amenorrhea or frequent prolonged bleeding
	Risk of expulsion in first year: 2%–10% Risk of perforation: <1 in 1000 insertions		

Abbreviations: AIDS, acquired immunodeficiency syndrome; FDA, US Food and Drug Administration; LNG, levonorgestrel.

[a] *Adapted from* Centers for Disease Control and Prevention. Summary chart of U.S. medical eligibility criteria for contraceptive use. 2012. Available at: http://www.cdc.gov/reproductivehealth/UnintendedPregnancy/USMEC.htm. Accessed February 11, 2015.

Adapted from Centers for Disease Control and Prevention. Summary chart of U.S. medical eligibility criteria for contraceptive use. 2010. Available at: http://www.cdc.gov/reproductivehealth/unintendedpregnancy/Docs/USMEC-Color-final.doc. Accessed November 30, 2010; with permission.

the first year of use compared with the rates of 0.2 for the LNG-IUD and 0.8 for the copper IUD.[1]

The most common complaint for women using the IUD (copper more than LNG) is dysmenorrhea and irregular bleeding. Other common complaints are similar to other hormonal methods: headaches, nausea, breast tenderness, depression, and vulvovaginitis.[8] Similarly the most common complaint with the subdermal implant is prolonged and irregular bleeding.[9] According to a recent Cochrane Review, nonsteroidal antiinflammatory drugs reduce bleeding and pain caused by intrauterine devices and tranexamic acid is a second-line treatment of excessive bleeding.[10]

Discontinuation of LARC methods has been studied extensively and rates were similar across the 3 types at 6 months: 7.3% of LNG-IUD users, 8.0% of copper IUD users, and 6.9% of subdermal implant users.[11] The most common reasons for IUD discontinuation were cramping or pain.[11] However, despite initial complaints of these symptoms, most women continued their IUD (79% at 2 years for LNG-IUD, and 77% for copper).[12] The subdermal implant had slightly worse continuation rates compared with the IUD, with only 69% of women continuing the implant at 2 years.[12]

Each of the LARCs can be removed at any time, and resumption of fertility is nearly immediate.[9,13] Postdiscontinuation rates at 1 year for the LNG-IUD and copper IUD are high and consistent with natural fertility rates (see **Table 1**), with median time to pregnancy approximately 2 to 4 months.[13] Rates of return to fertility for the implant vary, with 37% to 85% of women becoming pregnant within 1 year. The median time to pregnancy ranges from 3 to 8 months.[13]

CDC guidelines for postpartum contraceptive use state that progestin-only contraceptives (such as the LNG-IUD and implant) as well as the copper IUD can start immediately after delivery and are safe for women who are breastfeeding.[14] There is no difference in infant growth and development or in overall breastfeeding success between the two types of IUDs.[15]

Noncontraceptive benefits of IUD use include a reduction in cervical cancer risk (odds ratio, 0.55), possibly by triggering cellular immunity,[16] and a reduction in endometrial cancer (odds ratio, 0.39), possibly because of altered endometrial response to hormones caused by chronic inflammation.[17] Most women with the LNG-IUD also report decreased menorrhagia and those with endometriosis report decreased symptoms.[18] Some women are able to avoid hysterectomy for dysfunctional uterine bleeding with LNG-IUD use.[9,19]

Table 2 lists the contraindications to use for each LARC based on the CDC's Medical Eligibility Criteria for Contraceptive Use.[14] Some providers have been reluctant to use IUDs for adolescents or nulliparous women and women with history of ectopic pregnancy, sexually transmitted infections (STIs), or high-risk sexual behaviors.[20] Recent evidence has shown that the benefits of highly effective contraception far outweigh any perceived risks for these women[20,21]:

- There is no increased risk of perforation, difficultly in placement, or expulsion for nulliparous women compared with multiparous women.[20,22]
  - LNG-IUDs are not approved by the FDA for use in nulliparous women, whereas copper IUDs are, which may prevent insurance approval or use by state or federal organizations.[20]
- ACOG states that IUDs are safe to use in any age group, including adolescents,[22] especially to reduce the risk of rapid repeat pregnancy. They are recommended as first-line contraception agents.[9]
- Women with a history of ectopic pregnancy have no restriction in using IUDs for contraception.[8] Women who become pregnant with an IUD in situ have a 10-fold

increased risk that the pregnancy will be ectopic compared with women who become pregnant under other circumstances; nevertheless, the women's absolute risk for pregnancy is extremely low compared with using no contraception.[20]

- Beyond the first 20 days of IUD use, women with a history of STI are at no increased risk of PID with IUD use, suggesting that increased risk is caused by bacterial contamination at the time of insertion.[8]
- Women with active cervicitis caused by an STI should be treated before IUD placement.[8]

In the past, specific concerns about the subdermal implant were based on the impact on bone health and possible decreased efficacy in overweight or obese women. However, studies report that no decrease in bone mineral density is seen with the implant.[9] Also, there does not seem to be any decrease in effectiveness or increased rate of pregnancy in overweight or obese women.[23]

As noted earlier, ACOG recommends encouraging LARC use.[8] Despite recommendations from this and other organizations, studies show that less than half of physicians follow the evidence-based guidelines, with no difference in specialties (ie, family practice vs obstetrics-gynecology).[21,24] Based on the advantages of LARC options compared with other reversible methods, the authors agree that providers should consider LARC as first-line methods for most women.

OTHER FORMS OF CONTRACEPTION

Permanent Contraception: Female and Male Sterilization

Sterilization is a permanent and highly effective form of contraception and is a desirable option for many women. Since first performed in 1880, female sterilization has increased in popularity and is the second most commonly used form in the United States (23%), second only to oral contraceptives (28%).[25] This form of contraception is typically chosen by monogamous, married women after completion of childbearing; however, young nulliparous women may also choose this method.[26]

There are several current options for sterilization depending on timing and desirability by the patient. For women, these include an in-office procedure with hysteroscopic placement of coils (Essure) or outpatient surgery for occlusion of the fallopian tubes.[26] For men, this is an in-office vasectomy with local anesthetic. **Table 3** describes the procedure, efficacy, and complications for all 4 methods of sterilization: Essure, laparoscopic, minilaparotomy with partial salpingectomy, and vasectomy.

With proper counseling by health care professionals, regret is usually very low, especially in women older than 30 years.[26] Regret rates in women less than 30 years of age approach 20%.[27] Although contraceptive failure does occur (pregnancy rates 0.5% for Essure and tubal ligation, 0.15% for vasectomy),[1] sterilization should be considered irreversible. Couples who desire pregnancy after sterilization usually require in vitro fertilization.

According the CDC, the main contraindication to surgical female sterilization is related to medical risk of general anesthesia.[26]

A potential noncontraceptive benefit to tubal sterilization is a 34% reduction in risk of certain types of ovarian cancer, primarily endometrioid and serous cancers.[28] Some women also experience increased sexual satisfaction after sterilization.[29] One study found that women postprocedure were more likely to find sex pleasurable, were less likely to take too long to reach orgasm, and were less likely to experience vaginal dryness during sex.[30]

Male sterilization is the fourth most commonly used contraceptive method (after COCs, tubal sterilization, and condoms) among couples aged 15 to 44 years.[26,31]

Table 3
Female and male sterilization procedures

Method	Timing	Procedure	Efficacy	Complications
Hysteroscopic, Essure[26]	At least 6 mo postpartum	In-office pericervical block	Requires secondary backup for at least 3 mo until tubal occlusion confirmed	Misplacement of coils, lack of follow-up may result in unintended pregnancy
Laparoscopic	Anytime	Outpatient surgery	Immediately	Bowel, bladder, major vessel injury; use of general anesthesia
Minilaparotomy with partial salpingectomy	Can be immediately postpartum	Surgical suite; after cesarean section or after vaginal delivery with epidural in place	Immediately	Similar to laparoscopic risks: anesthesia, damage to surrounding structures
Male sterilization	Any point	Outpatient office procedure with local anesthesia	Azospermic by 3 mo, backup must be used until confirmed; 0.15% failure rate in the first year or 0.5 pregnancies per 1000 cases[62]	Local anesthetic risks

For men, vasectomy is performed in an office setting under local anesthesia with minimal risks and complications.[26]

There is a large gap in sterilization use between women and men, with 3 times as many women sterilized as men.[32] Female sterilization is effective with minimal side effects, but needs to be weighed against the safer and more cost-effective option of vasectomy for male partners or the newer LARC options.

Nonoral Hormonal Options: Injectable Progestin, Vaginal Ring, and the Patch

Many women have difficulty with remembering to take daily COCs, thus limiting the pill's efficacy.[33] Injectable progestin, vaginal rings, and transdermal patches were designed to increase ease in use and theoretically increase efficacy.[33] However, they have failure rates similar to those of COCs (see **Table 1**) and the differences between perfect use and typical use indicate that there is still significant user error and that these are not forgettable contraceptive methods.[1,33]

Medroxyprogesterone acetate (Depo-Provera) is an injectable long-acting progestin that is a reliable form of birth control for 11 to 12 weeks that can be given anytime during a woman's menstrual cycle. If the woman returns within 11 to 13 weeks for repeat injections, its perfect use efficacy is very good at 0.2%.[1] Women can be offered same-day injections if it can be reasonably assumed that she is not pregnant (ie, menses <5 days and negative urine pregnancy test).[34] If it has been greater than 5 days since menses and she has had unprotected intercourse greater than 5 days prior, the injection can be done with a backup recommended for the first 7 days. If a pregnancy does result, there no adverse side effects have been seen.[35]

As with the subdermal implant, amenorrhea, unpredictable bleeding, and approximately 2.0 kg weight gain are common side effects over the first year of therapy.[36] Women should be advised that, despite low levels of progestin detectable after 4 months, many women experience a long delay to return of ovulation; up to 10 to 12 months is reported.[13] This contraceptive method has several advantages: it requires only 4 clinic visits per year, and confers some protection against endometrial cancer and PID.[37]

The vaginal ring (Nuvaring) is a flexible, soft, transparent polymer ring. The circular tube releases a constant rate of etonogestrel plus estrogen over the course of 3 weeks.[38] The woman then removes the ring for 1 week for withdrawal bleeding. Because the hormones are absorbed vaginally, it has the advantage of avoiding gastrointestinal absorption and hepatic first-pass metabolism.[38] A 2013 Cochrane Review reported that the ring conferred better cycle control than COCs.[38] Users also reported less nausea, acne, irritability, and depression. Ten percent of vaginal ring users noted increased vaginal discharge, but there was no higher incidence of candidal infections or bacterial vaginosis.[39]

The transdermal patch (OrthoEvra) contains norelgestromin plus ethinyl estradiol. It is applied to the skin once a week for 3 weeks then removed for 1 week for withdrawal bleeding. It was first marketed in 2002 and overall effectiveness was not significantly different for the patch versus COCs, but compliance seemed to be better than COCs in 3 trials.[38] The transdermal delivery approach minimizes the peaks and troughs of hormone concentrations associated with daily oral administration and avoids hepatic first-pass metabolism.[40]

Patch users noted more side effects of breast discomfort, dysmenorrhea, nausea, and vomiting than with COCs.[38] Postmarketing studies revealed that the patches also had high detachment rates, especially when exposed to heat and humidity, potentially leading to contraceptive failure.[41] Case reports shortly after the product was released noted increased risk of venous thrombosis, but recent case-controlled trials showed no measurable increased risk with the patch compared with similar COCs.[42]

Barrier Methods: Male Condom, Female Condom, Diaphragm, and Cervical Cap

Male condoms are used worldwide for combined STI, human immunodeficiency virus (HIV), and pregnancy prevention. They are inexpensive, easily obtained, and their use is especially common among teenagers, adults 20 to 24 years old, and childless and never-married women.[31] Other barrier methods, such as the female condom, diaphragm, and cervical cap, are less widely used and account for less than 5% of contraception for users.[43] **Table 4** gives details of each of the most commonly used barrier methods.

Withdrawal

Perfect use pregnancy rates of withdrawal, or coitus interruptus, are twice the perfect use rates of condoms (4% vs 2%).[1,44] Withdrawal is used worldwide by as many as 38 million couples.[45] However, it is thought not to be an effective form of contraception, and is often used secondary to other forms of contraceptive. In one study of US women, withdrawal was most common among the youngest women, and use decreased with age.[44] However, although 41% of women aged 18 to 24 years used withdrawal, only 10% relied solely on this method. More commonly, young adults used withdrawal with condoms (17%) or highly effective methods (21%).[44]

Table 4
Barrier methods of contraception

Type of Barrier	Mechanism	How to Obtain	*Noncontraceptive* Benefits	Complications	Cautions
Male condom	Single-use sheath over erect penis just before insertion	OTC, free in many clinics and schools	Protection against HIV, HSV2, unclear HPV	Latex allergy Potential decrease in sensation for both partners; slipping and tearing	Decrease in effectiveness with heat, humidity, sunlight, and oil-based lubricants[63]
Female condom	Single-use sheath inserted into the vagina up to 8 h before intercourse	OTC, free in many clinics; \$2.50–\$4/condom on US market	Protection against HIV; nonlatex, no storage limitations	Easily displaced; makes noise during intercourse (lessened by lubricant)[43,63]	Placed similar to diaphragm, requires finger dexterity
Diaphragm	Shallow dome covers the cervix; placed up to 6 h before intercourse; needs to be left in place up to 6–8 h after last intercourse	Requires office visit with trained profession to fit during pelvic examination	Repeated intercourse without need to remove; if properly stored can be used for 1–2 y	Recommended to be used with spermicide; dyspareunia if too large; dislodged if too small; postcoital colonization by *Escherichia coli* and others in situ may increase risk for vaginitis; TSS >9 h	Obesity, arthritis may make placement and removal difficult Not recommended for women with vaginal abnormality: cystocele/rectocele
Cervical cap	Smaller, deeper, rigid dome over cervix held by suction; silicone; can be inserted up to 1 d before coitus and can be left in for 24 h	Requires office visit with trained profession to fit during pelvic examination[64]; FemCap (\$60–75 in US); Rx	Unlikely to be dislodged by partner	Recommend spermicide as adjunct; may cause discomfort during intercourse; foul smelling discharge if left in place for >2 d	Obesity, arthritis may make placement and removal difficult

Abbreviations: HPV, human papillomavirus; HSV2, herpes simplex virus 2; OTC, over the counter; Rx, prescription; TSS, toxic shock syndrome.

Data from Batár I, Sivin I. State-of-the-art of non-hormonal methods of contraception: I. Mechanical barrier contraception. Eur J Contracept Reprod Health Care 2010;15(2):67–88.

Fertility Awareness Methods

Fertility Awareness methods involve identification of the fertile days during the menstrual cycle (via cervical secretions, basal body temperature, or by charting days in the cycle), and avoiding intercourse or using barrier methods during these days.[46] Basal body temperature must be measured every day at the start of the day before any activity. The increase in progesterone level after ovulation causes a small increase in the baseline temperature, which can be detected. Intercourse should be avoided from the first day of a woman's menstrual period until the third consecutive day of increased temperature.[46]

In addition to increase in temperature, cervical mucus also becomes more transparent and slippery around the time of ovulation.[46] Avoidance of intercourse or backup contraceptive methods should be used during this change and for up to 4 days afterward to avoid pregnancy.[46] Calendar calculations, or the rhythm method, uses past cycle lengths to calculate fertile days, and is the least effective of the three methods.[46]

Planned abstinence for 7 to 17 days of the menstrual cycle may not be desirable for all couples. In addition, charting can be time consuming for women. However, there are no other side effects and these methods have low cost.[47] Efficacies, pregnancy rates, and continuation rates are difficult to study in these methods, but one study in Germany found that women who abstained from intercourse during fertile periods had a pregnancy rate of 0.6 per 100 women over 13 cycles. The investigators concluded that the symptothermal method, which combines temperature and cervical secretion observation, can be highly effective if practiced appropriately.[48]

IMPACT OF CONTRACEPTION ON SEXUAL FUNCTION AND DESIRE

Choosing a contraceptive method is a complex decision for women, who decide between multiple methods that vary by convenience, cost, efficacy, and noncontraceptive benefits. In addition, many women have questions about the impact of contraceptive methods on desire and sexual function. Men report that condoms decrease sexual pleasure, and studies show that the lower men rated their pleasure during protected vaginal intercourse, the less likely they were to use them.[49] Similarly for women, sexual side effects affect compliance.[50] **Table 1** shows the impact on sexual satisfaction for the contraceptive options discussed in this article. Interviews with 60 men and women aged 18 to 36 years indicate that there is great variability in the impact of contraception on sexual satisfaction. Some women experienced an increase in libido and sex drive, caused by the reliability of their contraception, whereas others had specific complaints because of their methods' adverse side effects (decreased pleasure with condom use; increased emotional liability with COCs).[50] It is important to counsel patients that contraception may affect sexual function and acknowledge that these effects could influence continuation.

EMERGENCY CONTRACEPTION OPTIONS

Emergency contraception is used after unprotected sexual intercourse (UPSI) to try to prevent pregnancy. Several different options are described in **Table 5**. In the past, increased doses of standard COCs were used off label to prevent pregnancy,[51] which is known as the Yuzpe method. Levonorgestrel regimens, such as Plan B and Plan B One-Step, are more commonly used now. They are effective when used within 72 hours after UPSI and have fewer estrogen-related side effects than the Yuzpe method.[52] Ulipristal (eg, ella and ellaOne) is a selective progesterone receptor modulator that can be used for up to 120 hours after the sexual encounter. It may be most

Table 5
Emergency contraception options

Method	Timing (h)	Efficacy (%)	Availability
Yuzpe method	Up to 72 after UPSI	52 to 85	By prescription
Levonorgestrel, split dose Plan B	Up to 72 after UPSI	52–85	By prescription
Levonorgestrel, single dose Plan B, One-Step	Up to 72 after UPSI	—	Avail OTC
Ulipristal Ella or ellaOne	Up to 120	>85	By prescription
Cu-IUD	Up to 120	>99	Provider visit

appropriate for women with body mass index greater than 25.[53,54] The copper IUD is appropriate for use as emergency contraception, especially if the woman also desires long-acting contraception afterward.[55]

No physical examination or pregnancy testing is needed to provide oral emergency contraception; it does not interrupt an established pregnancy and has no known adverse effects on the pregnancy or fetus if administered inadvertently.[56] Hormonal emergency contraception should be initiated as soon as possible after the UPSI to be most efficacious.[55] Studies show that advance provision of emergency contraception increases the rate and timeliness of use and does not increase the frequency of STI or change in routine contraceptive use.[57]

SUMMARY

A variety of contraception options are available in addition to traditional COC pills. LARC options such as IUDs and subcutaneous implants are preferred options because they are forgettable contraception. They are highly effective options and appropriate for most women, including adolescents, nulliparous women, and women with multiple sexual partners. Female and male sterilization are other highly effective options, but they are irreversible and require counseling to minimize regret. The contraceptive injection, patch, and ring do not require daily administration, but their typical use efficacy rates are lower than those of LARC methods and similar to those for COCs. Barrier methods, withdrawal, and fertility monitoring methods are practiced by many women but are much less effective than LARCs because of difficult perfect use. Emergency contraception can be used in the setting of contraception failure or nonuse and many groups are encouraging advanced provision for certain populations.

ACKNOWLEDGMENTS

The authors thank Stephen Johnson, who assisted with the literature review; Linda Baier, for the editorial suggestions; and Geriatrics Research Education and Clinical Center manuscript 15-007.

REFERENCES

1. Trussell J. Contraceptive failure in the United States. Contraception 2011;83(5): 397–404.
2. Frost JJ, Darroch JE, Remez L. Improving contraceptive use in the United States. Issues Brief (Alan Guttmacher Inst) 2008;(1):1–8.

3. CDC - winnable battles. Available at: http://www.cdc.gov/winnablebattles/. Accessed August 20, 2014.
4. Winner B, Peipert JF, Zhao Q, et al. Effectiveness of long-acting reversible contraception. N Engl J Med 2012;366(21):1998–2007.
5. Finer LB, Jerman J, Kavanaugh ML. Changes in use of long-acting contraceptive methods in the United States, 2007–2009. Fertil Steril 2012;98(4):893–7.
6. Secura GM, Allsworth JE, Madden T, et al. The contraceptive choice project: reducing barriers to long-acting reversible contraception. Am J Obstet Gynecol 2010;203(2):115.e1–7.
7. Gassman A. Center for drug evaluation and research: summary review, Skyla/levonorgestrel-Releasing intrauterine system. Available at: http://www.accessdata.fda.gov/drugsatfda_docs/nda/2013/203159Orig1s000SumR.pdf. Accessed November 4, 2014.
8. American College of Obstetricians and Gynecologists. ACOG practice bulletin No. 121: long-acting reversible contraception: implants and intrauterine devices. Obstet Gynecol 2011;118(1):184–96.
9. Espey E, Ogburn T. Long-acting reversible contraceptives: intrauterine devices and the contraceptive implant. Obstet Gynecol 2011;117(3):705–19.
10. Grimes DA, Hubacher D, Lopez LM, et al. Non-steroidal anti-inflammatory drugs for heavy bleeding or pain associated with intrauterine-device use. Cochrane Database Syst Rev 2006;(4):CD006034.
11. Grunloh DS, Casner T, Secura GM, et al. Characteristics associated with discontinuation of long-acting reversible contraception within the first 6 months of use. Obstet Gynecol 2013;122(6):1214–21.
12. O'neil-Callahan M, Peipert JF, Zhao Q, et al. Twenty-four-month continuation of reversible contraception. Obstet Gynecol 2013;122(5):1083–91.
13. Mansour D, Gemzell-Danielsson K, Inki P, et al. Fertility after discontinuation of contraception: a comprehensive review of the literature. Contraception 2011;84(5):465–77.
14. Division of Reproductive Health, National Center for Chronic Disease Prevention and Health Promotion, Centers for Disease Control and Prevention (CDC). U.S. selected practice recommendations for contraceptive use, 2013: adapted from the World Health Organization selected practice recommendations for contraceptive use, 2nd edition. MMWR Recomm Rep 2013;62(RR-05):1–60. Available at: http://www.cdc.gov/mmwr/preview/mmwrhtml/rr5904a1.htm.
15. Shaamash AH, Sayed GH, Hussien MM, et al. A comparative study of the levonorgestrel-releasing intrauterine system Mirena versus the Copper T380A intrauterine device during lactation: breast-feeding performance, infant growth and infant development. Contraception 2005;72(5):346–51.
16. Castellsagué X, Díaz M, Vaccarella S, et al. Intrauterine device use, cervical infection with human papillomavirus, and risk of cervical cancer: a pooled analysis of 26 epidemiological studies. Lancet Oncol 2011;12(11):1023–31.
17. Beining RM, Dennis LK, Smith EM, et al. Meta-analysis of intrauterine device use and risk of endometrial cancer. Ann Epidemiol 2008;18(6):492–9.
18. Grimes DA, Lopez LM, Manion C, et al. Cochrane systematic reviews of IUD trials: lessons learned. Contraception 2007;75(Suppl 6):S55–9.
19. Hubacher D, Grimes DA. Noncontraceptive health benefits of intrauterine devices: a systematic review. Obstet Gynecol Surv 2002;57(2):120–8.
20. Black K, Lotke P, Buhling KJ, et al. Intrauterine contraception for Nulliparous women: Translating Research into Action (INTRA) group. A review of barriers and myths preventing the more widespread use of intrauterine contraception

in nulliparous women. Eur J Contracept Reprod Health Care 2012;17(5): 340–50.
21. Callegari LS, Darney BG, Godfrey EM, et al. Evidence-based selection of candidates for the levonorgestrel intrauterine device (IUD). J Am Board Fam Med 2014;27(1):26–33.
22. Committee on Adolescent Health Care Long-Acting Reversible Contraception Working Group, The American College of Obstetricians and Gynecologists. Committee opinion no. 539: adolescents and long-acting reversible contraception: implants and intrauterine devices. Obstet Gynecol 2012;120(4):983–8.
23. Xu H, Wade JA, Peipert JF, et al. Contraceptive failure rates of etonogestrel subdermal implants in overweight and obese women. Obstet Gynecol 2012;120(1): 21–6.
24. Stubbs E, Schamp A. The evidence is in. Why are IUDs still out?: family physicians' perceptions of risk and indications. Can Fam Physician 2008;54(4):560–6.
25. Peterson HB. Sterilization. Obstet Gynecol 2008;111(1):189–203.
26. American College of Obstetricians and Gynecologists. ACOG practice bulletin no. 133: benefits and risks of sterilization. Obstet Gynecol 2013;121(2 Pt 1): 392–404.
27. Bartz D, Greenberg JA. Sterilization in the United States. Rev Obstet Gynecol 2008;1(1):23–32.
28. Cibula D, Widschwendter M, Májek O, et al. Tubal ligation and the risk of ovarian cancer: review and meta-analysis. Hum Reprod Update 2011;17(1):55–67.
29. Higgins J, Davis A. Sexuality and Contraception. In: Hatcher R, Trussell J, Nelson A, et al, editors. Contraceptive Technology, 20th Revised Edition. New York: Ardent Media; 2011. p. 1–28.
30. Smith A, Lyons A, Ferris J, et al. Are sexual problems more common in women who have had a tubal ligation? A population-based study of Australian women. BJOG 2010;117(4):463–8.
31. Guttmacher Institute. Contraceptive use in the United States. Available at: http://www.guttmacher.org/pubs/fb_contr_use.html. Accessed September 14, 2014.
32. Chandra A, Martinez GM, Mosher WD, et al. Fertility, family planning, and reproductive health of U.S. women: data from the 2002 National Survey of Family Growth. Vital Health Stat 23 2005;(25):1–160.
33. Grimes DA. Forgettable contraception. Contraception 2009;80(6):497–9.
34. Nelson AL, Katz T. Initiation and continuation rates seen in 2-year experience with same day injections of DMPA. Contraception 2007;75(2):84–7.
35. Borgatta L, Murthy A, Chuang C, et al. Pregnancies diagnosed during Depo-Provera use. Contraception 2002;66(3):169–72.
36. Vickery Z, Madden T, Zhao Q, et al. Weight change at 12 months in users of three progestin-only contraceptive methods. Contraception 2013;88(4):503–8.
37. Hofmeyr GJ, Singata M, Lawrie TA. Copper containing intra-uterine devices versus depot progestogens for contraception. Cochrane Database Syst Rev 2010;(6):CD007043.
38. Lopez LM, Grimes DA, Gallo MF, et al. Skin patch and vaginal ring versus combined oral contraceptives for contraception. Cochrane Database Syst Rev 2013;(4):CD003552.
39. Lete I, Cuesta MC, Marin JM, et al. Vaginal health in contraceptive vaginal ring users - a review. Eur J Contracept Reprod Health Care 2013;18(4):234–41.
40. Massaro M, Di Carlo C, Gargano V, et al. Effects of the contraceptive patch and the vaginal ring on bone metabolism and bone mineral density: a prospective, controlled, randomized study. Contraception 2010;81(3):209–14.

41. Jick SS, Hagberg KW, Kaye JA, et al. The risk of unintended pregnancies in users of the contraceptive patch compared to users of oral contraceptives in the UK general practice research database. Contraception 2009;80(2):142–51.
42. Jick SS, Hagberg KW, Kaye JA. ORTHO EVRA and venous thromboembolism: an update. Contraception 2010;81(5):452–3.
43. Batár I, Sivin I. State-of-the-art of non-hormonal methods of contraception: I. Mechanical barrier contraception. Eur J Contracept Reprod Health Care 2010;15(2):67–88.
44. Jones RK, Lindberg LD, Higgins JA. Pull and pray or extra protection? Contraceptive strategies involving withdrawal among US adult women. Contraception 2014;90:416–21.
45. Ortayli N, Bulut A, Ozugurlu M, et al. Why withdrawal? Why not withdrawal? Men's perspectives. Reprod Health Matters 2005;13(25):164–73.
46. Grimes DA, Gallo MF, Grigorieva V, et al. Fertility awareness-based methods for contraception. Cochrane Database Syst Rev 2004;(4):CD004860.
47. Grimes DA, Gallo MF, Grigorieva V, et al. Fertility awareness-based methods for contraception: systematic review of randomized controlled trials. Contraception 2005;72(2):85–90.
48. Frank-Herrmann P, Heil J, Gnoth C, et al. The effectiveness of a fertility awareness based method to avoid pregnancy in relation to a couple's sexual behaviour during the fertile time: a prospective longitudinal study. Hum Reprod 2007;22(5):1310–9.
49. Randolph ME, Pinkerton SD, Bogart LM, et al. Sexual pleasure and condom use. Arch Sex Behav 2007;36(6):844–8.
50. Fennell J. "And Isn't that the point?": pleasure and contraceptive decisions. Contraception 2014;89(4):264–70.
51. Ellertson C, Webb A, Blanchard K, et al. Modifying the Yuzpe regimen of emergency contraception: a multicenter randomized controlled trial. Obstet Gynecol 2003;101(6):1160–7.
52. Piaggio G, von Hertzen H. Ulipristal acetate for emergency contraception? Lancet 2010;375(9726):1607–8 [author reply: 1608].
53. Glasier AF, Cameron ST, Fine PM, et al. Ulipristal acetate versus levonorgestrel for emergency contraception: a randomised non-inferiority trial and meta-analysis. Lancet 2010;375(9714):555–62.
54. Glasier A, Cameron ST, Blithe D, et al. Can we identify women at risk of pregnancy despite using emergency contraception? Data from randomized trials of ulipristal acetate and levonorgestrel. Contraception 2011;84(4):363–7.
55. American College of Obstetricians and Gynecologists. ACOG practice bulletin no. 112: Emergency contraception. Obstet Gynecol 2010;115(5):1100–9.
56. Gemzell-Danielsson K, Rabe T, Cheng L. Emergency contraception. Gynecol Endocrinol 2013;29(Suppl 1):1–14.
57. Bosworth MC, Olusola PL, Low SB. An update on emergency contraception. Am Fam Physician 2014;89(7):545–50.
58. Lopez LM, Newmann SJ, Grimes DA, et al. Immediate start of hormonal contraceptives for contraception. Cochrane Database Syst Rev 2012;(12):CD006260.
59. Battaglia C, Morotti E, Persico N, et al. Clitoral vascularization and sexual behavior in young patients treated with drospirenone–ethinyl estradiol or contraceptive vaginal ring: a prospective, randomized, pilot study. J Sex Med 2014;11(2):471–80.
60. Amy JJ, Tripathi V. Contraception for women: an evidence based overview. BMJ 2009;339:b2895.
61. Wu JP, Pickle S. Extended use of the intrauterine device: a literature review and recommendations for clinical practice. Contraception 2014;89(6):495–503.

62. Coward RM, Badhiwala NG, Kovac JR, et al. Impact of the 2012 American Urological Association vasectomy guidelines on post-vasectomy outcomes. J Urol 2014;191(1):169–74.
63. Macaluso M, Blackwell R, Jamieson DJ, et al. Efficacy of the male latex condom and of the female polyurethane condom as barriers to semen during intercourse: a randomized clinical trial. Am J Epidemiol 2007;166(1):88–96.
64. Sivin I, Batár I. State-of-the-art of non-hormonal methods of contraception: III. Intrauterine devices. Eur J Contracept Reprod Health Care 2010;15(2):96–112.
65. Sanders J, Smith N, Higgins J. The Intimate Link: A Systematic Review of Highly Effective Reversible Contraception and Women's Sexual Experience. Clin Obstet Gynecol 2014;57(4):777–89.

Menopause

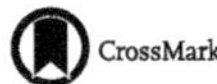

Traci A. Takahashi, MD, MPH[a,*], Kay M. Johnson, MD, MPH[b]

KEYWORDS

- Menopause • Hot flashes • Vulvovaginal atrophy • Vasomotor symptoms
- Hormone therapy • Estrogen

KEY POINTS

- Hot flashes and menstrual irregularity are hallmarks of the menopausal transition.
- Genitourinary symptoms predominate in the postmenopause phase.
- Although various treatment options are available, systemic estrogen is the most effective treatment of vasomotor symptoms, and vaginal estrogen is the most effective treatment of vulvovaginal atrophy.
- Estrogen therapy is safe for most women; it should be prescribed at the lowest effective dose and for the shortest period of time necessary to control symptoms.

DEFINITION OF MENOPAUSE

Menopause is defined retrospectively as the cessation of spontaneous menses for 12 months. Worldwide, most women enter menopause between the ages of 49 and 52 years.[1] In the United States, the average age of menopause is 51 years. An estimated 6000 US women reach menopause each day, and with increasing life expectancy, will spend approximately 40% of their lives in the postmenopause phase. Factors associated with earlier menopause include smoking, lower body mass index, nulliparity, and lower educational attainment.[2,3]

Although menopause is often seen as a single point in time, correlating with the cessation of ovarian production of oocytes, the menopausal transition actually occurs over several years and is a dynamic period when women experience

Dr. T.A. Takahashi and Dr. K.M. Johnson are staff physicians at VA Puget Sound Health Care System. The authors have nothing to disclose. The views expressed in this article are those of the authors and do not necessarily represent the views of the Department of Veterans Affairs or University of Washington.

[a] Department of Medicine, University of Washington School of Medicine, and VA Puget Sound Health Care System, 1660 South Columbian Way, S-123-PCC, Seattle, WA 98108, USA; [b] Department of Medicine, University of Washington School of Medicine, and VA Puget Sound Health Care System, 1660 South Columbian Way, S-111-HSM, Seattle, WA 98108, USA

* Corresponding author.

E-mail address: traci@u.washington.edu

Med Clin N Am 99 (2015) 521–534
http://dx.doi.org/10.1016/j.mcna.2015.01.006 medical.theclinics.com
0025-7125/15/$ – see front matter Published by Elsevier Inc.

predictable changes to their menstrual cycle. The Stages of Reproductive Aging Workshop staging system (STRAW+10) is considered the gold standard for characterizing the changes associated with reproductive aging. This staging system consists of three phases (reproductive, menopausal transition, and postmenopause), and includes seven stages within the phases. It describes the typical duration, menstrual cycle characteristics, hormone levels, antral follicle count, and symptoms for each stage.[4]

PHYSIOLOGY OF MENOPAUSE

Women are born with their full complement of oocytes and during their reproductive years, these oocytes are gradually depleted through ovulation and atresia. The decreased numbers of oocytes secrete less inhibin B, decreasing the ovarian negative feedback on follicle-stimulating hormone (FSH). The resultant increase in FSH level leads to more follicular recruitment and an accelerated follicular loss, with preservation of estradiol levels in early menopausal transition. Eventually, the depletion of follicles results in variability in the ovarian response to FSH, widely fluctuating estrogen levels, and loss of the normal reproductive cycle. When all the ovarian follicles are depleted, the ovary is unable to respond to even high levels of FSH and estrogen levels decline. The postmenopausal period is characterized hormonally by an elevated FSH (>30 mIU/mL) and low estradiol levels (**Box 1**).[5]

VASOMOTOR SYMPTOMS

Hot flashes and night sweats are common, affecting 65% of women.[6] Women experience hot flashes as spontaneous sensations of warmth, usually felt on the chest, neck, and face, often associated with perspiration and then a chill, and sometimes with palpitations and anxiety. They usually last less than 5 minutes but sometimes last up to 30 minutes. They are sometimes triggered by warm environments, stress, or hot food and beverages.[6] Night sweats are hot flashes that occur at night and often interfere with sleep. The precise cause of vasomotor symptoms is not known but is thought to be related to low estrogen levels (and possibly changes in FSH and inhibin B), which affect endorphin concentrations in the hypothalamus.

Box 1
Signs and symptoms of menopause

Menopausal Transition

- Menstrual irregularity
- Hot flashes
- Night sweats
- Sleep disruption

Postmenopause

- Vaginal dryness
- Vulvovaginal atrophy
- Lower urinary tract symptoms
- Dyspareunia

The normal thermoregulatory zone (the core temperature range within which a person can maintain their temperature without resorting to symptomatic vasodilation or sweating) in the hypothalamus seems to be narrowed in menopause, so that vasodilation and sweating are triggered at a lower temperature.

Vasomotor symptoms typically persist for 4 years, but this is variable.[7] In fact, 29% of 60-year-old women have persistent hot flashes.[6] A meta-analysis of two longitudinal and several cross-sectional studies concluded that vasomotor symptoms generally begin 2 years before menopause, peak 1 year after menopause, and then diminish over the next 10 years.[7]

EVALUATION OF VASOMOTOR SYMPTOMS

Vasomotor symptoms in a woman in her late 40s to mid-50s do not require laboratory tests for confirmation unless there is reason to suspect another cause. Careful history taking can generally rule out other causes (**Box 2**).

Panic attacks and high stress can cause symptoms similar to hot flashes. Interestingly, in a large longitudinal study, anxiety symptoms at baseline were strongly associated with later vasomotor symptoms.[8]

Measuring an FSH level is generally not helpful to confirm the diagnosis of perimenopausal vasomotor symptoms. Although levels rise and fall predictably with the menstrual cycle in premenopausal women, they fluctuate greatly during the perimenopause. FSH is persistently elevated (>30 mIU/mL) after menopause, but by then menstruation has stopped and the diagnosis is obvious. FSH levels can be helpful when evaluating premature menopause (amenorrhea before age 40), or occasionally to look for evidence of menopause in women who are amenorrheic for other reasons (eg, hysterectomy without oophorectomy, or levonorgestrel intrauterine device use).

Box 2
Other causes of hot flashes

- Alcohol consumption
- Carcinoid syndrome
- Dumping syndrome
- Hyperthyroidism
- Narcotic withdrawal
- Pheochromocytoma
- Panic attacks/high stress
- Medications, including
  - Tamoxifen
  - Raloxifene
  - Danazol
  - Leuprolide
  - Goserelin

Data from Grady D. Clinical practice. Management of menopausal symptoms. N Engl J Med 2006;355(22):2338–47; and Col NF, Fairfield KM, Ewan-Whyte C, et al. In the clinic. Menopause. Ann Intern Med 2009;150(7):ITC4-1–15; [quiz: ITC4-16].

TREATMENT OF VASOMOTOR SYMPTOMS

Studies have consistently shown a very strong placebo effect, so placebo-controlled randomized trials are required to assess efficacy of any treatment.

Lifestyle Modifications

Lowering the room temperature, dressing in layers, keeping a fan nearby, and avoiding hot drinks, caffeine, and hot or spicy foods can be helpful to manage hot flash symptoms.[9] Smoking is associated with frequency of vasomotor symptoms, providing another reason to encourage smoking cessation in perimenopausal women.[8,9]

Hormonal Treatment

Estrogen therapy (ET) is the most effective intervention for menopausal hot flashes and also improves vaginal and urogenital atrophic symptoms. Oral estrogen decreases hot flash frequency by 75% relative to placebo.[10]

Estrogen for vasomotor symptoms can be prescribed orally, transdermally, or in a vaginal ring (**Table 1**). A progestin must be added to prevent endometrial hyperplasia and cancer unless the patient has had a hysterectomy. The progesterone is given separately in a tablet, via a levonorgestrel-releasing intrauterine device, or combined with the estrogen in a tablet or patch. It can be given either continuously (daily, as in the conjugated equine estrogen [CEE] + medroxyprogesterone acetate [MPE] tablet or the estradiol + norethindrone patch) or sequentially (as in the CEE + MPE dose pack, where the progesterone is included in the tablets for days 14–28). Low-dose oral contraceptive pills containing only 20 μg ethinyl estradiol plus a progesterone are not only effective for hot flashes, but also provide contraception and cycle control for perimenopausal women. Because 5 μg of ethinyl estradiol is equivalent to CEE 0.625 mg, they are four times stronger than standard hormone-replacement therapy (HRT) and should be avoided in women who smoke, are obese, have migraines, or have hypertension. Other than oral contraceptive pills, the only treatment listed in **Table 1** that is effective for contraception is the levonorgestrel intrauterine system.

Oral HRT undergoes first pass hepatic metabolism, which promotes prothrombotic hemostatic changes.[11] In case control studies, transdermal estrogen is associated with a significantly lower risk of deep venous thrombosis compared with the equivalent dose of oral estrogen.[12]

Ultra-low-dose estrogen formulations are also available and are effective for treating hot flashes in some women. They are available as transdermal gels, emulsions, patch, or spray.

Duration of Therapy, Perioperative Management, and Side Effects

Short-term HRT (up to 5 years) is reasonable for most patients with disabling hot flashes. Vasomotor symptoms decrease after menopause for many women, so it is reasonable to try discontinuing hormone therapy every 6 to 12 months and restarting if necessary. Tapering versus abruptly stopping does not prevent hot flash recurrence.[13,14] However, some women may prefer tapering.

Whether HRT should be held before surgery to avoid perioperative venous thromboembolism (VTE) is controversial because of lack of compelling evidence that HRT increases the risk of VTE greater than that associated with surgery. One expert recommends holding HRT only in patients with other strong risk factors, such as prior VTE or anticipated prolonged immobility,[15] and others recommend stopping HRT for 4 to 6 weeks before surgery for women undergoing procedures associated with moderate or high risk for VTE.[16]

Table 1
Some forms of hormone therapy for menopausal symptoms (numerous brands available)

		Available Doses
Estrogen		
Oral	CEE	0.3, 0.45, **0.625**, 0.9, 1.25 mg/d
	17β-estradiol	0.5, **1**, 2 mg/d
Transdermal patch	17β-estradiol	0.025, 0.0375, **0.05**, 0.075, 0.1 mg/d Applied weekly or twice weekly, depending on the brand
Vaginal ring	Estradiol acetate	0.05 or 0.1 mg/d (inserted every 90 d)
Progestin		
Oral	MPA	2.5, 5.0, 10 mg/d
	Micronized progesterone	100 or 200 mg/d
Intrauterine system	Levonorgestrel	14 or 20 μg/d
Combined estrogen + progestin		
Oral sequential progestin	CEE and MPA	**0.625 mg** CEE + 5.0 mg MPA
Oral continuous progestin	CEE and MPA	**0.625 mg** CEE + 2.5 or 5.0 mg MPA 0.45 mg CEE + 2.5 mg MPA 0.3 mg or 0.45 CEE + 1.5 mg MPA
Oral contraceptive pills	Ethinyl estradiol + norethindrone, levonorgestrel, or drospirenone	20 μg ethinyl estradiol + norethindrone 1 mg or levonorgestrel 0.1 mg or drospirenone 3 mg
Transdermal patch	17β-estradiol + norethindrone	**0.05 mg** estradiol + 0.14 or 0.25 mg norethindrone twice weekly, or
	17β-estradiol + levonorgestrel	0.045 mg estradiol + 0.015 mg levonorgesterol applied weekly

BOLD: equivalent doses of estrogen. Other available oral estrogens not listed include estradiol acetate, esterified estrogen, estropipate, and conjugated synthetic estrogens. Other available oral estrogen + progesterone combinations not listed include estradiol/norethindrone, ethinyl estradiol/norethindrone, and estradiol/drosperinone.

Abbreviations: CEE, conjugated equine estrogens; MPA, medroxyprogesterone acetate.

Side effects of ET include breast tenderness, vaginal bleeding, and nausea and some women experience mood symptoms and bloating with progestin therapy. Contraindications are listed in **Box 3**.

Interpreting the Risks Identified by the Women's Health Initiative

Estrogen was used for many years for treatment of vasomotor symptoms, and also taken by millions of women in hopes of preventing chronic illness, including osteoporosis and cardiovascular disease. In 2002 the initial results from the Women's Health Initiative (WHI) suggested overall harms exceeded benefits of estrogen for prevention of disease. Both ET and estrogen and progesterone therapy (EPT) decreased the risk of osteoporosis, but were associated with an increased risk of stroke, venous

Box 3
Contraindications to hormonal therapy

- History of breast or endometrial cancer
- Atypical ductal hyperplasia of the breast
- History of venous thromboembolic disease
- History of coronary artery disease or stroke
- Unexplained vaginal bleeding
- Uncontrolled hypertension
- Migraine headaches (may increase risk of stroke)
- Active liver disease (decreases estrogen metabolism)
- Immobilization
- Active gallbladder disease
- Porphyria (may be exacerbated)
- Hypertriglyceridemia (may increase venous thromboembolic disease)

Data from Al-Safi ZA, Santoro N. Menopausal hormone therapy and menopausal symptoms. Fertil Steril 2014;101(4):905–15.

thrombosis, gallbladder disease, and incontinence. EPT was also associated with an increase in invasive breast cancer and coronary artery disease. After the release of these data, most women stopped HRT for disease prevention, and were wary of taking it even for severe vasomotor symptoms.

When considering HRT for perimenopausal women, who are almost always in their late 40s to early 50s, it is important to remember that their personal risk of complications is much lower than the absolute risks documented in the WHI. The WHI enrolled primarily older women (mean age, 63). According to the Endocrine Society, for 1000 women ages 50 to 59 taking ET for 5 years, two to three cases of stroke and/or VTE would be expected, and about 14 cases of gallbladder disease. Adding progesterone also increases the risk of breast cancer, but this risk may be much smaller than a woman may anticipate (about 7 cases per 1000)[17]. Using HRT for only a year or two may have lower risks. Providing these data is important so patients can make informed choices about their options. Because most would experience an improvement in their vasomotor symptoms, the quality of life benefits may outweigh the risks for many women.[18] Further analysis of WHI data also revealed an important age effect: women starting HRT within 10 years of the onset of menopause had a reduced risk of coronary artery disease, compared with those who started later.[6,18] The US Preventive Services Task Force and other organizations recommend against the use of HRT for the prevention of chronic conditions in average-risk postmenopausal women (Grade D recommendation).[19]

Nonhormonal Prescription Treatment of Hot Flashes

Although less effective than estrogen, the selective serotonin reuptake inhibitors paroxetine (10–20 mg per day) and fluoxetine (20 mg per day) and the serotonin-norepinephrine reuptake inhibitor venlafaxine (75 or 150 mg per day) have been shown to decrease hot flash frequency. Potential side effects are dry mouth and nausea. Paroxtine decreases the most effective metabolite of tamoxifen and should not be prescribed to women taking it for breast cancer treatment.[11] Gabapentin, 900 mg per day, also decreases hot flash frequency and severity[6] and its tendency to sedate may make it useful at bedtime. Clonidine has some efficacy but has difficult-to-tolerate side effects (dry mouth, insomnia, drowsiness).[20] **Fig. 1** summarizes the effectiveness of estrogen, nonestrogen prescription medications, and two herbal supplements for hot flash treatment.[6]

Nonprescription Treatments

Alternative therapies are tried by 50% to 75% of postmenopausal women. They are not regulated by the Food and Drug Administration and are not well studied. Most evidence suggests that alternative therapies, such as soy, black cohosh, and acupuncture, are no more effective than placebo for hot flashes.[21,22] Phytoestrogens (eg, isoflavones in red clover and soy) are plant-derived nonsteroidal compounds that bind to estrogen receptors. Randomized trials do not demonstrate the efficacy of red clover isoflavone extracts and reveal mixed results for soy isoflavone extracts.[19] Women with a personal or strong family history of hormone-dependent cancers (breast, uterine, or ovarian), thromboembolic events, or cardiovascular events should not use soy-based therapies.[23]

GENITOURINARY SYNDROME OF MENOPAUSE

Genitourinary syndrome of menopause encompasses vulvovaginal atrophy (VVA) and lower urinary tract symptoms associated with menopause and aging.[24]

Vulvovaginal Atrophy

In premenopausal women, the lining of the vagina is thickened, rugated, well-vascularized, and lubricated. After menopause, when estrogen levels decline, the vaginal lining thins and becomes dry and pale. The vagina becomes less elastic and

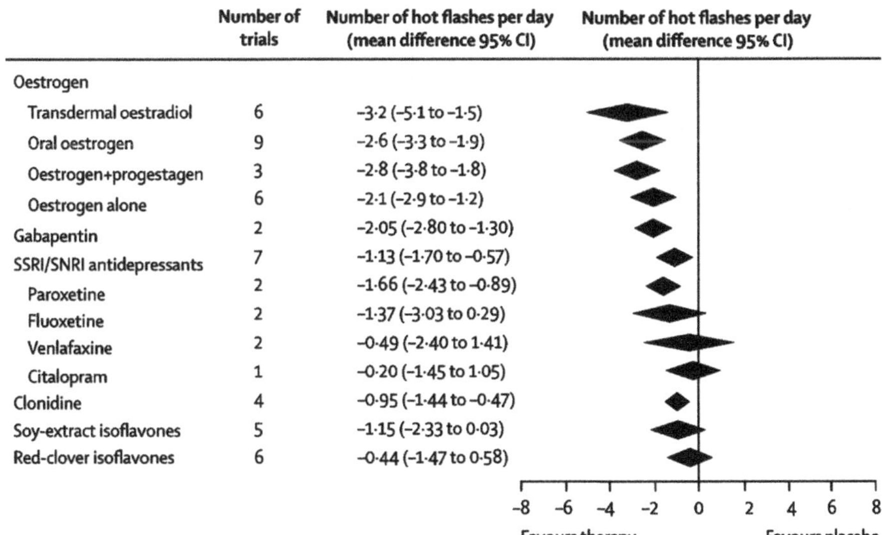

Fig. 1. Nonhormonal treatments for hot flashes. CI, confidence interval; SNRI, serotonin-norepinephrine reuptake inhibitor; SSRI, selective serotonin reuptake inhibitor. (*From* Nelson HD. Menopause. Lancet 2008;371(9614):764.)

can narrow and shorten. Atrophic vaginitis, or inflammation of the vagina, can occur, resulting in brownish or yellow discharge. A shift in the vaginal bacteria to less acid-producing bacilli results in a higher pH, typically greater than 5.0. On wet mount microscopy, white blood cells outnumber epithelial cells, parabasal cells (immature epithelial cells with large nuclei) are present, and there are few or no lactobacilli.[25] These changes to the vagina and vulva can result in a variety of symptoms that can negatively impact a woman's quality of life and sexual function (**Box 4**).

An estimated 45% of postmenopausal women experience symptoms of VVA.[26] Vaginal dryness is the most commonly reported symptom, followed by dyspareunia and irritation.[27,28] Despite the high prevalence of symptoms related to VVA in post-menopausal women, 44% of women do not seek care for their symptoms and few health care providers initiate discussion of vaginal symptoms. When evaluating post-menopausal women who report symptoms of vaginal or vulvar itching, irritation, and vaginal discharge, clinicians should consider other conditions that can cause those symptoms, in addition to VVA (**Box 5**).[27]

Treatment of Vulvovaginal Atrophy

Nonprescription therapies

Lubricants are used primarily before intercourse to reduce friction and irritation, whereas moisturizers can be used more regularly for vaginal dryness. Several formulations exist that are water-based, silicone-based, or oil-based (**Box 6**).[25] Because oil-based lubricants can degrade condoms, women should be counseled about the reduced protection of condoms against sexually transmitted infections and pregnancy.

Prescription therapies

Vaginal estrogen Local application of estrogen in the vagina is more effective than systemic hormones (oral or transdermal) in alleviating VVA symptoms; up to 80% of women experience an improvement in symptoms,[29,30] which typically occurs within 1 to 3 months of starting therapy. Various effective preparations are available in the United States (**Table 2**).[31]

Box 4
Genitourinary symptoms

Vaginal Symptoms

- Dryness
- Itching
- Irritation
- Discharge
- Dyspareunia

Lower Urinary Tract Symptoms

- Frequency
- Burning
- Dysuria
- Recurrent urinary tract infections
- Nocturia

Box 5
Differential diagnosis for symptoms of vulvovaginal atrophy

- Vaginal infections (bacterial vaginosis, *Candida*, *Trichomonas*)
- Contact dermatitis/irritation from lubricants, moisturizers, soaps, condoms
- Lichen sclerosis
- Lichen planus
- Malignancy: vulvar cancer or vulvar intraepithelial neoplasm
- Paget disease
- Desquamative inflammatory vaginitis
- Trauma
- Foreign body

Data from Management of symptomatic vulvovaginal atrophy: 2013 position statement of the North American Menopause Society. Menopause 2013;20(9):888–902. [quiz: 903–4]; and Mac Bride MB, Rhodes DJ, Shuster LT. Vulvovaginal atrophy. Mayo Clin Proc 2010;85(1):87–94.

Clinicians should prescribe the lowest dose of vaginal estrogen that alleviates symptoms. Low-dose vaginal estrogen (≤50 μg of estradiol or ≤0.3 mg of conjugated estrogens) has minimal systemic absorption and women using it for less than a year generally do not need endometrial surveillance or progesterone.[25] Monitoring for endometrial hyperplasia or use of progesterone for endometrial protection may be appropriate for women at increased risk of endometrial cancer, or when using vaginal estrogen higher than recommended dosing. Any vaginal bleeding requires evaluation for endometrial hyperplasia or cancer.[25]

Potential side effects of topical estrogen include breast pain, vaginal bleeding, and perineal pain, which seem to be dose related. Low-dose vaginal estrogen has not been associated with deep venous thrombosis.[31] Because there is some systemic absorption of vaginal estrogen, women with a history of breast cancer should discuss its use with their oncologist. Women with undiagnosed vaginal bleeding or with endometrial cancer should not use vaginal ET.

Ospemifene (Osphena) Ospemifene is a selective estrogen receptor modulator that was approved by the Food and Drug Administration in 2013 for treatment of moderate to severe dyspareunia from VVA. It acts as an estrogen agonist on the vaginal epithelium but has little or no estrogen effect on breast tissue and endometrium. Ospemifene, 60 mg daily, significantly reduced dyspareunia and vaginal dryness in women with VVA. Hot flushes occurred in 7.2% of those taking ospemifene compared with 2% of those in the placebo group. There was no increase in risk of VTE, although the studies may not have been powered to detect this.[32–34]

Urinary Symptoms

Postmenopausal women can develop lower urinary tract symptoms of urgency, frequency, dysuria, nocturia, and urinary incontinence. It is unclear whether these lower urinary tract symptoms are caused by aging or by low estrogen.

Up to 10% of postmenopausal women report having a urinary tract infection within the past 12 months.[35,36] It has been hypothesized that low estrogen alters the vaginal flora and pH, allowing enteric coliforms to colonize more easily and increasing

Box 6
Examples of nonhormonal therapeutic options for dyspareunia secondary to VVA

Lubricants

Water-based

- Astroglide liquid
- Astroglide gel liquid
- Astroglide
- Just Like Me
- K-Y Jelly
- Pre-Seed
- Slippery Stuff
- Liquid Silk

Silicone-based

- Astroglide X
- ID Millennium
- K-Y Intrigue
- Pink
- Pjur Eros

Oil-based

- Elégance Women's Lubricants
- Olive oil

Moisturizers

Replens

Me Again

Vagisil

Feminease

K-Y SILK-E

Luvena

Silken Secret

Courtesy of The North American Menopause Society, Mayfield Heights, OH; with permission.

susceptibility to urinary tract infections. Although systemic estrogen has not been shown to reduce the incidence of recurrent urinary tract infections, several studies have shown a reduction with vaginal estrogen.[37]

OTHER COMMON CONDITIONS DURING MENOPAUSE

Depression

Longitudinal studies have found that women are two to four times more likely to experience depressive symptoms during the menopausal transition compared with premenopause. Depressive symptoms have been associated with hormonal fluctuations,

Table 2
Vaginal estrogen preparations for VVA

	Type of Estrogen	Strength	Recommended Regimen
Premarin cream	Conjugated estrogens	0.625 mg/g cream	0.5–2 g cream twice weekly
Estrace cream	Estradiol	100 μg/g cream	1–4 g cream daily for 1–2 wk then reduce to one-half initial dose for 1–2 wk then 0.5–1 g one to three times a week
Estring estrogen ring	Estradiol	7.5 μg estradiol per day for 90 d	One ring intravaginal every 90 d
Vagifem vaginal tablet	Estradiol	10 μg estradiol per tablet	One tablet intravaginal daily for first 2 wk then twice weekly

and with the presence of vasomotor symptoms.[38,39] It remains unclear whether ET should be recommended to alleviate depressive symptoms. Small randomized controlled trials have found transdermal estrogen to be more effective than placebo in improving symptoms of depression during the menopausal transition.[40,41]

Cognitive Function

Although up to 40% of women report episodes of forgetfulness during the perimenopausal period, any cognitive decline noted in observational studies has been subtle and transient.[42,43] Similarly, it has been difficult to establish whether older women later in menopause have higher rates of dementia compared with men because of differences in survival.[44] The effect of hormone therapy on cognitive function may be variable, depending on when it is initiated during menopause. Analyses of pooled data from the ET and the EPT arms of the WHI show that hormone therapy initiated in women 65 years and older increased the risk of developing probable dementia, and resulted in more cognitive decline and greater brain atrophy. The decrease in cognitive function was small and of unclear clinical significance.[45–51] In contrast, the WHI Memory Study of Younger Women evaluated the effect of hormone therapy on cognitive function in women aged 50 to 55 years and did not find a sustained benefit or decline.[52]

Cardiovascular Disease, Osteoporosis, and Malignancy

These are important issues and more prevalent among postmenopausal women. These issues are addressed elsewhere in this issue.

SUMMARY

Hot flashes and menstrual irregularity are hallmarks of the menopausal transition, although vasomotor symptoms can persist for years in some women. Genitourinary symptoms predominate in the postmenopause phase and can impact sexual function and quality of life. Although various treatment options are available, systemic estrogen is the most effective treatment of vasomotor symptoms, and vaginal estrogen is the most effective treatment of VVA, using the lowest dose of estrogen to alleviate symptoms. Other common conditions in menopause include cardiovascular disease, depression, and cognitive dysfunction. The understanding of the relationship between menopause, HRT, and these conditions continues to evolve.

REFERENCES

1. Morabia A, Costanza MC. International variability in ages at menarche, first livebirth, and menopause. World Health Organization collaborative study of neoplasia and steroid contraceptives. Am J Epidemiol 1998;148(12):1195–205.
2. Gold EB, Bromberger J, Crawford S, et al. Factors associated with age at natural menopause in a multiethnic sample of midlife women. Am J Epidemiol 2001; 153(9):865–74.
3. Parazzini F, Progetto Menopausa Italia Study Group. Determinants of age at menopause in women attending menopause clinics in Italy. Maturitas 2007; 56(3):280–7.
4. Harlow SD, Gass M, Hall JE, et al. Executive summary of the Stages of Reproductive Aging Workshop + 10: addressing the unfinished agenda of staging reproductive aging. J Clin Endocrinol Metab 2012;97(4):1159–68.
5. Hall JE. Neuroendocrine changes with reproductive aging in women. Semin Reprod Med 2007;25(5):344–51.
6. Nelson HD. Menopause. Lancet 2008;371(9614):760–70.
7. Politi MC, Schleinitz MD, Col NF. Revisiting the duration of vasomotor symptoms of menopause: a meta-analysis. J Gen Intern Med 2008;23(9):1507–13.
8. Gold EB, Colvin A, Avis N, et al. Longitudinal analysis of the association between vasomotor symptoms and race/ethnicity across the menopausal transition: study of women's health across the nation. Am J Public Health 2006;96(7):1226–35.
9. Col NF, Fairfield KM, Ewan-Whyte C, et al. In the clinic. menopause. Ann Intern Med 2009;150(7):ITC4-1–ITC4-15 [quiz: ITC4–16].
10. Maclennan AH, Broadbent JL, Lester S, et al. Oral oestrogen and combined oestrogen/progestogen therapy versus placebo for hot flushes. Cochrane Database Syst Rev 2004;(4):CD002978.
11. Al-Safi ZA, Santoro N. Menopausal hormone therapy and menopausal symptoms. Fertil Steril 2014;101(4):905–15.
12. Canonico M, Oger E, Plu-Bureau G, et al. Hormone therapy and venous thromboembolism among postmenopausal women: impact of the route of estrogen administration and progestogens: the ESTHER study. Circulation 2007;115(7):840–5.
13. Haimov-Kochman R, Barak-Glantz E, Arbel R, et al. Gradual discontinuation of hormone therapy does not prevent the reappearance of climacteric symptoms: a randomized prospective study. Menopause 2006;13(3):370–6.
14. Grady D, Sawaya GF. Discontinuation of postmenopausal hormone therapy. Am J Med 2005;118(Suppl 12B):163–5.
15. Ueng J, Douketis JD. Prevention and treatment of hormone-associated venous thromboembolism: a patient management approach. Hematol Oncol Clin North Am 2010;24(4):683–94, vii-viii.
16. Golob AL, Julka R. Perioperative medication management. In: Wong CJ, Hamlin NP, editors. The perioperative medicine consult handbook. New York: Springer; 2013. p. 21–7.
17. Santen RJ, Allred DC, Ardoin SP, et al. Executive summary: postmenopausal hormone therapy: an Endocrine Society scientific statement. J Clin Endocrinol Metab 2010;95(Suppl 1):S1–66.
18. Manson JE. Current recommendations: what is the clinician to do? Fertil Steril 2014;101(4):916–21.
19. Moyer VA, U.S. Preventive Services Task Force. Menopausal hormone therapy for the primary prevention of chronic conditions: U.S. preventive services task force recommendation statement. Ann Intern Med 2013;158(1):47–54.

20. Nelson HD, Vesco KK, Haney E, et al. Nonhormonal therapies for menopausal hot flashes: systematic review and meta-analysis. JAMA 2006;295(17):2057–71.
21. Newton KM, Reed SD, LaCroix AZ, et al. Treatment of vasomotor symptoms of menopause with black cohosh, multibotanicals, soy, hormone therapy, or placebo: a randomized trial. Ann Intern Med 2006;145(12):869–79.
22. Dodin S, Blanchet C, Marc I, et al. Acupuncture for menopausal hot flushes. Cochrane Database Syst Rev 2013;(7):CD007410.
23. Goodman NF, Cobin RH, Ginzburg SB, et al, American Association of Clinical Endocrinologists. American Association of Clinical Endocrinologists medical guidelines for clinical practice for the diagnosis and treatment of menopause: executive summary of recommendations. Endocr Pract 2011;17(6):949–54.
24. Portman DJ, Gass ML, Vulvovaginal Atrophy Terminology Consensus Conference Panel. Genitourinary syndrome of menopause: new terminology for vulvovaginal atrophy from the International Society for the Study of Women's Sexual Health and the North American Menopause Society. Menopause 2014;21(10):1063–8.
25. Management of symptomatic vulvovaginal atrophy: 2013 position statement of the North American Menopause Society. Menopause 2013;20(9):888–902 [quiz: 903–4].
26. Santoro N, Komi J. Prevalence and impact of vaginal symptoms among postmenopausal women. J Sex Med 2009;6(8):2133–42.
27. Kingsberg SA, Wysocki S, Magnus L, et al. Vulvar and vaginal atrophy in postmenopausal women: findings from the REVIVE (REal women's VIews of treatment options for menopausal vaginal ChangEs) survey. J Sex Med 2013;10(7):1790–9.
28. Simon JA, Kokot-Kierepa M, Goldstein J, et al. Vaginal health in the United States: results from the vaginal health: insights, views & attitudes survey. Menopause 2013;20(10):1043–8.
29. Cardozo L, Bachmann G, McClish D, et al. Meta-analysis of estrogen therapy in the management of urogenital atrophy in postmenopausal women: second report of the hormones and urogenital therapy committee. Obstet Gynecol 1998;92 (4 Pt 2):722–7.
30. Long CY, Liu CM, Hsu SC, et al. A randomized comparative study of the effects of oral and topical estrogen therapy on the vaginal vascularization and sexual function in hysterectomized postmenopausal women. Menopause 2006;13(5): 737–43.
31. Suckling J, Lethaby A, Kennedy R. Local oestrogen for vaginal atrophy in postmenopausal women. Cochrane Database Syst Rev 2006;(4):CD001500.
32. Bachmann GA, Komi JO, Ospemifene Study Group. Ospemifene effectively treats vulvovaginal atrophy in postmenopausal women: results from a pivotal phase 3 study. Menopause 2010;17(3):480–6.
33. Portman DJ, Bachmann GA, Simon JA, Ospemifene Study Group. Ospemifene, a novel selective estrogen receptor modulator for treating dyspareunia associated with postmenopausal vulvar and vaginal atrophy. Menopause 2013;20(6): 623–30.
34. Simon J, Portman D, Mabey RG Jr, et al. Long-term safety of ospemifene (52-week extension) in the treatment of vulvar and vaginal atrophy in hysterectomized postmenopausal women. Maturitas 2014;77(3):274–81.
35. Brown JS, Vittinghoff E, Kanaya AM, et al. Urinary tract infections in postmenopausal women: effect of hormone therapy and risk factors. Obstet Gynecol 2001;98(6):1045–52.
36. Foxman B, Barlow R, D'Arcy H, et al. Urinary tract infection: self-reported incidence and associated costs. Ann Epidemiol 2000;10(8):509–15.

37. Perrotta C, Aznar M, Mejia R, et al. Oestrogens for preventing recurrent urinary tract infection in postmenopausal women. Cochrane Database Syst Rev 2008;(2): CD005131.
38. Cohen LS, Soares CN, Vitonis AF, et al. Risk for new onset of depression during the menopausal transition: the Harvard study of moods and cycles. Arch Gen Psychiatry 2006;63(4):385–90.
39. Freeman EW, Sammel MD, Lin H, et al. Symptoms associated with menopausal transition and reproductive hormones in midlife women. Obstet Gynecol 2007; 110(2 Pt 1):230–40.
40. Schmidt PJ, Nieman L, Danaceau MA, et al. Estrogen replacement in perimenopause-related depression: a preliminary report. Am J Obstet Gynecol 2000;183(2):414–20.
41. Soares CN, Almeida OP, Joffe H, et al. Efficacy of estradiol for the treatment of depressive disorders in perimenopausal women: a double-blind, randomized, placebo-controlled trial. Arch Gen Psychiatry 2001;58(6):529–34.
42. Meyer PM, Powell LH, Wilson RS, et al. A population-based longitudinal study of cognitive functioning in the menopausal transition. Neurology 2003;61(6): 801–6.
43. Greendale GA, Huang MH, Wight RG, et al. Effects of the menopause transition and hormone use on cognitive performance in midlife women. Neurology 2009; 72(21):1850–7.
44. Barrett-Connor E, Laughlin GA. Endogenous and exogenous estrogen, cognitive function, and dementia in postmenopausal women: evidence from epidemiologic studies and clinical trials. Semin Reprod Med 2009;27(3):275–82.
45. Shao H, Breitner JC, Whitmer RA, et al. Hormone therapy and Alzheimer disease dementia: new findings from the cache county study. Neurology 2012;79(18): 1846–52.
46. Resnick SM, Espeland MA, An Y, et al. Effects of conjugated equine estrogens on cognition and affect in postmenopausal women with prior hysterectomy. J Clin Endocrinol Metab 2009;94(11):4152–61.
47. Espeland MA, Rapp SR, Shumaker SA, et al. Conjugated equine estrogens and global cognitive function in postmenopausal women: women's health initiative memory study. JAMA 2004;291(24):2959–68.
48. Rapp SR, Espeland MA, Shumaker SA, et al. Effect of estrogen plus progestin on global cognitive function in postmenopausal women: the women's health initiative memory study: a randomized controlled trial. JAMA 2003;289(20):2663–72.
49. Shumaker SA, Legault C, Kuller L, et al. Conjugated equine estrogens and incidence of probable dementia and mild cognitive impairment in postmenopausal women: women's health initiative memory study. JAMA 2004;291(24):2947–58.
50. Whitmer RA, Quesenberry CP, Zhou J, et al. Timing of hormone therapy and dementia: the critical window theory revisited. Ann Neurol 2011;69(1):163–9.
51. Espeland MA, Brunner RL, Hogan PE, et al. Long-term effects of conjugated equine estrogen therapies on domain-specific cognitive function: results from the women's health initiative study of cognitive aging extension. J Am Geriatr Soc 2010;58(7):1263–71.
52. Espeland MA, Shumaker SA, Leng I, et al. Long-term effects on cognitive function of postmenopausal hormone therapy prescribed to women aged 50 to 55 years. JAMA Intern Med 2013;173(15):1429–36.

Cardiovascular Risk Factors and Disease in Women

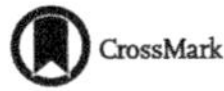

Sharon K. Gill, MD

KEYWORDS

• ASCVD • Heart disease • Stroke • Risk factors • Women • Prevention

KEY POINTS

- Use American Heart Association (AHA) and American College of Cardiology (ACC) guidelines and calculator to assess atherosclerotic cardiovascular disease (ASCVD) risk.
- Use evidence-based recommendations to counsel women on risk reduction strategies.
- Statin medications reduce risk for women at elevated risk but have important adverse effects to discuss with patients.
- Women have unique cardiovascular disease (CVD) risk factors, including hypertensive disorders of pregnancy, polycystic ovarian syndrome (PCOS), and migraine.

DEFINITIONS

Cardiovascular Disease

CVD means damage to or narrowing of arteries due to atherosclerosis. Therefore, it is a systemic disease that can lead to a variety of end-organ manifestations:

- Coronary artery disease (CAD) with or without acute coronary syndrome
- Heart failure (ischemic)
- Arrhythmia (atrial fibrillation)
- Stroke (especially related to carotid artery stenosis and cerebrovascular disease)
- Peripheral vascular disease (PVD)
- Aortic aneurysm
- Chronic kidney disease (CKD)

For purposes of discussing risk factors and primary prevention, CVD does not include valvular disease, pericarditis, endocarditis, nonischemic cardiomyopathy, or other arrhythmia (eg, supraventricular tachycardia).

No financial or other disclosures.
Women's Health Program, VA Puget Sound, 1660 South Columbian Way, Seattle, WA 98108, USA
E-mail addresses: Sharon.gill@va.gov; Sgill@aya.yale.edu

Med Clin N Am 99 (2015) 535–552
http://dx.doi.org/10.1016/j.mcna.2015.01.007
0025-7125/15/$ – see front matter Published by Elsevier Inc.

Statin

Statin is a medication class that inhibits HMG CoA reductase, thus blocking a key step in cholesterol synthesis. Originally used primarily to lower cholesterol, especially low-density lipoprotein (LDL), recently it has been found to lower overall ASCVD risk via incompletely understood beneficial effects on endothelial function, inflammation, and plaque stabilization.[1]

Primary Prevention

Primary prevention refers to preventing development of a disease state that a person does not already have. In cases of ASCVD, it refers to preventing a first coronary event or stroke in a person not known to have ASCVD.

Secondary Prevention

Secondary prevention refers to preventing subsequent events or symptoms in a person known to have a disease.

Polycystic Ovary Syndrome

PCOS is a heterogeneous disorder of unknown etiology characterized by hyperandrogenism and anovulation, which present as insulin resistance, menstrual irregularity, infertility, obesity, hirsutism, and/or acne.

Number Needed to Treat

Number needed to treat (NNT) is a statistical representation of the likelihood of beneficial effect of a treatment, or "How many patients do I need to treat before I can expect to prevent 1 adverse outcome?" It is calculated from the absolute risk reduction: 1/(adverse outcome rate with placebo – adverse outcome rate with treatment). For example, in a randomized controlled trial, if that study's adverse outcome occurred in 5% of patients in the medication-treated group and 10% of patients in the placebo group, then NNT = 20.

Number Needed to Harm

Number needed to harm (NNH) is a statistical representation of the likelihood of a patient experiencing an adverse effect of an intervention, calculated from absolute harm reduction: 1/(adverse event rate with treatment – adverse event rate with placebo).

INTRODUCTION

CVD and stroke are the most frequent causes of death in women. Knowledge among women themselves has improved (from 30% to 56% from 1997 to 2012), but this still leaves approximately half of women unaware that they are at highest risk of dying from heart disease or stroke as opposed to other causes, such as cancer (**Table 1**).[2]

Reducing cardiovascular risk in women may initially evoke questions, such as "When should we start aspirin in a diabetic woman?" and, "In whom should we start a statin?" These are important questions, but addressing CVD prevention completely must start much earlier, with questions for young women, such as, "Are your periods regular?" and "Did you have high blood pressure during pregnancy?" Obesity, smoking, PCOS, migraine history, and pregnancy complications should all be considered when assessing current and future cardiovascular risk and advising young women about choices that lead to lower versus higher risk later in life. For all women, the usual culprits must be addressed: obesity, smoking, hypertension (HTN), and

Table 1
Causes of death in women

	Women (%)	Men (%)
Heart disease + stroke	29.7	29.1
Heart disease	23.5	24.9
Cancer	22.1	24.4
Stroke	6.2	4.2
Chronic lower respiratory diseases	5.9	5.3
Alzheimer disease	4.7	2.1
Unintentional injuries	3.6	6.2
Diabetes	2.7	2.9
Suicide	0.7	2.5
Influenza and pneumonia	2.1	1.9
Kidney disease	2.1	2.0
Septicemia	1.5	1.3

From Centers for Disease Control. Deaths, percent of total deaths, and death rates for the 15 leading causes of death in selected age groups, by race and sex: United States, 2011. Available at: http://www.cdc.gov/nchs/data/dvs/LCWK3_2011.pdf. Accessed September 14, 2014.

diabetes. This article reviews current evidence on ASCVD risk factors as they pertain to women and presents information that is most useful for educating and counseling women on what they can do to reduce their risk of an ASCVD event.

RISK FACTOR ASSESSMENT

In November 2013, the AHA and ACC released new guidelines for assessing risk of ASCVD and treating based on multiple risk factors.[3,4] The approach to risk factor assessment and modification shifted focus from treat to target (LDL cholesterol) to overall risk factor assessment (**Box 1**).[5]

Using albeit a controversial calculation, 10-year and lifetime risk of an ASCVD event can be calculated based on well-established and readily available risk factors. An ASCVD event comprises nonfatal myocardial infarction (MI), coronary heart disease (CHD)-related death, or stroke (fatal or nonfatal). A person who meets high-risk criteria or whose 10-year ASCVD event risk exceeds 7.5% should receive a recommendation for statin medication. Statin therapy is estimated to reduce 10-year ASCVD risk by 30% for moderate-intensity and 45% for high-intensity statin. For example, if 10-year ASCVD event risk for a nondiabetic is 12%, taking a statin reduces 10-year risk to approximately 8%. Additionally, the calculator can be used as part of a clinic visit to demonstrate the effect of risk factor modification on an individual's ASCVD 10-year and lifetime risk level (eg, quitting smoking or exercising to control blood

Box 1
Why the change from low-density lipoprotein numbers to risk factors?

- There is no scientific basis to support clinical benefit from treating to a target LDL number.
- Available evidence does not demonstrate safety of treating to target LDL.
- Treatment based on individual risk factors is simpler, is safer, and has an evidence base to support effectiveness on clinical outcomes.

pressure [BP]). The calculator is available via the AHA Web site in multiple formats (http://my.americanheart.org/cvriskcalculator) (**Box 2**, **Table 2**, **Box 3**).

Diabetes is a stronger predictor of CVD in women than in men.[6,7] Women who smoke even a small amount (1–4 cigarettes per day) double their CAD risk.[8] In women, low high-density lipoprotein (HDL) seems a stronger predictor of CVD than high LDL.[9,10] Because there is no current evidence that raising HDL via medication has a meaningful effect on lowering ASCVD risk, and recent evidence is mounting for excess harm with niacin, the ability to focus interventions for women based on this information is limited.[11–13] Exercise and heart-healthy diet may have some beneficial effect on HDL, and these lifestyle interventions are globally recommended for general ASCVD risk reduction.

Lifetime risk calculation is not linked to specific medication or other treatment recommendations; rather, it can be useful in young adults to highlight the importance of risk factor modification. For example, a 35-year-old woman who is overweight, has newly diagnosed diabetes, and smokes but has normal BP and cholesterol values can be counseled that her lifetime ASCVD risk would drop from 50% to 27% if she quit smoking and lost enough weight to reverse the early diabetes. A sedentary 35-year-old woman who smokes and has a systolic BP 130 (untreated) could reduce her lifetime ASCVD risk from 39% to 8% if she quit smoking and lowered her BP to under 120 via regular exercise and weight loss; this profile represents "optimal risk factors."[14–21] **Box 4** illustrates risk reduction counseling in terms of added disease-free years of life with optimized risk factors.[22]

Special Considerations for Older Women

- There are not enough women (or men) ages 75 years or older in studies to make strong conclusions about statin use.
- For secondary prevention, use a moderate-intensity instead of a high-intensity statin.
- Consider starting statin for primary prevention, depending on comorbidities.
- Continue statin if already taking and tolerating.

Box 2
Data needed for statin recommendation assessment with the American Heart Association calculator

History of preexisting ASCVD (CAD, PVD, or stroke)

Age

Gender

Race

Total cholesterol

HDL cholesterol

Systolic BP

Use of hypertensive medications

Diabetes

Smoking (current)

Notes on the risk factors: women overall have a lower risk of an ASCVD event. Race is represented only by black or white. Hispanic Americans and Asian Americans generally have lower risk than whites, so using "white" is the best estimate but may overestimate risk.

Table 2
Race/ethnicity and cardiovascular disease–related causes of death in women

Race/Ethnicity	Heart Disease (%)	Stroke (%)	Diabetes (%)	Kidney Disease (%)	Hypertension (%)
Black	24.1	6.4	4.6	3.4	2.1
White	23.5	6.2	2.4	1.9	—
Asian/Pacific Islander	21.3	8.5	3.7	2.3	1.9
Hispanic	20.9	6.0	4.9	2.4	—
American Indian/Alaska Native	16.8	4.3	6.0	2.6	—
All races	23.5	6.2	2.7	2.1	—

From Centers for Disease Control, Leading Causes of Death in Females. 2010 Data. Available at: http://www.cdc.gov/women/lcod/. Accessed September 14, 2014.

- Do not calculate ASCVD risk score for women over 75; even with optimal risk factors, their 10-year ASCVD risk is 12% or more.
- Atrial fibrillation substantially increases stroke risk; use the $CHADS_2$ or CHA_2DS_2-VASc calculator to quantify this risk and make an anticoagulation recommendation.[23,24] Female gender is a risk factor for stroke, particularly in women over 65, and is included as a risk factor in the newer CHA_2DS_2-VASc calculation. The 2014 American Stroke Association (ASA)/AHA stroke prevention guidelines for women recommend screening for atrial fibrillation in women 65 and older to prevent stroke. Initial screen is pulse check, followed by ECG if abnormal.[25]

Additional Risk Factors

Even though these additional tests are not used to calculate a risk number nor should they be done routinely for risk assessment, the AHA/ACC guidelines recommend considering these other factors/tests if the risk calculation is borderline or unclear:

- Primary LDL cholesterol ≥160 mg/dL or other evidence of genetic hyperlipidemias
- Family history of premature ASCVD with onset less than 55 years of age in a first-degree male relative or less than 65 years of age in a first-degree female relative

Box 3
Algorithm for determining statin recommendation

Patient already has ASCVD → *Recommend high-intensity statin*

LDL ≥190 → *Recommend high-intensity statin*

Calculate 10-year ASCVD event risk for patients ages 40–75 years and not in one of the high-risk groups listed previously:

Patients without diabetes

Less than 7.5% risk → *Do not recommend statin*

≥7.5% Risk → *Recommend moderate- or high-intensity statin*

Patients with diabetes

Less than 7.5% risk → *Recommend moderate-intensity statin*

≥7.5% Risk → *Recommend high-intensity statin*

Box 4
Patient counseling example

A 45-year-old woman has a 55.6% risk of any CVD event in her lifetime. This woman would live up to 14 years longer free of CVD events if she had an optimal risk factor profile instead of 2 or more major risk factors:

- BP greater than 160 → less than 120
- Total cholesterol greater than 240 → less than 180
- Diabetes YES → NO
- Smoking YES → NO

If this 45-year-old woman were a smoker with a new diagnosis of diabetes, then quitting smoking and losing approximately 10% of her body weight would likely add 14 CVD-free years to her life.

- High-sensitivity C-reactive protein (hs-CRP) ≥2 mg/L
- Coronary artery calcium (CAC) score ≥300 Agatston units or ≥75th percentile for age, gender, and ethnicity (for additional information, see http://www.mesa-nhlbi.org/CACReference.aspx)
- Ankle-brachial index (ABI) less than 0.9
- High lifetime risk of ASCVD

Other Disorders That Increase Atherosclerotic Cardiovascular Disease Risk

These chronic diseases increase ASCVD risk, but are not specifically addressed in the AHA/ACC guideline/calculation.

- Obesity (body mass index [BMI] ≥30) is more prevalent in women than in men (37% vs 34%). More women than men are obese in all age groups and across all races/ethnicities. Non-Hispanic black women have the highest rates at 57% versus the lowest rates in Asian women at 11%.[26] Although obesity is not considered in calculations of risk factors, it is the major underlying disorder for future development of HTN, diabetes, and unfavorable lipid profile. Diet and exercise for weight loss are critical interventions addressed in 2 additional AHA/ACC guidelines.[27,28]
- Rheumatologic diseases (eg, rheumatoid arthritis and lupus) are more prevalent in women than men and are independently associated with 59% higher risk of CAD than in the unaffected population.[29] Chronic inflammatory disorders are also associated with increased risk of other CVDs, including heart failure, atrial fibrillation, and stroke.
- Chronic kidney disease: a glomerular filtration rate reduction of 10 mL/min/1.73 m^2 correlates with a 5% increased risk of CVD. This study included 55% women, with no difference between men and women in effect of renal disease on ASCVD risk.[30]
- Sleep apnea is well established as increasing risk of HTN and other cardiovascular outcomes. Prevalence of sleep apnea is 9% in women compared with 24% in men. Sleep apnea is, however, estimated as undiagnosed in 90% of women with moderate to severe sleep apnea, suggesting that women frequently do not have classic symptoms of obstructive sleep apnea. Women often present with atypical symptoms, such as insomnia, fatigue (not sleepiness), depression/anxiety, decreased libido, palpitations, ankle edema, and/or nocturia.[31–34]

RISK FACTORS UNIQUE TO WOMEN

Polycystic Ovarian Syndrome

Women with PCOS are at increased risk for obesity, diabetes, HTN, and ultimately CVD.[35,36] PCOS confers double the risk of diabetes and elevated cholesterol levels 18 to 20 years from baseline, independent of obesity.[37] After making a diagnosis of PCOS, women should have more aggressive CVD risk factor management[38]:

- BP and BMI measured regularly, per usual guidelines
- Lipids measured at diagnosis (this is likely earlier than otherwise indicated)
- Oral glucose tolerance test, if possible, or fasting glucose and hemoglobin A_{1C} measured at diagnosis. If a woman has impaired glucose tolerance, then screen for diabetes every year. If she has normal glucose tolerance, then screen for diabetes at least every 2 years and more often if other risk factors are present.

Menopause

Postmenopausal women are at higher risk of ASCVD events than premenopausal women; however, menopause itself does not seem to be the culprit. Rather, other CVD risk factors increase with age. Menopause can have a negative impact on cardiovascular risk factors; early menopause seems to be associated with increased risk of CHD events.[39,40] Within a year of menopause, total cholesterol, LDL, and apolipoprotein B have been shown to increase substantially in women, a change noted across ethnicities and geography.[41] Although other risk factors for CVD, such as diabetes and HTN, increase in older women, it is not clear if menopause itself increases the prevalence of these risk factors versus aging alone. Alternatively, estrogen seems to play a protective role in premenopausal women, such that premenopausal women have a lower risk of CVD compared with men of a similar age.

In premenopausal women, estrogen is thought to alter the lipid profile favorably by increasing HDL and reducing vascular injury and atherosclerosis. The effect of postmenopausal hormone therapy on cardiovascular risk is complex and understanding its impact on CVD has evolved over the past decade. Analyses of the Women's Health Initiative (WHI) cohort have found that hormone therapy initiated within 10 years of menopause significantly reduces CAC, a marker of atherosclerosis and a risk factor for future cardiovascular events.[42] In addition, an unrelated secondary analysis of the WHI found a nonsignificant trend toward reduced CHD events and mortality in younger women receiving hormone therapy compared with older women.[43] More recent follow-up analysis shows a persistent increase in thrombotic stroke risk (approximately 15%, barely statistically significant) and neutral CHD risk in most groups. In women ages 50 to 59, estrogen alone (for women without a uterus) may be protective, whereas combination therapy trends toward increased CHD risk.[44] At this time, there is not enough evidence to support the use of hormone therapy to reduce CVD risk, particularly when other interventions that reduce CVD risk are underutilized by women. I continue to advise women to use hormone therapy sparingly, at the lowest dose, for the shortest period of time and for intolerable vasomotor symptoms and to inform women that there may be some increased risk of ASCVD.

Pregnancy Complications

ASCVD risk assessment and management include pregnancy planning. Planned pregnancies along with risk factor reduction prior to pregnancy can reduce women's CVD risk long term.[45] The following list describes the magnitude of effect of these risk factors and risk factor reduction on pregnancy outcomes and long-term ASCVD risk.

- Preeclampsia confers a 4-fold increased risk of HTN later in a woman's life, triples the risk of a CVD event in her lifetime, and doubles her future stroke risk. Evidence supports this association but does not explain if the association is due to a common underlying condition or actual endothelial damage done by preeclampsia. Consider screening for high BP, obesity, smoking, and high cholesterol starting 1 year after delivery (limited evidence).[46]
- Obesity prior to pregnancy greatly increases risk of multiple complications, including gestational diabetes (adjusted odds ratio [OR] 6.5), HTN of pregnancy (adjusted OR 7.9), and preeclampsia (adjusted OR 3.7). In turn, these pregnancy complications increase risk of diabetes and HTN later in life and ultimately raise ASCVD risk.[47] Weight loss prior to pregnancy makes a difference. Among women whose weight changed from one pregnancy to the next, those who lost 10 or more pounds reduced their risk of gestational diabetes by 40%. Those who gained 10 or more pounds increased their risk by 50%.[48]
- Gestational diabetes increases risk of developing type 2 diabetes later in life. Within 5 to 15 years after pregnancy, 15% to 60% of these women develop diabetes.[49]
- Preterm delivery is independently associated with future hospitalization related to CVD (adjusted hazard ratio [HR] 1.4).[50]
- Multiple miscarriages are an independent risk factor for future MI (adjusted HR 5.1), as is stillbirth (adjusted HR 3.4) (**Fig. 1**).[51]

Stroke Risk Factors

Stroke risk factors generally are the same as for CHD, but young women have several unique stroke risk factors. Their strokes generally are thrombotic, and the elevated risk ceases to be a factor if condition/therapy is discontinued (eg, pregnancy or oral contraceptive pills [OCPs]). Migraine with aura, however, confers a lifelong 2.5-fold elevated risk of stroke.[52] Frequency of migraine directly correlates with higher stroke risk, but only minimal evidence supports reducing migraine frequency with medications to reduce stroke risk. Women with migraine with aura who smoke have a 9-fold increased risk of stroke; these women should be strongly encouraged to stop smoking (AHA/ASA guideline).[25]

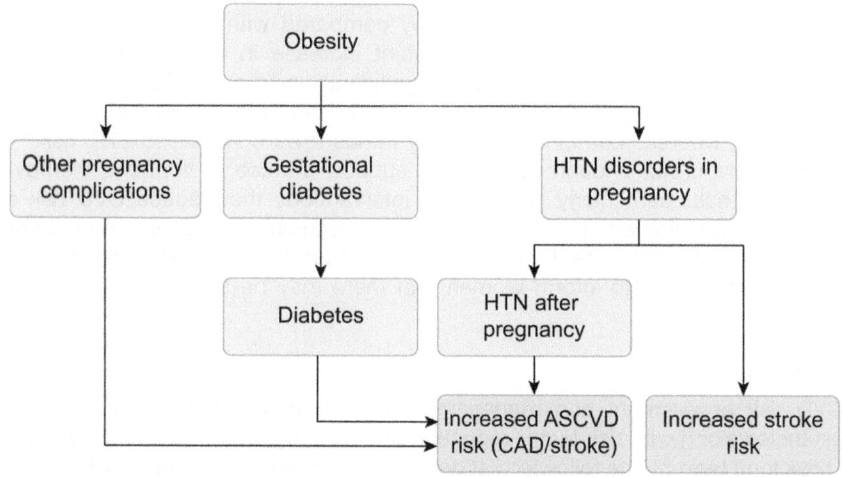

Fig. 1. Cascade of complications from prepregnancy obesity.

Oral Contraceptives

Combination estrogen/progestin OCP use contributes to thrombotic stroke and MI risk in young women, but is NOT an independent risk factor for ASCVD risk long--term.[53–55] Stroke risk for young women increases greatly when OCPs are combined with other risk factors. Women taking OCPs should be advised to manage their modifiable stroke risk factors (OR = OR for stroke compared with women with each risk factor NOT taking OCPs)[56]:

- OCPs + migraine/aura = OR 7.02
- OCPs + HTN = OR 7.6
- OCPs + smoking (at any age) = OR 4.4
- OCPs + hyperlipidemia = OR 10.8
- OCPs + diabetes = OR 5.3
- OCPs + obesity = OR 4.6
- OCPs + thrombophilia = OR for stroke 11–200 (lupus anticoagulant worst)
  - Do not screen for thrombophilia, prevalence is too low.
  - Do obtain personal and family VTE history; check serum markers only if significant positive history.

RISK FACTOR MODIFICATION—PHARMACOLOGIC

Statins have a large body of evidence supporting their role in reducing ASCVD risk. They lower LDL cholesterol and to a lesser degree triglycerides, but recent studies have shown reduced CVD outcomes independent of lipid profile changes (**Table 3**).[4]

Statin Adverse Effects

Many randomized controlled trials have demonstrated statin effectiveness with reducing cardiovascular events, but they suffer from a fundamental challenge to compliance: statin benefit cannot be felt by the patient taking the medication, but the adverse effects often can. Liver toxicity is feared but exceedingly rare and occurs only in patients with underlying liver disease. Hepatic transaminases should be checked prior to starting a statin, but monitoring transaminases in asymptomatic patients is not indicated.[57] Mild muscle aches are common and not harmful in themselves, but any patient experiencing new pain or discomfort should be evaluated with history, physical examination, and laboratory measurements to rule out more serious myopathy or rhabdomyolysis and the statin stopped. Alternative diagnoses must also be considered, such as vitamin D or B_{12} deficiency, thyroid disease, radicular pain, alcohol-related

Table 3
Relative potency of statins

Atorvastatin	Fluvastatin	Lovastatin	Pravastatin	Rosuvastatin	Simvastatin	↓ Low-Density Lipoprotein (%)
—	40 mg	20 mg	20 mg	—	10 mg	30
10 mg	**80 mg**	**40 mg**	**40 mg**	—	**20 mg**	38
20 mg	—	**80 mg**	**80 mg**	**5 mg**	**40 mg**	41
40 mg	—	—	—	**10 mg**		47
80 mg	—	—	—	*20 mg*	—	55
	—	—	—	*40 mg*	—	63

Bold, moderate-intensity statin.
Italics, high-intensity statin.

myopathy, myositis, or PVD. Whether a statin can be restarted depends on diagnostic evaluation, clinical response to stopping the medication, patient preference, and thoughtful counseling about alternative statin and/or dosing schedules.

Myalgia

Myalgia is muscle ache, heaviness, cramp, weakness, or fatigue without creatine kinase (CK) elevation. Statin-induced myalgia usually is symmetric, is diffuse, and affects lower more than upper extremities. It may resolve after the first few weeks of therapy; in those who discontinue the statin, myalgia should resolve within 2 weeks of stopping the medication. Studied incidence of myalgia ranges from 1% to 25%, with many studies having the same rate of myalgia in the placebo arm as the statin arm. Actual rates in the general population (many of whom are excluded from trials) are likely higher.[1,58] Higher prevalence in women is suggested in some studies, one of which showed that 60% of myalgia patients were women.[59] No treatment for statin myalgia is supported by strong evidence, but the following may relieve statin myalgia for some patients:

- Coenzyme Q10 may be helpful; this is supported only by weak evidence. Because statins block the common pathway for cholesterol and coenzyme Q10 production, it makes physiologic sense that adding back the enzyme could mitigate adverse effects. Clinical trials have not reported adverse effects significant enough for stopping therapy. The usual dose is 100 mg per day; cost ranges from $20 to $60/month.[60]
- Alternative dosing regimens may help patients tolerate statins without myalgia. Such regimens are possible with a long-acting statin (atorvastatin, rosuvastatin, or fluvastatin). Dosing with double dose every other day may reduce myalgia as well as cost and yields similar LDL reduction. Weekly rosuvastatin has been studied in patients with prior statin intolerance; 70% of patients tolerated this regimen, with an LDL reduction of 23%. Whether these dosing regimens result in reduction of ASCVD events has not yet been studied.[61]

Myopathy

Myopathy refers to muscle symptoms with CK elevation. This occurs in 0.1% to 0.5% of patients on a statin during randomized controlled trials and may also be under-representative of incidence in general population.[62]

Rhabdomyolysis

Rhabdomyolysis is a rare and serious disorder, usually defined as muscle symptoms with CK elevation greater than 10 times the upper limit of normal and creatinine elevation. Women represented approximately 54% of cases in 1 retrospective cohort study, which is not a significant difference.[63] This same study showed an NNH greater than 20,000 per year on statin monotherapy but an NNH of 484 in older diabetic patients on statin and fibrate, emphasizing the risks of combination therapy and underlying comorbidities. Monitoring CK in asymptomatic patients is not recommended.[4]

Cognitive decline

Cognitive decline is experienced by some patients who take a statin, but this effect resolves after discontinuation of the medication. Clinical trial evidence is conflicting on the incidence.[57]

Hyperglycemia/diabetes

Hyperglycemia/diabetes occurs in a small percentage of patients on statins.[64,65] The incidence and magnitude of the effect, however, are both small, and the beneficial effect far outweighs the harm. Because this is a particularly distressing and ironic complication for many patients, it may be helpful to present this in terms of NNT versus NNH. These statistics should be interpreted with caution, because they come from 2 different studies but do illustrate the approximate difference in magnitude of benefit versus harm:

NNH = 225 patients treated for 4 years to cause 1 new case of diabetes
NNT = 30 patients for 5 years to prevent 1 CVD event or death

Other Pharmaceutical Agents

Triglycerides

Elevated triglyceride levels correlate with higher ASCVD risk, with this association stronger in women than in men. Convincing evidence is still lacking, however, for a causal link between reducing triglyceride levels with targeted medications (eg, fibrates) and clinical outcomes.[66–68]

Niacin

There is no benefit on cardiovascular outcomes when niacin is added to statin therapy in patients on statin, and there is a higher incidence of adverse events when niacin is added to statin.[11,12]

Aspirin

US Preventive Services Task Force (USPSTF) recommendations (2009) for aspirin for primary prevention of CVD are currently being reviewed. Daily aspirin reduces stroke risk in women at high risk of stroke but does not reduce CHD risk. Daily aspirin (81 mg) should be recommended for women ages 55 to 79 when the benefit of reducing ischemic stroke risk outweighs potential harm of increasing gastrointestinal (GI) bleeding risk. Precise calculations of stroke risk and bleeding risk are not a realistic part of a typical clinic visit, so an overall assessment of ASCVD and bleeding risk factors should guide this decision. The American Diabetes Association and the AHA have similar recommendations based on CVD versus bleeding risk factors.[69] Because the guidelines are not exactly the same, I recommend daily aspirin for women ages 55 to 79 based on the overall risk profile and preferences of the patient. I recommend aspirin for a woman with known ASCVD equivalent (diabetes, PVD, atrial fibrillation, or left ventricular hypertrophy) or 2 other risk factors (high BP, smoking, dyslipidemia, family history of premature CVD, and kidney disease). I tend not to recommend daily aspirin in patients who frequently use nonsteroidal antiinflammatory medications (NSAIDs), have a history of GI bleeding or peptic ulcer disease, or have advanced cirrhosis. For example, I recommend aspirin for smokers with high BP and strong family history, even if they sometimes use NSAIDs, but do not recommend aspirin for cirrhotic patients with known varices who smoke and have HTN.

Antihypertensive medications

Therapy recommendations for antihypertensive medications were revised by the Eighth Joint National Committee; there are no different recommendations for women versus men.[70]

- Treatment goal for adults 60 years or older is more permissive than for adults under 60 years old: $\leq$150/90. If the patient's blood pressure is <140/90 (previously recommended treatment goal), and is tolerating her current medication without adverse effect, then, there is no need to change therapy.
- There is no change to general population treatment goal; this is still $\leq$140/90.
- Diabetics and patients with CKD now have the same goal as general population: $\leq$140/90.

- Initial medication choices have a few significant differences compared to prior guidelines. The following recommendations apply to both diabetics and patients without diabetes:
  - For nonblack patients, first line therapy: thiazide, calcium channel blocker, angiotensin-converting enzyme inhibitor (ACEI), or angiotensin II receptor blocker (ARB)
  - For black patients, first line therapy: thiazide or calcium channel blocker (note ACEI and ARB are NOT on this list)
  - For CKD patients, treatment regimen should include ACEI or ARB, regardless of race (**Table 4**).

RISK FACTOR MODIFICATION—NONPHARMACOLOGIC STRATEGIES

- Diet: With minor variations, the USPSTF and AHA/ACC both recommend a diet rich in fruits, vegetables, whole grains/legumes, low-fat dairy products, nuts, and seafood.[71] Please see recent review of lifestyle interventions for diabetes treatment.[72]
- Physical activity: ACC/AHA lifestyle guidelines recommend at least 150 minutes per week of moderate-intensity exercise, in episodes of at least 10 minutes.
- Vitamins and supplements: patients should save their money and eat more vegetables.
  Vitamin E: according to the USPSTF D recommendation, the harms of vitamin E supplements outweigh benefits.[73]
  Multivitamins: according to the USPSTF I recommendation, there is no evidence to recommend for or against multivitamins (**Table 5**).

FUTURE CONSIDERATIONS

- New potential risk factors: the USPSTF cites insufficient evidence to assess benefit/harm balance for the following nontraditional risk factors (2009)[75]:
  - Hs-CRP: higher levels of CRP are associated with higher ASCVD risk. Statins reduce CRP levels. Therefore, there may be a future role for incorporating CRP measurements into risk factor calculations and statin recommendations, but currently the evidence does not support this.[76]

Table 4
Choosing an antihypertensive medication based on patient preference and comorbidity

Medication	May Also Benefit	Avoid If
Thiazides	Venous insufficiency, some kidney stones	Gout, urinary incontinence, hypercalcemia
Lisinopril	Diabetic renal protection	Asthma (cough), pregnancy possible
Losartan	Gout (lowers uric acid), renal protection	Pregnancy possible
Propranolol	Anxiety, migraine prevention	Asthma, very high BP (not very effective)
Amlodipine	Raynaud phenomenon, stable angina	Venous insufficiency (edema)
Nifedipine	Raynaud phenomenon	Venous insufficiency (edema)
Verapamil	Cluster headache	Bradycardia
Spironolactone	Hirsutism	Pregnancy possible
Clonidine	Anxiety, vasomotor symptoms	Nonadherent (rebound HTN)

Table 5
US Preventive Services Task Force recommendations for atherosclerotic cardiovascular disease screening in women

Screening Test	Recommendation Grade	Bottom Line
Abdominal aortic aneurysm	I: insufficient evidence to assess benefit/harm balance for asymptomatic adults at intermediate–high risk	Women over age 65 who are smokers and/or have family history of abdominal aortic aneurysm are at increased risk of abdominal aortic aneurysm; evidence is insufficient[74] but screening women at very high risk could be considered.
Peripheral artery disease with ABI	I: insufficient evidence to assess benefit/harm balance	For asymptomatic patients, time is better spent on more evidence-based preventive strategies.
Carotid artery stenosis with duplex	D: harms outweigh benefits. Low prevalence, high false-positive rate of duplex, harms from intervention.	Multiple organizations recommend AGAINST screening asymptomatic individuals without risk factors.
ECG	D: harms outweigh benefits in asymptomatic patients at low ASCVD risk I: insufficient evidence to assess benefit/harm balance for asymptomatic adults at intermediate–high risk.	For asymptomatic patients, time is better spent on more evidence-based preventive strategies.
BP	A: strong evidence supports annual BP screening.	Screen all adults 18 and older for high BP. Interval not specified.
Dyslipidemia (nonfasting blood draw IS acceptable); this recommendation is currently under review.	A: strongly recommends screening women 45 or older if they have CVD risk factors B: recommends screening women 20–40 years old if they have CVD risk factors	Risk factors = diabetes, CHD/peripheral artery disease, smoking, HTN, obesity, positive family history (male relative <50, female relative <60). Screening interval not supported by evidence.
Tobacco cessation counseling	A: strongly recommends asking all adults about tobacco use and counseling on cessation; offering pharmacotherapy.	Minimal (<3 min) counseling interventions are effective to increase quit rates. Time well spent.
Diabetes	B: recommends screening all adults if BP >135/80. Fasting glucose or hemoglobin A_{1C} acceptable.	Screening interval not specified. ADA recommends every 3 y (expert opinion).
Obesity (BMI $\geq$30)	B: recommends screening all adults for obesity and offering/referring for intervention.	Screening interval not specified.
Healthful diet and physical activity	B: recommends offering or referring overweight/obese adults with CVD risk factors for intensive behavioral counseling interventions.	Risk factors = HTN, dyslipidemia, impaired fasting glucose, and metabolic syndrome.

    - ABI
    - Leukocyte count
    - Fasting blood glucose level
    - Periodontal disease
    - Carotid intima-media thickness
    - CAC score on electron-beam CT
    - Homocysteine level
    - Lipoprotein(a) level
- A multitude of lipid subclasses, apolipoproteins, and other novel biomarkers have been and are being studied as independent risk factors for ASCVD. This line of research is promising, but none has yet shown reliable predictable effect and an effect of intervention on lowering risk.[77]

SUMMARY

CAD and stroke predominantly affect older women as opposed to younger women, but the risk factors that contribute to ASCVD risk often start in very young women. Additionally, young women with PCOS, with migraine, and who use OCPs have short-term increases in thrombotic complications that can result in coronary events or stroke. Attention should be focused on risk reduction in women of all ages. Screening for and discussing diabetes, HTN, obesity, smoking, migraine, PCOS, and pregnancy complication history and carefully discussing the pros and cons of hormone and statin medications are all part of reducing cardiovascular risk for women.

REFERENCES

1. Desai CS, Martin SS, Blumenthal RS. Non-cardiovascular effects associated with statins. BMJ 2014;349:g3743.
2. Mosca L, Hammond G, Mochari-Greenberger H, et al. Fifteen-year trends in awareness of heart disease in women: results of a 2012 American Heart Association national survey. Circulation 2013;127:1254–63.
3. Goff DC, Lloyd-Jones D, Bennett G, et al. 2013 ACC/AHA Guideline on the Assessment of Cardiovascular Risk: A Report of the American College of Cardiology/American Heart Association Task Force on Practice Guidelines. Circulation 2014;129:S49–73.
4. Stone NJ, Robinson JG, Lichtenstein AH, et al. 2013 ACC/AHA Guideline on the Treatment of Blood Cholesterol to Reduce Atherosclerotic Cardiovascular Risk in Adults: A Report of the American College of Cardiology/American Heart Association Task Force on Practice Guidelines. Circulation 2014;129:S1–45.
5. Hayward RA, Krumholz HM. Three reasons to abandon low-density lipoprotein targets: an open letter to the adult treatment panel IV of the National Institutes of Health. Circ Cardiovasc Qual Outcomes 2012;5:2–5.
6. Barrett-Connor EL, Cohn BA, Wingard DL, et al. Why is diabetes mellitus a stronger risk factor for fatal ischemic heart disease in women than in men? JAMA 1991;265:627–31.
7. Singer DE, Nathan DM, Anderson KM, et al. Association of HbA1c with prevalent cardiovascular disease in the original cohort of the Framingham Heart Study. Diabetes 1992;41:202–8.
8. Willett WC, Green A, Stampfer M, et al. Relative and absolute excess risks of coronary heart disease among women who smoke cigarettes. N Engl J Med 1987;317:1309–14.

9. Jacobs DR Jr, Meban IL, Bangdiwala SI, et al. High density lipoprotein cholesterol as a predictor of cardiovascular disease mortality in men and women: the follow-up study of the Lipid Research Clinics Prevalence Study. Am J Epidemiol 1990;131(1):32–47.
10. Mora S, Buring JE, Ridker PM, et al. Association of high-density lipoprotein cholesterol with incident cardiovascular events in women, by low-density lipoprotein cholesterol and apolipoprotein B100 levels. Ann Intern Med 2011;155: 742–50.
11. AIM-HIGH Investigators. Niacin in patients with low HDL cholesterol levels receiving intensive statin therapy. N Engl J Med 2011;365(24):2255–67.
12. The HPS2-THRIVE Collaborative Group. Effects of extended-release niacin with laropiprant in high-risk patients. N Engl J Med 2014;371:203–12.
13. Anderson TJ, Boden WE, Desvigne-Nickens P, et al. Safety profile of extended-release niacin in the AIM-HIGH trial. N Engl J Med 2014;371:288–90.
14. Mosca L, Appel LJ, Benjamin EJ, et al. Evidence-based guidelines for cardiovascular disease prevention in women. Circulation 2004;109:672–93.
15. Mosca L, Banka CL, Benjamin EJ, et al. Evidence-based guidelines for cardiovascular disease prevention in women: 2007 update. Circulation 2007;115: 1481–501.
16. Chobanian AV, Bakris GL, Black HR, et al. The seventh report of the Joint National Committee on Prevention, Detection, Evaluation, and Treatment of High Blood Pressure: the JNC 7 report. JAMA 2003;289:2560–71.
17. Reaven PD, Barrett-Connor E, Edelstein S. Relation between leisure-time physical activity and blood pressure in older women. Circulation 1991;83:559–65.
18. Whelton SP, Chin A, Xin X, et al. Effect of aerobic exercise on blood pressure. Ann Intern Med 2002;136(7):493–503.
19. Blumenthal JA, Sherwood A, Gullette EC, et al. Exercise and weight loss reduce blood pressure in men and women with mild hypertension: effects on cardiovascular, metabolic, and hemodynamic functioning. Arch Intern Med 2000;160(13): 1947–58.
20. Gordon NF, Scott CB, Levine BD. Comparison of single versus multiple lifestyle interventions: are the antihypertensive effects of exercise training and diet-induced weight loss additive? Am J Cardiol 1997;79:763–7.
21. Kawachi I, Colditz GA, Stampfer MJ, et al. Smoking cessation and time course of decreased risks of coronary heart disease in middle-aged women. Arch Intern Med 1994;154:169–75.
22. Wilkins JT, Ning H, Berry J, et al. Lifetime risk and years lived free of total cardiovascular disease. JAMA 2012;308(17):1795–801.
23. Gage BF, Waterman AD, Shannon W, et al. Validation of clinical classification schemes for predicting stroke: results from the National Registry of Atrial Fibrillation. JAMA 2001;285(22):2864–70.
24. Lip GY, Nieuwlaat R, Pisters R, et al. Refining clinical risk stratification for predicting stroke and thromboembolism in atrial fibrillation using a novel risk factor-based approach: the Euro Heart Survey on Atrial Fibrillation. Chest 2010; 137(2):263–72.
25. Bushnell CB, McCullough LD, Awad IA, et al. Guidelines for the prevention of stroke in women: a statement for healthcare professionals from the American Heart Association/American Stroke Association. Stroke 2014;45: 1545–88.
26. Ogden CL, Carroll MD, Kit BK, et al. Prevalence of childhood and adult obesity in the United States, 2011-2012. JAMA 2014;311(8):806–14.

27. Eckel RH, Jakicic JM, Ard JD, et al. 2013 AHA/ACC guideline on lifestyle management to reduce cardiovascular risk: a report of the American College of Cardiology American Heart Association Task Force on Practice Guidelines. Circulation 2014;129:S76–99.
28. Jensen MD, Ryan DH, Apovian CM, et al. 2013 AHA/ACC/TOS Guideline for the Management of Overweight and Obesity in Adults: A Report of the American College of Cardiology/American Heart Association Task Force on Practice Guidelines and The Obesity Society. Circulation 2014;129:S102–38.
29. Aviña-Zubieta JA, Choi HK, Sadatsafavi M, et al. Risk of cardiovascular mortality in patients with rheumatoid arthritis: a meta-analysis of observational studies. Arthritis Rheum 2008;59:1690–7.
30. Manjunath G, Tighiouart H, Ibrahim H, et al. Level of kidney function as a risk factor for atherosclerotic cardiovascular outcomes in the community. J Am Coll Cardiol 2003;41(1):47–55.
31. Tamanna S, Geraci S. Major sleep disorders among women. South Med J 2013; 106(8):470–8.
32. Shepertycky MR, Banno K, Kryber MH. Differences between men and women in the clinical presentation of patients diagnosed with obstructive sleep apnea syndrome. Sleep 2005;28:309–14.
33. Hajduk IA, Strollo PJ Jr, Jasani R, et al. Prevalence and predictors of nocturia in obstructive sleep apnea-hypopnea syndrome (OSAHS) – a retrospective study. Sleep 2003;1:61–4.
34. Bradley TD, Floras JS. Obstructive sleep apnoea and its cardiovascular consequences. Lancet 2009;373:82–93.
35. Randeva HS, Tan BK, Weickert MO, et al. Cardiometabolic aspects of the polycystic ovary syndrome. Endocr Rev 2012;33:812–41.
36. Trikudanathan S. Polycystic ovarian syndrome. Med Clin N Am 2015;99:221–35.
37. Wang ET, Calderon-Margalit R, Marcelle I, et al. Polycystic ovary syndrome and risk for long-term diabetes and dyslipidemia. Obstet Gynecol 2011;117(1):6–13.
38. Salley KE, Wickham EP, Cheang KI, et al. Glucose intolerance in polycystic ovary syndrome–a position statement of the Androgen Excess Society. J Clin Endocrinol Metab 2007;92:4546.
39. Colditz GA, Willett WC, Stampfer MJ, et al. Menopause and the risk of coronary heart disease in women. N Engl J Med 1987;316:1105–10.
40. Atsma F, Bartelink ME, Grobbee DE, et al. Postmenopausal status and early menopause as independent risk factors for cardiovascular disease: a meta-analysis. Menopause 2006;13(2):265–79.
41. Matthews KA, Crawford SL, Chae CU, et al. Are changes in cardiovascular disease risk factors in midline women due to chronological aging or to the menopausal transition? J Am Coll Cardiol 2009;54(25):2366–73.
42. Manson JE, Allison MA, Rossouw JE, et al. Estrogen therapy and coronary-artery calcification. N Engl J Med 2007;356:2591–602.
43. Rossouw JE, Ross LP, Manson JE, et al. Postmenopausal hormone therapy and risk of cardiovascular disease by age and years since menopause. JAMA 2007; 297(13):1465–77.
44. Manson JE, Chlebowski RT, Stefanick ML, et al. Menopausal hormone therapy and health outcomes during the intervention and extended poststopping phases of the Women's Health Initiative randomized trials. JAMA 2013;310(13):1353–68.
45. Romundstad PR, Magnussen EB, Smith GD, et al. Hypertension in pregnancy and later cardiovascular risk: common antecedents? Circulation 2010;122(6): 579–84.

46. Bellamy L, Casas JP, Hingorani AD, et al. Pre-eclampsia and risk of cardiovascular disease and cancer in later life: systematic review and meta-analysis. BMJ 2007;335(7627):974–7.
47. Doherty DA, Magann EF, Francis J, et al. Pre-pregnancy body mass index and pregnancy outcomes. Int J Gynaecol Obstet 2006;95:242–7.
48. Glazer NL, Hendrickson AF, Schellenbaum GD, et al. Weight change and the risk of gestational diabetes in obese women. Epidemiology 2004;15:733–7.
49. Kim C, Newton KM, Knopp RH. Gestational diabetes and the incidence of type 2 diabetes: a systematic review. Diabetes Care 2002;25:1862–8.
50. Kessous R, Shoham-Vardi I, Pariente G, et al. An association between preterm delivery and long-term maternal cardiovascular morbidity. Am J Obstet Gynecol 2013;209(4):368.e1–8.
51. Kharazmi E, Dossus L, Rohrmann S, et al. Pregnancy loss and risk of cardiovascular disease: a prospective population-based cohort study (EPIC-Heidelberg). Heart 2011;97(1):49–54.
52. Spector JT, Kahn SR, Jones MR, et al. Migraine headache and ischemic stroke risk: an updated meta-analysis. Am J Med 2010;123:612–24.
53. Lidegaard Ø, Løkkegaard E, Jensen A, et al. Thrombotic stroke and myocardial infarction with hormonal contraception. N Engl J Med 2012;366:2257–66.
54. Merz CN, Johnson BD, Berga S, et al. Past oral contraceptive use and angiographic coronary artery disease in postmenopausal women: data from the National Heart, Lung, and Blood Institute-sponsored Women's Ischemia Syndrome Evaluation. Fertil Steril 2006;85:1425–31.
55. Chasan-Taber L, Willett WC, Manson JE, et al. Prospective study of oral contraceptives and hypertension among women in the United States. Circulation 1996;94:483–9.
56. Kemmeren JM, Tanis BC, van den Bosch MA, et al. Risk of arterial thrombosis in relation to oral contraceptives (RATIO) study: oral contraceptives and the risk of ischemic stroke. Stroke 2002;33(5):1202–8.
57. Important safety label changes to cholesterol-lowering statin drugs. In: FDA Drug Safety Communication. 2012. Available at: http://www.fda.gov/Drugs/DrugSafety/ucm293101.htm. Accessed November 29, 2014.
58. Fernandez G, Spatz ES, Jablecki C, et al. Statin myopathy: a common dilemma not reflected in clinical trials. Cleve Clin J Med 2011;78(6):393–403.
59. Parker BA, Capizzi JA, Grimaldi AS, et al. Effect of statins on skeletal muscle function. Circulation 2013;127(1):96–103.
60. Wyman M, Leonard M, Morledge T. Coenzyme Q10: a therapy for hypertension and statin-induced myalgia? Cleve Clin J Med 2010;77(7):435–42.
61. Ruisinger JF, Backes JM, Gibson CA, et al. Once-a-week rosuvastatin (2.5 to 20mg) in patients with a previous statin intolerance. Am J Cardiol 2009;103(3):393–4.
62. Kashani A, Phillips CO, Foody JM, et al. Risks associated with statin therapy: a systematic overview of randomized clinical trials. Circulation 2006;114(25):2788–97.
63. Graham DJ, Staffa JA, Shatin D, et al. Incidence of hospitalized rhabdomyolysis in patients treated with lipid-lowering drugs. JAMA 2004;292:2585–90.
64. Sattar N, Preiss D, Murray HM, et al. Statins and risk of incident diabetes: a collaborative meta-analysis of randomised statin trials. Lancet 2010;375(9716):735–42.
65. Scandinavian Simvastatin Survival Study Group. Randomised trial of cholesterol lowering in 4444 patients with coronary heart disease: the Scandinavian Simvastatin Survival Study (4S). Lancet 1994;344(8934):1383–9.

66. Hokanson JE, Austin MA. Plasma triglyceride level as a risk factor for cardiovascular disease independent of high-density lipoprotein cholesterol level: a meta-analysis of population-based prospective studies. J Cardiovasc Risk 1996;3:213–9.
67. Jun M, Foote C, Lv J, et al. Effects of fibrates on cardiovascular outcomes: a systematic review and meta-analysis. Lancet 2010;375(9729):1875–84.
68. Nordestgaard BG, Varbo A. Triglycerides and cardiovascular disease. Lancet 2014;384:626–35.
69. Pignone M, Alberts MJ, Colwell JA, et al. Aspirin for primary prevention of cardiovascular events in people with diabetes: a position statement of the American Diabetes Association, a scientific statement of the American Heart Association, and an expert consensus document of the American College of Cardiology Foundation. Circulation 2010;121:2694–701.
70. James PA, Oparil S, Carter BL, et al. 2014 Evidence-based guideline for the management of high blood pressure in adults: report from the panel members appointed to the 8th Joint National Committee (JNC-8). JAMA 2014;311(5):507–20.
71. LeFevre ML. Behavioral counseling to promote a healthful diet and physical activity for cardiovascular disease prevention in adults with cardiovascular risk factors: U.S. Preventive Services Task Force recommendation statement. Ann Intern Med 2014;161(8):587–93.
72. Evert AB, Riddel MC. Lifestyle intervention: nutrition therapy and physical activity. Med Clin N Am 2015;99:69–85.
73. Moyer VA. Vitamin, mineral, and multivitamin supplements for the primary prevention of cardiovascular disease and cancer: U.S. Preventive Services Task Force recommendation statement. Ann Intern Med 2014;160(8):558–64.
74. U.S. Preventive Services Task Force, Screening for Abdominal Aortic Aneurysm. Available at: http://www.uspreventiveservicestaskforce.org/uspstf/uspsaneu.htm. Accessed September 14, 2014.
75. U.S. Preventive Services Task Force, Coronary Heart Disease: Screening Using Non-Traditional Risk Factors. Available at: http://www.uspreventiveservicestaskforce.org/uspstf/uspscoronaryhd.htm. Accessed November 29, 2014.
76. Ridker PM, Cannon CP, Morrow D, et al. C-reactive protein levels and outcomes after statin therapy. N Engl J Med 2005;352(1):20–8.
77. Ridker PM. LDL cholesterol: controversies and future therapeutic directions. Lancet 2014;384:566–8.

Common Vaginal and Vulvar Disorders

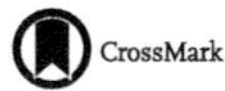

Andrea Prabhu, MD[a,*], Carolyn Gardella, MD[a,b]

KEYWORDS

• Vulva • Vagina • Diagnosis • Treatment

KEY POINTS

- Vaginal and vulvar conditions are common and cause significant distress for patients.
- The symptoms often overlap and may include itching, burning, pain, and dyspareunia.
- Because of the overlap in symptoms, we recommend obtaining a history, physical examination, and appropriate testing rather than empirical treatment.

INTRODUCTION

Problems related to the vulva and the vagina are responsible for more than 10 million office visits each year.[1,2] It is important to have a systematic approach to patients with these concerns. The vagina contains a rich diversity of bacterial organisms. The vaginal pH is usually 4.0 to 4.5 and is regulated primarily by the creation of lactic acid by *Lactobacillus*. The vulva is made primarily of stratified squamous epithelium. This article outlines conditions that cause a disruption in these 2 environments.

FUTURE CONSIDERATIONS

Further research in women's health to optimize diagnosis and treatment. For example, in patients for whom estrogen is contraindicated, finding an alternative and equally effective treatment for atrophy. We have a limited understanding of the complexity of the vaginal ecosystem (and diseases such as bacterial vaginosis [BV]), and this is an area of active research.

Further education of patients and providers as to good vulvar hygiene guidelines is essential.

PATIENT HISTORY

The patient should be asked about location and duration of symptoms, abnormal discharge, itching, burning, pain, soreness, odor, dyspareunia, bleeding, and dysuria.

[a] Division of Women's Health, Department of Obstetrics and Gynecology, University of Washington, Box 356460, Seattle, WA 98195, USA; [b] Department of Gynecology, VA Puget Sound Medical Center, 1600 South Columbian Way, Seattle, WA 98108, USA
* Corresponding author. 1959 Northeast Pacific Street, Box 356460, Seattle, WA 98195.
E-mail address: azins@uw.edu

Med Clin N Am 99 (2015) 553–574
http://dx.doi.org/10.1016/j.mcna.2015.01.008 medical.theclinics.com

A sexual and menstrual history should be obtained. The patient's medication list should be reviewed with special notes of recent antibiotics, antifungals, over-the-counter treatments, and contraception. Other sources of pelvic pain should be covered, including pelvic inflammatory disease, urinary tract infections, and gastrointestinal changes. Hygiene habits must be covered. Many times patients who are symptomatic may be overzealous in washing the genitals. Ask patients about soaps, detergents, creams, and douching. Also ask about contact or irritant exposures (**Box 1**).

SYMPTOMS

Symptoms of vulvar and vaginal irritation may overlap. Women frequently experience itching, burning, pain, and/or dyspareunia (painful intercourse).

Box 1
Common vulvar irritants

- Body fluids
  - Abnormal/excessive vaginal discharge
  - Feces
  - Semen
  - Sweat
  - Urine
- Excessive bathing
  - Soap
  - Detergents
  - Bubble baths
- Feminine hygiene products
  - Pantiliners
  - Benzocaine
- Heat
- Dyes
- Medications
  - Alcohol-based creams and gels
  - Imiquimod
  - Phenol
  - Propylene glycol
  - Spermicides
  - Podophyllin
  - Trichloroacetic acid
  - Topical antibiotics
  - Topical anesthetics
  - Topical antifungals

PHYSICAL EXAMINATION

Knowledge of normal female anatomy is important to be able to describe accurately areas of lesions and also to educate the patient on her own anatomy. For any lower genital tract symptoms, an evaluation of the vulva and vagina should be performed. A magnifying glass or colposcope may also be helpful in the examination (**Fig. 1**).

DIAGNOSTIC TESTING AND IMAGING STUDIES

The test of the vaginal secretions with nitrazine paper to measure the pH is an excellent place to start narrowing the differential diagnosis of abnormal vaginal discharge. In premenopausal women, the vaginal pH is typically between 4.0 and 4.5. Elevation of pH may be owing to presence of red blood cells, semen, amniotic fluid in pregnant women, an increase in white blood cells, atrophy, trichomoniasis, and BV.

Performing a wet mount of secretions ideally obtained from the vaginal sidewall is an important skill for the office clinician. A potassium hydroxide preparation can help to identify yeast hyphae and spores. The normal saline wet mount can help to identify clue cells to aid in the diagnosis of BV, Trichomonads, sperm, parabasal cells, and white blood cells. The following elements should be reported on your wet mount: white blood cells, red blood cells, bacteria, epithelial cells, yeast, clue cells, and *Trichomonas*.

A whiff test should be performed by adding potassium hydroxide to a slide with discharge on it. A strong ammonia smell is a positive test. We also report the vaginal pH and note any excessive numbers of parabasal cells.

Additional Testing

Discharge may also be sent out for other tests such as *Gonorrhea* and *Chlamydia* nucleic acid amplification testing, fungal culture, and *Trichomonas* polymerase chain reaction. We do not recommend routine bacterial cultures of vaginal secretions because they are often nonspecific.

Vulvar biopsy is important in cases where vulvar dystrophy or cancer may be suspected. The most abnormal area should be biopsied. If there are ulcers and erosions, biopsy the edge. Beware of biopsies near the urethra or the clitoris. Concerning findings on examination include raised white lesions, nonhealing ulcers, or pigmented lesions with abnormal coloring or irregular borders. Lesions not responding to typical treatment also should be considered for biopsy (**Boxes 2** and **3**).

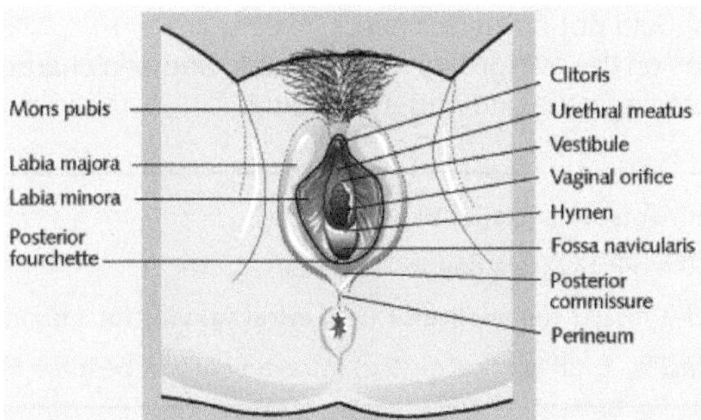

Fig. 1. Vulvar anatomy. (*From* Panay N, Horton-Szar D. Vulvar disease. In: Panay N, Horton-Szar D, editors. Crash course: obstetrics & gynecology. Philadelphia: Mosby; 2007. p. 129–32; with permission.)

Box 2
Vulvar punch biopsy steps

1. Obtain informed consent and verify any drug allergies before beginning.
2. Cleanse the skin with povidone iodine or chlorhexidine.
3. Inject 1% lidocaine with epinephrine in a small wheal.
4. Stretch the skin perpendicular to the skin tension lines with your nondominant hand.
5. Place the punch biopsy perpendicular to the surface and slowly twist with minimal pressure.
6. Life with Adson forceps and cut the base with an Iris scissors.
7. If a 3-mm punch biopsy or smaller is taken, usually hemostasis is achieved with silver nitrate. A stitch is used for larger lesions.
8. Instruct the patient on postprocedure hygiene.

DIFFERENTIAL DIAGNOSIS

Bacterial Vaginosis

BV is characterized by increased vaginal discharge with a fishy odor. Patients may present with white–yellow discharge noted on their underwear. Often they have tried douching to remove the increased discharge and odor. Women with BV do not tend to have associated itching, but may describe mild vaginal burning. They do not tend to have associated pain. Important findings on pelvic examination include homogenous discharge throughout the vagina, fishy odor, minimal vaginal or cervical erythema, and lack of cervical motion tenderness.

Diagnosis relies on pH testing, amine whiff test, and microscopic examination of the vaginal discharge via wet mount. The slide is evaluated using 40× lens for the presence of clue cells. BV is diagnosed if 3 of 4 "Amsel criteria" are met:

1. Increased, homogenous, thin white vaginal discharge
2. 20 percent of the epithelial cells on wet mount should be clue cells
3. Vaginal fluid pH of greater than 4.5, or
4. Fishy odor of vaginal discharge before or after the addition of 10% KOH (the whiff test).

Many clinics do not have ready access to real-time, provider-performed microscopy. In these cases, vaginal fluid can be sent to a laboratory for Gram stain diagnosis. DNA probe-based test for high concentrations of *Gardnerella vaginalis* (Affirm VP III, Becton Dickinson, Sparks, MD) and the OSOM BV Blue test have acceptable performance characteristics compared with Gram stain. Vaginal culture is not helpful and should not be performed.

Treatment focuses on the overgrowth of anaerobic bacteria characteristic of BV and is provided to relieve vaginal signs and symptoms.

Recommended Treatments for Bacterial Vaginosis

Metronidazole 500 mg PO twice a day for 7 days *or*

Metronidazole gel 0.75%, 1 full applicator (5 g) intravaginally for 5 nights *or*

Clindamycin cream 2%, 1 full applicator (5 g) intravaginally at bedtime for 7 days.

Metronidazole can have an disulfiram-like reaction with alcohol, so patients should be counseled to avoid drinking alcohol until 24 hours after treatment is completed.

Box 3
Common causes of vulvar pruritus and irritation

1. Acute
   a. Contact dermatitis
      i. Allergic
      ii. Irritant
   b. Infections
      i. Candidiasis
      ii. Bacterial vaginosis
      iii. Human papilloma virus
      iv. Molluscum contagiosum
      v. Trichomoniasis
      vi. Scabies
2. Chronic
   a. Contact dermatitis
      i. Allergic
      ii. Irritant
   b. Vulvar dystrophies
      i. Lichen planus
      ii. Lichen sclerosus
      iii. Lichen simplex chronicus
      iv. Psoriasis
   c. Infections
      i. Candidiasis
      ii. Human papilloma virus
   d. Neoplasia
      i. Paget disease
      ii. Vulvar cancer
   e. Atrophy

From Rodriguez MI, Leclair CM. Benign vulvar dermatoses. Obstet Gynecol Surv 2012;67(1):56; with permission.

Other side effects may include nausea or a metallic taste. Women should avoid sex or use condoms during treatment.

Data are limited regarding efficacy of alternative treatments with oral tinidazole or oral clindamycin.

Prevention and Management of Recurrence

Although BV is related to sexual activity, treatment of male partners does not prevent recurrence.[3] BV seems to be common among lesbian partners, but studies regarding partner treatment in this population have not been performed. Further study of partner treatment to prevent recurrence among heterosexual and homosexual women is an area of active research.

Planned follow-up is unnecessary if symptoms resolve. Recurrent BV is common and there are limited data regarding best treatment practices. If symptoms persist, retreatment with the same medication or with an alternative medication may be helpful. For women with frequent recurrences of BV, treatment with metronidazole gel twice a week for 4 to 6 months decreases recurrences for the duration of treatment.[4] Limited data suggest oral nitroimidazole followed by intravaginal boric acid and suppressive metronidazole gel may be effective.[5]

Other Considerations

Asymptomatic BV noted on routine physical examination, or as a comment on a pap smear, does not require treatment unless the patient is planning a pregnancy, gynecologic procedure, or surgery, or is at high risk for human immunodeficiency virus acquisition, such as part of serodiscordant couple. BV in pregnancy is associated with late miscarriage and preterm birth. BV increases the risk of postprocedure or postoperative infection, and of human immunodeficiency virus acquisition.

Researchers using molecular techniques are making groundbreaking observations about the microbiome characteristic of BV that are expected to lead to a paradigm shift in how we diagnose and treat BV.[6–8] Currently available probiotics for the treatment of BV are not beneficial and are not recommended.[9] Douching also should be discouraged because it disrupts the vaginal ecosystem, and can transport vaginal bacteria to the uterus to increase the risk of pelvic inflammatory disease.

TRICHOMONIASIS

Women infected with *Trichomonas vaginalis* present with vaginal discharge without odor, with or without itching. However, 70% to 85% of infected women have slight to no symptoms.[10] Untreated infections may last for months to years. *Trichomonas* is easily passed to sex partners and is more common in women over the age of 40, African Americans, patients at sexually transmitted disease clinics, and prisoners.[11] On physical examination, the vagina and cervix may be erythematous, and a yellow to green frothy discharge is present.

Diagnosis previously relied on identification of Trichomonads on wet mount of vaginal fluid. However, the sensitivity of wet mount is 80% at best, and decreases dramatically if the sample is not evaluated within 10 minutes of collection. Therefore, the US Centers for Disease Control and Prevention now recommends molecular testing to detect Trichomonads. The available tests use nucleic acid amplification and have excellent sensitivity and specificity and can be used on urine or vaginal fluid.[12,13] Test approved by the US Food and Drug Administration and their performance characteristics are listed in **Table 1**.

Treatment for *Trichomonas*

- Metronidazole 2 g orally in a single dose *or*
- Tinidazole 2 g orally in a single dose *or*
- Metronidazole 500 mg orally twice a day for 7 days

Partners should be concurrently treated to decrease the risk of reinfection.[14] All persons with known exposure to *T vaginalis* should be treated with or without a

Table 1
FDA approved nucleic acid amplification tests for trichomonas

FDA + Test	Point of Care	Method	Sensitivity (%)	Specificity (%)
APTIMA TV	No	RNA by transcription medicated amplification	95–100	98–99
OSOM Trich Rapid Test	Yes 10 min	Antigen detection	71–99	99–100
Affirm VP III	Yes 45 min	Nucleic acid probe hybridization	63–93	99.9–100

Abbreviation: FDA, US Food and Drug Administration.

diagnostic test. Partners should not have intercourse until treatment is completed and symptoms resolved. Rescreening is recommended for all sexually active women within 3 months after the initial treatment.[15]

Recurrent cases of Trichomonas need to be distinguished from treatment failures. The majority of recurrent cases result from reexposure to an infected partner and can be treated with single dose medication again. Resistant trichomonas species are emerging, with 4% to 10% of cases resistant to metronidazole and 1% of cases resistant to tinidazole.[16] If you suspect a treatment failure rather than reinfection after single-dose therapy with metronidazole, either retreat with a 7-day course or prescribe tinidazole.[17] If you suspect that your patient has a strain that is antibiotic resistant, samples should be sent to the US Centers for Disease Control and Prevention for testing (Telephone (404) 718-4141, http://www.cdc.gov/std).

VULVOVAGINAL CANDIDIASIS

Vulvovaginal candidiasis (VVC) typically is caused by *Candida albicans*. Women with VVC present with symptoms including pruritis, vaginal soreness, pain with intercourse, dysuria, and/or abnormal vaginal discharge. On physical examination, the vulva and vagina may seem to be erythematous and the discharge has a curdlike consistency that adheres to the vaginal sidewalls. Occasionally, physical findings can be subtle, including vulvar fissures with minimal vaginal discharge.

Microscopy remains the primary method to detect vulvovaginal Candida and should be performed on all patients presenting with symptoms consistent with yeast. A swab is used to collect discharge from the vaginal sidewall. The swab is rolled across a slide and a drop of 10% KOH is applied to lyse cellular debris that might obscure visualization of budding yeast, hyphae, or pseudohyphae (**Fig. 2**). Yeast culture is indicated only if there is concern that the yeast species may be atypical and, therefore, azole resistant. pH testing, if performed, is less than 4.5.

Treatment should be offered to symptomatic women with Candida detected on wet mount. If wet mount is negative but symptoms are present, a culture for yeast can be considered. If culture is not available, empiric treatment is reasonable. Intravaginal or oral azole therapy is the mainstay of treatment. Many topical over-the-counter options are available and are equally effective, clearing about 90% of cases of uncomplicated VVC with short course therapy. Single-dose fluconazole 150 mg orally is effective, providing treatment levels for 3 days owing to the long half-life of fluconazole.

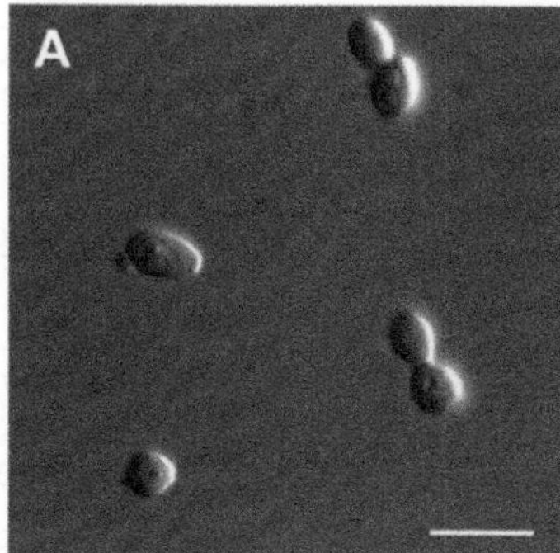

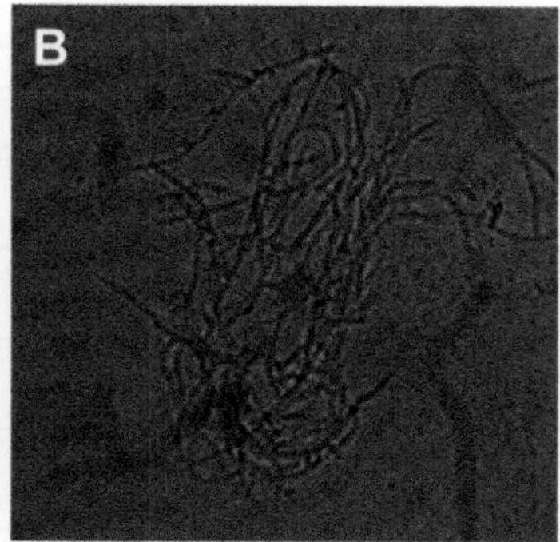

Fig. 2. (*A*) Yeast buds and (*B*) hyphae (Candida albicans). ([*A*] *From* Sudbery P, Gow N, Berman J. The distinct morphogenic states of Candida albicans. Trends Microbiol 2004;12(7):317–24; with permission; [*B*] *From* Sobel JD. Vulvovaginal candidosis. Lancet 2007;369(9577): 1961–71; with permission.)

Complicated Vulvovaginal Candidiasis

Approximately 10% of cases of VVC are considered "complicated," defined as recurrent VVC, particularly severe VVC, non-*C albicans* VVC, or host with uncontrolled diabetes, debilitation or immunosuppression.

Recurrent VVC generally is defined as 4 or more episodes of symptomatic VVC in 1 year.[18] Vaginal cultures should be collected because 10% to 20% of these patients will have non-*C albicans* species. For those with recurrent *C. albicans*, a longer duration of azole therapy can improve mycologic control before initiating maintenance therapy. For example, 7 to 10 days of topical therapy or 150 mg oral dose of fluconazole every third day for a total of 3 doses is commonly used, followed by oral fluconazole 100 to 200 mg once a week for 6 months. There is no need to check liver function tests in otherwise healthy women.[19]

Severe VVC is treated with 7 to 14 days of topical azole or oral fluconazole 150 mg every 3 days for several doses. Non-*C albicans* VVC can be treated with intravaginal nystatin once daily for 7 to 14 days or with intravaginal boric acid 600 mg in gelatin capsules nightly for 14 days.[20,21]

ATROPHIC VAGINITIS

Atrophic vaginitis is a common vaginal condition that can affect women of many ages. It primarily affects women who are in low estrogen states, such as menopause (natural or surgical), breastfeeding, and sometimes as a result of medications.

Symptoms

Atrophic vaginitis presents in women with vulvar burning, itching, and dryness. Pain with intercourse and dysuria also may be present.

Test Results

On physical examination, the vaginal epithelium seems to be a light pink, with decreased rugation. Diagnosis can be made by symptoms and physical examination findings alone. The presence of parabasal cells on wet mount supports but is not necessary for the diagnosis. Parabasal cells are cuboidal epithelial cells.

Differential Diagnosis

The differential diagnosis includes lichen planus, BV, and desquamative inflammatory vaginitis.

Treatment

Topical estrogen is the treatment of choice. Options include intravaginal estrogen cream once nightly for 14 days followed by twice weekly maintenance therapy for 6 to 12 months or an intravaginal estrogen ring that is changed every 3 months by the patient. The intravaginal ring provides the lowest dose of systemic estrogen and is well tolerated. Local estrogen therapy has lower risks of thromboembolic events than oral estrogen therapy. Treatment with patients who have breast cancer should be coordinated with the patient's medical oncologist. Vaginal estrogen can also be provided in a tablet form. This is also used nightly for 14 days followed by twice weekly maintenance therapy.

At a follow-up in 6 to 12 weeks, we confirm that symptoms have improved and that the patient is using the therapy as prescribed. We stress that intravaginal estrogen should not be used daily after the initial 14-day course because it could cause endometrial hyperplasia.

DISORDERS OF THE BARTHOLIN'S GLAND

The Bartholin's glands exit near the hymenal ring near the vestibule.

Symptoms

A Bartholin cyst is usually asymptomatic until it reaches a threshold of several centimeters. At this point, the patient feels pain or pressure, especially while sitting.

Test Results

No specific tests are generally needed. However, if the patient has a Bartholin's mass, this should be biopsied owing to risk of carcinoma. This is more common in women after menopause.

Differential Diagnosis

The differential diagnosis includes keratin cyst, mucous cyst, and perirectal or vulvar abscess.

Treatment

Unless the Bartholin gland's cyst is symptomatic, no treatment is needed. Symptomatic cysts and abscesses require drainage. Word catheters are commonly used for this purpose. Simple incision and drainage is not recommended as first-line treatment because of the risk of recurrence. Women over the age of 40 have a higher chance of Bartholin's gland carcinoma, so a biopsy should be considered at the time of any procedure. An alternative to the Word catheter is marsupialization of the cyst. Excision of the Bartholin's gland is rarely performed owing to risk of scarring, hematoma, infection, and dyspareunia and is generally reserved for recurrent cases.

Management

While the patient is symptomatic, we also recommend using Sitz baths to keep the area clean. This therapy can also be soothing for the area. Some patients require topical analgesics. Small abscesses may be treated with warm Sitz baths and antibiotics (**Fig. 3**).

VULVAR INTRAEPITHELIAL NEOPLASIA/CONDYLOMA

Vulvar intraepithelial neoplasia (VIN) is associated with the human papilloma virus.

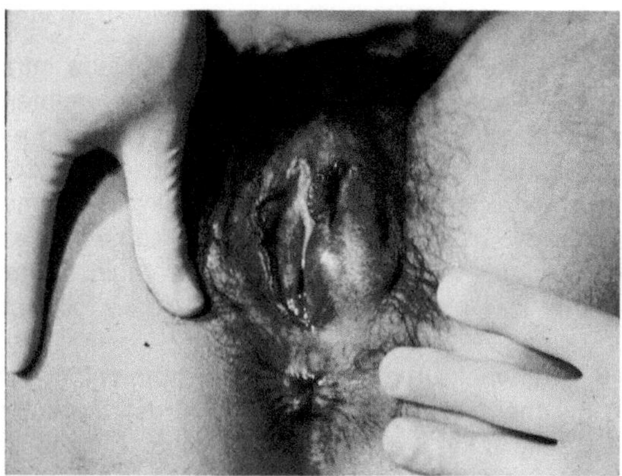

Fig. 3. Left Bartholin's gland cyst.

Symptoms

Patient may have no symptoms; some patients experience itching, pain, or both.

Test Results

Diagnosis is made primarily through visual inspection of the vulva. Vulvar biopsy helps to confirm the diagnosis. Raised lesions of concern may be biopsied. Acetic acid application causes the lesions to have a classic acetowhite appearance.

Differential Diagnosis

The differential diagnosis includes *Molluscum contagiosum*, nevi, and melanoma.

Treatment

The management of VIN depends on the severity of the disease. Biopsy specimens are graded VIN-1 (low grade) to VIN-3 (high grade). Condyloma may be treated with liquid nitrogen, trichloroacetic acid, excision, or laser. VIN-2 and VIN-3 are treated more commonly with surgical excision or laser therapy. Imiquimod is also more frequently. Imiquimoid is applied 3 times weekly on alternative days for 6 to 10 hours and then rinsed off with mild soap and water. Total duration of treatment should be 16 weeks or less if there is total clearance of warts (**Fig. 4**).

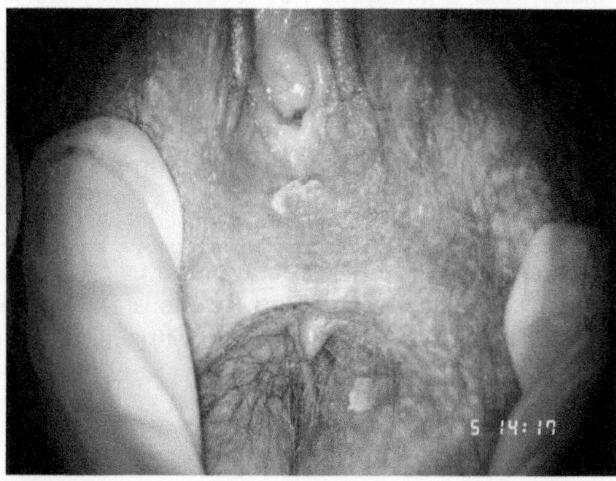

Fig. 4. Vulvar intraepithelial neoplasia (condyloma).

GENITAL HERPES SIMPLEX VIRUS

Herpes simplex virus (HSV) is the most common cause of vulvar ulcers in the United States. There are 2 serotypes of HSV: HSV1 and HSV2. HSV2 is more commonly associated with genital outbreaks; however, HSV1 can also affect the vulva in about 20% of cases.[22]

Symptoms

Symptoms depend on the timing for the herpes outbreak. The primary infection for genital herpes can cause fevers, dysuria, burning, and pruritus. Vesicles are seen on the vulva, which are painful. They are often found in clusters. Pain may be severe enough that patients present with urinary retention. Immunocompromised patients (such as patients in pregnancy, with human immunodeficiency virus, and with cancer) may develop a disseminated infection, which can be lethal. Patients with a prior herpes outbreak may have recurrent disease at any time. Generally, the extent of discomfort and lesions is less during secondary outbreaks. Patients may experience prodromal symptoms before a recurrence, including burning, tingling, or pruritus before the appearance of lesions.

Test Results

For visible lesions, active vesicles should be unroofed and a swab for viral polymerase chain reaction can be run. To see if patients have ever been exposed to HSV, immunoglobulin G antibody testing can be performed.

Differential Diagnosis

Many different conditions can cause ulcers, the most common of which includes aphthous ulcers, Behçet disease, chancroid, Crohn disease, pemphigoid, systemic lupus erythematosus, and syphilis (**Table 2**). For patients with recurrent disease, prophylactic medication can be used to decrease the number of episodes. Education of the patient is also important. Most HSV transmission occurs during asymptomatic viral shedding (**Figs. 5** and **6**).

Table 2
Treatment for Herpes Simplex Virus in immunocompetent patients

Type of Treatment	Acyclovir	Valacyclovir
First episode	200 mg 5 times daily × 7–10 d or 400 mg TID × 7–10 d	1 g BID × 7–10 d
Recurrent episode	400 mg TID × 5 d or 800 mg BID × 5 d or 800 mg PO TID × 2 d	500 mg PO BID × 3 d or 1 g PO daily × 5 d
Suppression	400 mg PO BID	500 mg PO daily or 1 g PO daily

Data from Workowski KA, Berman SM. Sexually transmitted diseases treatment guidelines, 2006. Centers for Disease Control and Prevention. MMWR Recomm Rep 2006;55:1–94. [Erratum appears in MMWR Morb Mortal Wkly Rep 2006;55:997].

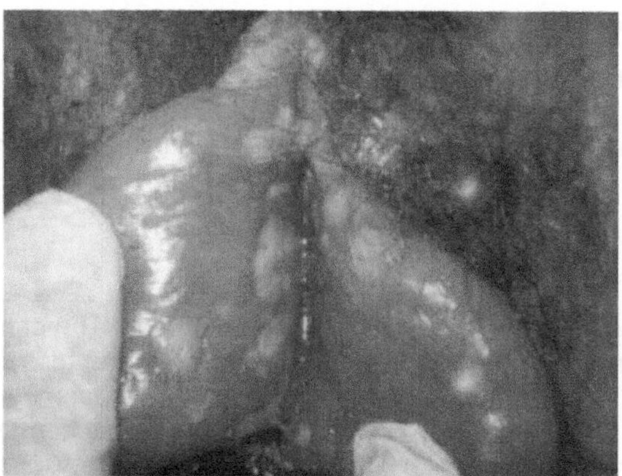

Fig. 5. Herpes simplex virus infection.

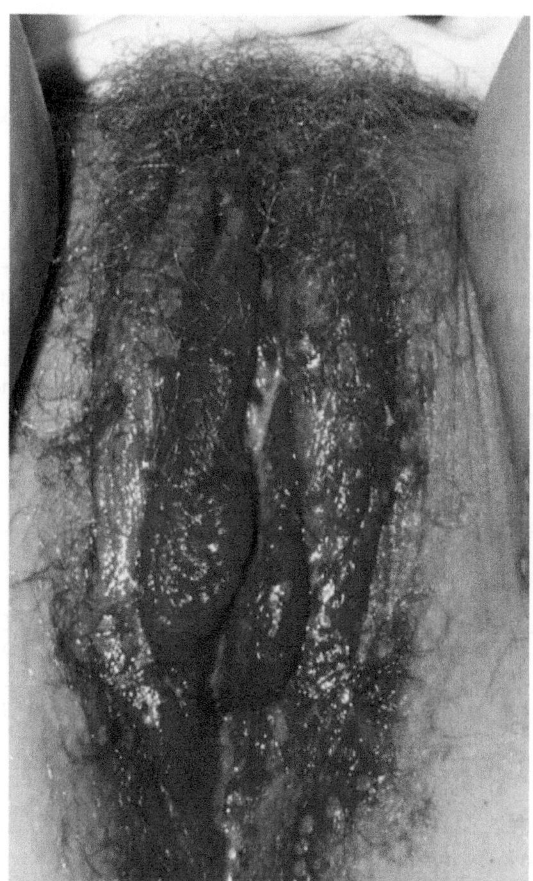

Fig. 6. Primary herpes simplex virus infection.

DERMATITIS

It is estimated that about 22% of vulvar itching cases are due to dermatitis.

Symptoms

Patients may experience itching, burning, stinging, pain, and dyspareunia. The skin may have small fissures.

Test Results

Patch testing may be done to identify any allergens.

Differential Diagnosis

- Allergic contact dermatitis
- Atopic dermatitis
- Candidiasis
- Erythrasma
- Extramammary Paget disease
- Irritant contact dermatitis
- Lichen simplex chronicus

Box 4
Vulvar hygiene guidelines

1. Clothing
   a. White, cotton underwear; no thongs
   b. Avoid pantyhose or remove middle insert
   c. Avoid tight-fitting or synthetic clothes
   d. Remove wet clothes or swimsuits quickly
   e. Consider "sensitive" laundry detergent
   f. Avoid dryer sheets
   g. Consider underwear-only cycle with additional water-only rinse
2. Bathing and hygiene
   a. Avoid bath soaps, salts, oils, gels, lotions, and perfumes
   b. Pat dry or use hairdryer on cool setting
   c. No douching
   d. Avoid deodorized pads and tampons
   e. No shaving; trimming of the pubic hair is recommended
3. Toileting
   a. White, unscented toilet paper
   b. Avoid medicated wipes for bowel movements
   c. Consider use of A&D ointment to protect the skin from incontinence
   d. Sitz baths or Pericare bottles can be used to help clean
4. Sex
   a. Use a water-based lubricant or a neutral oil as a lubricant
   b. Discuss contraceptive choices

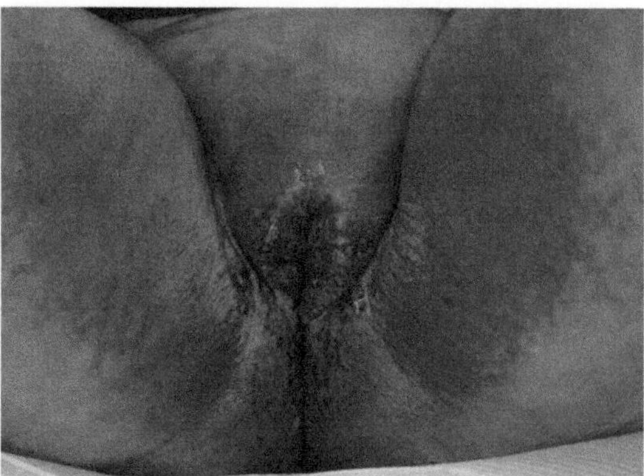

Fig. 7. Allergic contact dermatitis. Contact dermatitis from benzocaine 20% available in an over-the-counter product to help with itching. This medication caused erosions and ulcers and allergic contact dermatitis. (*Courtesy of* Lynette J. Margesson, MD, FRCPC, Manchester, NH.)

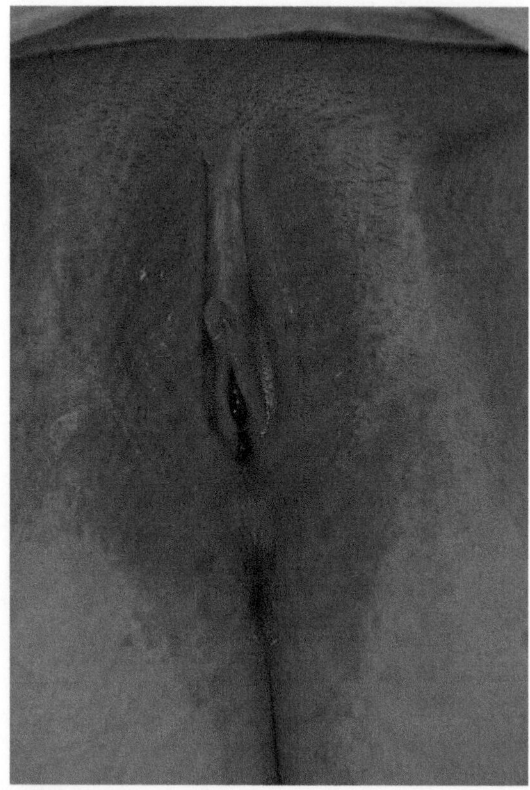

Fig. 8. Irritant dermatitis. Irritant contact dermatitis from cleansing wipes and pads in a younger woman. (*Courtesy of* Lynette J. Margesson, MD, FRCPC, Manchester, NH.)

- Psoriasis
- Seborrheic dermatitis
- Squamous cell carcinoma in situ
- Tinea cruris

Treatment

The most essential step in this diagnosis is to identify the offending agent and remove it. Next, for patients with itching, it is important to break the itching–scratching cycle (see section on lichen simplex chronicus). To help restore the barrier function of the skin, vegetable shortening, a neutral oil (eg, coconut oil) or plain petrolatum can be used. Inflammation may be reduced with a short course of topical steroids. We recommend following vulvar hygiene guidelines to minimize any other exposures (**Box 4**; **Figs. 7–9**).

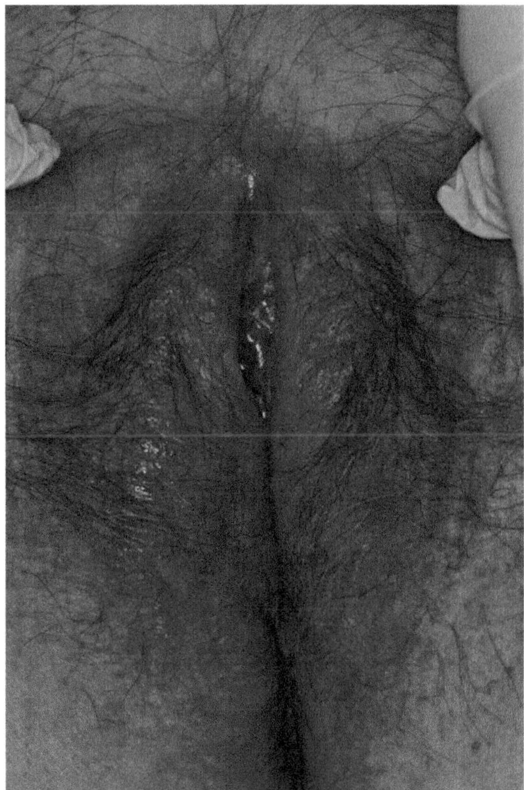

Fig. 9. Irritant contact dermatitis. Severe contact dermatitis from overusing soaps, wipes, and facecloths. The skin is thin owing to her low estrogen state of menopause. It is important to know that more than one condition may be present. This patient has lichen planus on the inner aspects of the vulva and contact dermatitis on the outside. (*Courtesy of* Lynette J. Margesson, MD, FRCPC, Manchester, NH.)

LICHEN SIMPLEX CHRONICUS

Lichen simplex chronicus is the end result of a chronic itch and scratch cycle.

Symptoms

The patient presents with intense pruritus. Sometimes she may scratch enough to cause bleeding or pain.

Test Results

In any areas with concerning pigment changes or raised lesions, a vulvar biopsy may be performed to confirm the diagnosis. This diagnosis is often made with visual inspection, which reveals changes in pigmentation (hypopigmentation or hyperpigmentation), thickening of the skin called *lichenification*, scaling, and excoriations. The key is to try to identify the underlying initiating cause of the itching (eg, irritant exposures, VIN, yeast, or lichen sclerosus).

Differential Diagnosis

The differential diagnosis includes Candidiasis, lichen sclerosus, VIN, Paget disease, and psoriasis.

Treatment

Treatment is focused on decreasing any inflammation present with a short course of topical steroids. Treatment of the underlying condition is also necessary. Patients should be seen in follow-up to ensure improvement in symptoms and physical examination. Additionally, this allows the practitioner to watch for other underlying causes (**Figs. 10** and **11**).

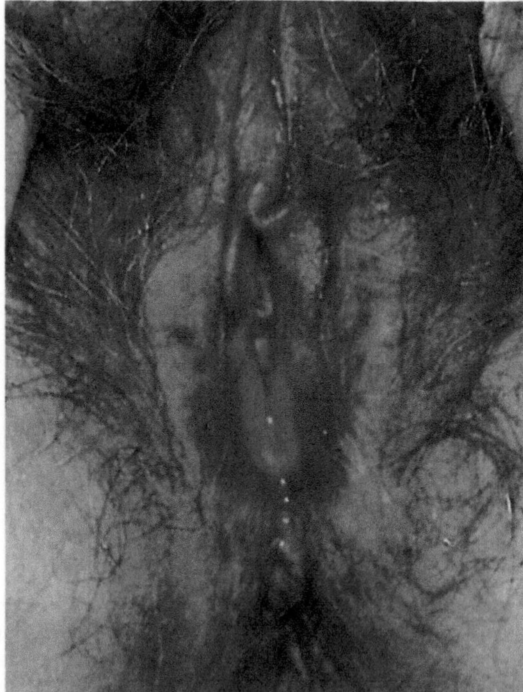

Fig. 10. Lichenification in lichen simplex chronicus.

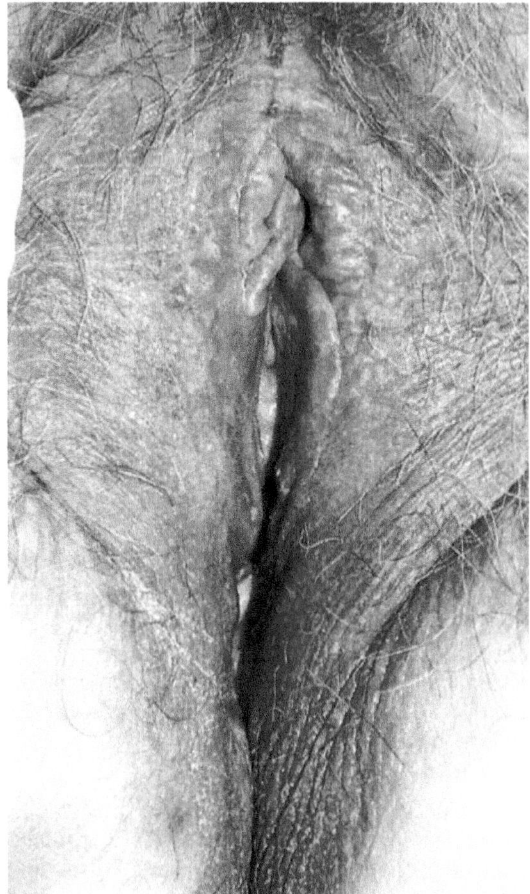

Fig. 11. Lichenification in lichen simplex chronicus. Note the coarse, leathery texture. The pigment changes are variable.

LICHEN PLANUS

Lichen planus an inflammatory skin condition currently thought to be autoimmune in nature. It can affect both the skin and mucosal (oral, vaginal, gastrointestinal) surfaces. The prevalence is about 1 in 4000 women. Patients with lichen planus may have other autoimmune disorders such as type I diabetes mellitus and Hashimoto thyroiditis. It is not well understood.

Symptoms

Patients may be asymptomatic. Other patients may present with pain, dyspareunia, bleeding with intercourse, vaginal narrowing or shortening, hair loss, a pruritic rash, and/or gingival bleeding and pain.

Test Results

Vulvar biopsy is performed to confirm the diagnosis. Visual inspection may reveal "polygonal purple papules" in classic lichen planus. Erosive lichen planus shows erythematous maculae from the vestibule and extending into the vagina. The gums may show a lacey white reticular pattern known as "Wickham's striae."

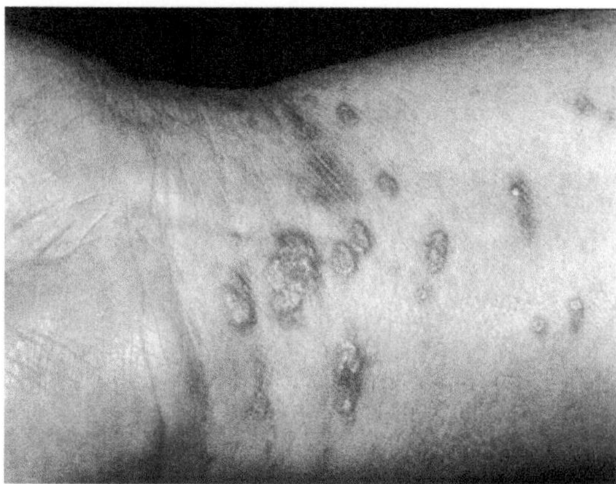

Fig. 12. Violaceous polygonal purple papules classic for lichen planus.

Differential Diagnosis

The differential diagnosis includes bullous diseases (pemphigus, cicatricial, pemphigoid), Behçet syndrome, Crohn disease, desquamative inflammatory vaginitis, and lichen sclerosus.

Treatment

Ultrapotent topical steroids (such as clobetasol or halobetasol) are used to control inflammation. Vaginal hydrocortisone suppositories may be used for vaginal disease. Triamcinolone paste may be used for oral disease.

Management

Patients with systemic lichen planus may require oral prednisone course. For esophageal manifestations, dilation may be required. We recommend dental care with a dentist familiar with the condition. Once stabilized, we recommend vulvar examinations every 6 to 12 months (**Figs. 12–15**).

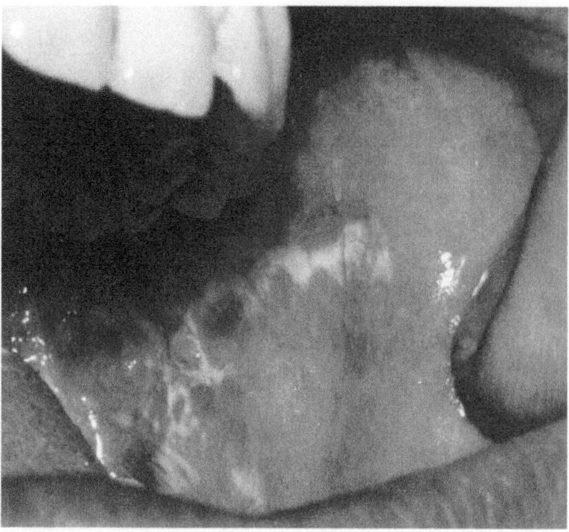

Fig. 13. Wickham's striae.

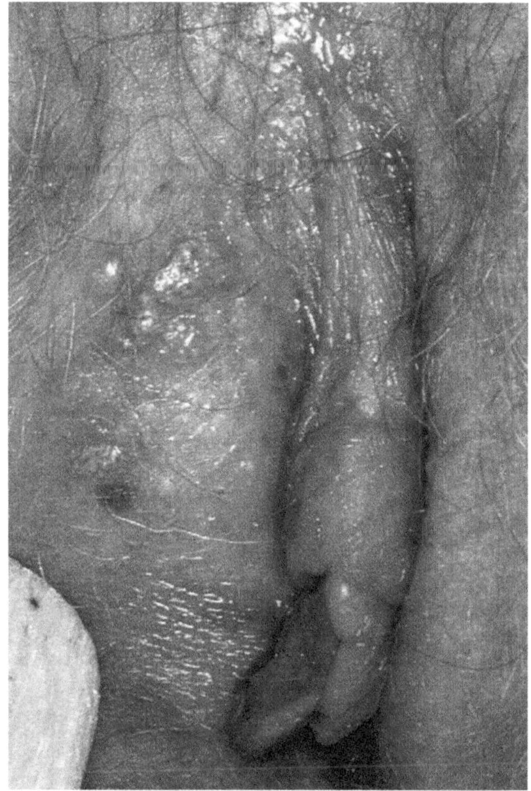

Fig. 14. Classic cutaneous vulvar lichen planus with violaceous papules.

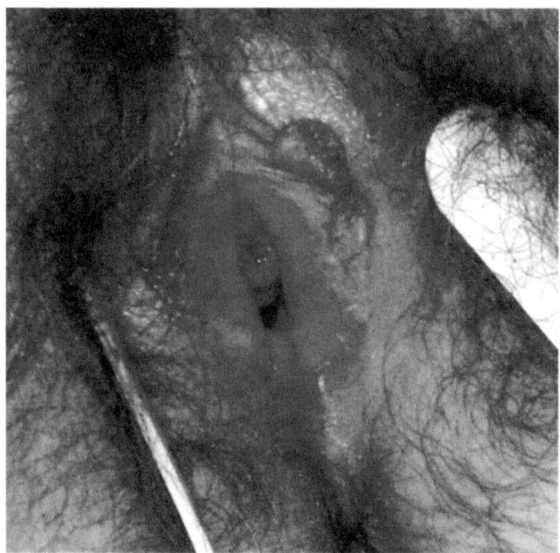

Fig. 15. Erosive lichen planus involving the mucosa.

LICHEN SCLEROSUS

Lichen sclerosus an inflammatory skin condition currently thought to be autoimmune in nature. It primarily affects skin surfaces. The prevalence is between 1 in 300 and 1 in 1000 women.[23] Patients with lichen sclerosus may have other autoimmune disorders, such as alopecia, vitiligo, and hypothyroidism.[24] It is not well understood. Lichen sclerosus can affect women of any age, although it is more commonly seen in prepubescent girls and women after the age of 50.

Symptoms

Patients may be asymptomatic. Other patients may present with itching, irritation, burning, pain, tearing, and dyspareunia. Narrowing of the introitus is also common. In severe cases, the stream of urine may change as the labia minora fuse.

Test Results

Vulvar biopsy may be performed to confirm the diagnosis. Visual inspection may reveal hypopigmentation, "parchment paper" thin appearance to the skin, and a classic "figure-of-8" distribution around the vulva and perianal area. Ecchymoses or fissures may be seen.

Differential Diagnosis

The differential diagnosis includes bullous diseases (pemphigus, cicatricial, pemphigoid), Behçet syndrome, Crohn disease, desquamative inflammatory vaginitis, and lichen planus.

Treatment

Ultrapotent topical steroids (such as clobetasol or halobetasol) are used to control inflammation.[25] Second-line therapies may be used such as tacrolimus. Surgery may be necessary for release of labial adhesions or dilation of the urethra. Once stabilized, we recommend vulvar examinations every 6 to 12 months. Nonhealing areas or areas not responding to topical steroids should be considered for biopsy.

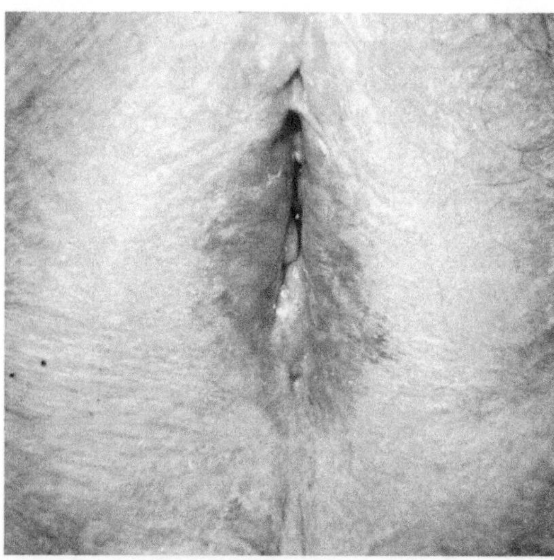

Fig. 16. Lichen sclerosus. Note the loss of architecture with the agglutination of labia minora. The skin has pigment changes and a "parchment paper" crinkled appearance.

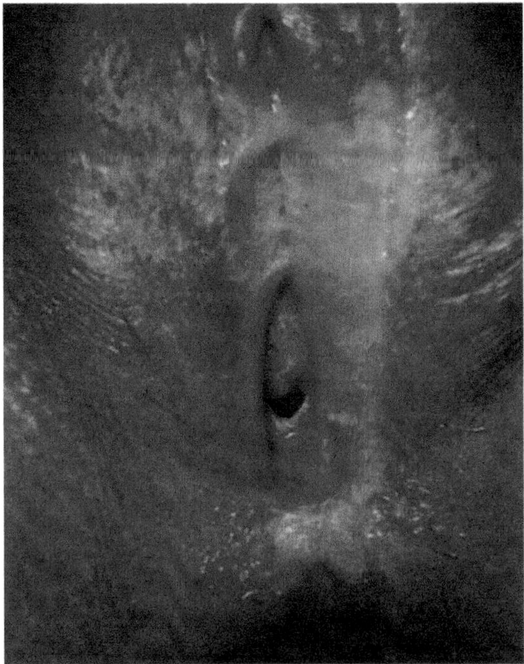

Fig. 17. Lichen sclerosus. Note the loss of architecture with the agglutination of labia minora. The skin is hypopigmented. There is also a band of agglutination superiorly and some narrowing of the vaginal introitus.

This is because women with lichen sclerosus are at an increased risk (4%–5%) of vulvar squamous cell carcinoma (**Figs. 16** and **17**).[24]

REFERENCES

1. Thorstensen KA, Birenbaum DL. Recognition and management of vulvar dermatologic conditions: lichen sclerosus, lichen planus, and lichen simplex chronicus. J Midwifery Womens Health 2012;57(3):260–75.
2. Paavonen J, Stamm WE. Sexually transmitted diseases. Lower genital tract infections in women. Infect Dis Clin North Am 1987;1(1):179–98.
3. Mehta SD. Systematic review of randomized trials of treatment of male sexual partners for improved bacteria vaginosis outcomes in women. Sex Transm Dis 2012;39(10):822–30.
4. Sobel JD, Ferris D, Schwebke J, et al. Suppressive antibacterial therapy with 0.75% metronidazole vaginal gel to prevent recurrent bacterial vaginosis. Am J Obstet Gynecol 2006;194(5):1283–9.
5. Reichman O, Akins R, Sobel JD. Boric acid addition to suppressive antimicrobial therapy for recurrent bacterial vaginosis. Sex Transm Dis 2009;36(11):732–4.
6. Fredricks DN, Fiedler TL, Marrazzo JM. Molecular identification of bacteria associated with bacterial vaginosis. N Engl J Med 2005;353(18):1899–911.
7. Fredricks DN, Fiedler TL, Thomas KK, et al. Changes in vaginal bacterial concentrations with intravaginal metronidazole therapy for bacterial vaginosis as assessed by quantitative PCR. J Clin Microbiol 2014;52(8):3137.

8. Hillier SL. The complexity of microbial diversity in bacterial vaginosis. N Engl J Med 2005;353(18):1886–7.
9. Senok AC, Verstraelen H, Temmerman M, et al. Probiotics for the treatment of bacterial vaginosis. Cochrane Database Syst Rev 2009;(4):CD006289.
10. Centers for Disease Control and Prevention. Trichomoniasis – CDC fact sheet. Available at: http://www.cdc.gov/std/trichomonas/stdfact-trichomoniasis.htm. Accessed November 3, 2014.
11. Sutton M, Sternberg M, Koumans EH, et al. The prevalence of Trichomonas vaginalis infection among reproductive-age women in the United States, 2001-2004. Clin Infect Dis 2007;45(10):1319–26.
12. Schwebke JR, Hobbs MM, Taylor SN, et al. Molecular testing for Trichomonas vaginalis in women: results from a prospective U.S. clinical trial. J Clin Microbiol 2011;49(12):4106–11.
13. Lawing LF, Hedges SR, Schwebke JR. Detection of trichomonosis in vaginal and urine specimens from women by culture and PCR. J Clin Microbiol 2000;38(10):3585–8.
14. Sena AC, Miller WC, Hobbs MM, et al. Trichomonas vaginalis infection in male sexual partners: implications for diagnosis, treatment, and prevention. Clin Infect Dis 2007;44(1):13–22.
15. Forna F, Gulmezoglu AM. Interventions for treating trichomoniasis in women. Cochrane Database Syst Rev 2003;(2):CD000218.
16. Kirkcaldy RD, Augostini P, Asbel LE, et al. Trichomonas vaginalis antimicrobial drug resistance in 6 US cities, STD Surveillance Network, 2009-2010. Emerg Infect Dis 2012;18(6):939–43.
17. Sobel JD, Nyirjesy P, Brown W. Tinidazole therapy for metronidazole-resistant vaginal trichomoniasis. Clin Infect Dis 2001;33(8):1341–6.
18. O'Connor MI, Sobel JD. Epidemiology of recurrent vulvovaginal candidiasis: identification and strain differentiation of *Candida albicans*. J Infect Dis 1986; 154(2):358–63.
19. Sobel JD. Recurrent vulvovaginal candidiasis. A prospective study of the efficacy of maintenance ketoconazole therapy. N Engl J Med 1986;315(23):1455–8.
20. Sobel JD. Management of patients with recurrent vulvovaginal candidiasis. Drugs 2003;63(11):1059–66.
21. Sobel JD, Chaim W, Nagappan V, et al. Treatment of vaginitis caused by *Candida glabrata*: use of topical boric acid and flucytosine. Am J Obstet Gynecol 2003; 189(5):1297–300.
22. Boardman LA, Colleen Kennedy Stockdale. ACOG Clinical Updates in Women's Health Care: Vulvar Disorders. ACOG 2009.
23. Edwards L, Lynch PJ. Genital dermatology atlas. 2nd edition. Baltimore: Lippincott Williams and Wilkins; 2011.
24. Smith YR, Haefner HK. Vuvlar lichen sclerosus: pathophysiology and treatment. Am J Clin Dermatol 2004;5:105–25.
25. Cooper SM, Gao XH, Powell JJ, et al. Does treatment of vulvar lichen sclerosus influence its prognosis? Arch Dermatol 2004;140:702–6.

Prevalence and Management of Chronic Hepatitis C Virus Infection in Women

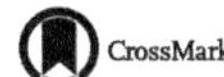

Lauren A. Beste, MD, MSc[a,b,*], Hollye C. Bondurant, PharmD[c], George N. Ioannou, BMBCh, MS[d,e]

KEYWORDS

• Viral hepatitis • Women • Pregnancy • Antiviral therapy

KEY POINTS

- Women should be tested for hepatitis C virus if they have risk factors for exposure, including birth year between 1945 and 1965.
- Routine hepatitis C virus testing is not recommended in pregnancy, except for women with risk factors for exposure.
- Hepatitis C virus infection does not clearly confer adverse risk during pregnancy, except in patients with cirrhosis.
- Premenopausal women must be carefully counseled about the risks of pregnancy and breast feeding during hepatitis C virus treatment.
- Highly effective hepatitis C virus antiviral therapies are rapidly emerging. All women with hepatitis C virus should be assessed for treatment candidacy.

Disclosures: The authors have no relevant disclosures.
The views expressed in this article are those of the authors and do not necessarily reflect the position or policy of the Department of Veterans Affairs. This material is the result of work supported by resources from the VA Puget Sound Health Care System (Seattle, Washington).
[a] Primary Care Service, Health Services Research and Development, VA Puget Sound Health Care System, 1660 South Columbian Way, S-111-GI, Seattle, WA 98108, USA; [b] Department of Internal Medicine, Division of General Internal Medicine, University of Washington, WA, USA; [c] Pharmacy Service, VA Puget Sound Health Care System, 1660 South Columbian Way, Seattle, WA 98108, USA; [d] Hospital and Specialty Medicine Service, VA Puget Sound Health Care System, 1660 South Columbian Way, Seattle, WA 98108, USA; [e] Department of Internal Medicine, Division of Gastroenterology, University of Washington, WA, USA
* Corresponding author.
E-mail address: Lauren.beste@va.gov

Med Clin N Am 99 (2015) 575–586
http://dx.doi.org/10.1016/j.mcna.2015.01.009
0025-7125/15/$ – see front matter Published by Elsevier Inc.

medical.theclinics.com

EPIDEMIOLOGY AND MANAGEMENT OF HEPATITIS C VIRUS IN WOMEN

Hepatitis C virus (HCV) is the most common blood-borne pathogen in the United States, chronically infecting an estimated 1% of the population, including roughly 970,000 women.[1] HCV is the nation's leading cause of cirrhosis, liver failure, hepatocellular carcinoma, and liver transplantation. HCV typically remains asymptomatic for 2 to 4 decades until cirrhosis, hepatocellular carcinoma, or liver failure occurs. Therefore, despite a decline in the number of new HCV infections in the United States since 1990, the burden of HCV-related complications is projected to continue increasing over the next 20 years.[2]

Women account for approximately 35.8% of cases of chronic HCV.[1] The course of HCV and its complications varies between women and men. In addition, women with HCV face unique risks related to antiviral treatment during pregnancy and breast feeding and the potential for vertical transmission to their offspring. The following review describes the epidemiology, disease progression, and treatment of HCV in women.

TRANSMISSION OF HEPATITIS C VIRUS IN WOMEN

HCV is spread by blood contact. The main modes of transmission include intravenous or intranasal drug use, blood product transfusion before 1990, and percutaneous exposures such as needle stick injuries. **Table 1** describes the US prevalence of HCV infection in selected risk groups for men and women.

Unlike hepatitis B virus or human immunodeficiency virus (HIV), sexual transmission of HCV between serodiscordant heterosexual partners is rare, with an incidence of 0.07% per year (or 1 in every 190,000 sexual contacts).[3] Therefore, from an HCV perspective, most women in long-term monogamous heterosexual relationships can safely maintain their current practices. Women who are concerned about HCV transmission or who have other risk factors that increase their chances of acquiring HCV (eg, HIV, multiple partners, injection drug use) should be counseled about safe sex practices with barrier methods. The rate of HCV transmission between female sexual partners is unknown, but is likely to be exceptionally low.

Table 1
US prevalence of HCV infection in selected groups

	HCV Infection Prevalence	
Population[a]	(%)	Range (%)
1945–1965 birth cohort	3.25	2.80–3.76[b]
History of injection drug use	79	72–86
Unexplained abnormal aminotransferase levels	15	10–18
Hemophilia with receipt of clotting factors before 1987	87	74–90
Organ transplant or blood product transfusion before 1990	6	5–9
Children born to HCV-infected mothers	5	0–25
Chronic hemodialysis	10	0–64
Men who have sex with men	4	2–18
HIV	25	15–30

[a] Includes both men and women.
[b] Presented as a 95% confidence interval.
Data from Refs.[7,28,29]

Vertical Transmission of Hepatitis C Virus

Based on systematic review of 77 prospective cohort studies of HCV-infected pregnant women, the overall rate of mother-to-infant transmission is 1.7% for antibody-positive women (indicating past exposure but not necessarily viremia) and 4.3% for women with documented HCV viremia.[4] Women with HIV/HCV co-infection have a 19.4% rate of vertical transmission.[4] Risk factors for vertical transmission include high HCV viral load, HIV co-infection, prolonged rupture of membranes, and invasive fetal monitoring such as the use of scalp electrodes.[5] Meta-analysis suggests that cesarean section does not reduce the risk of vertical transmission in HCV mono-infected women.[6] Based on the lack of evidence, professional society guidelines do not currently recommend specific interventions to prevent HCV vertical transmission.

Hepatitis C Virus Transmission and Breast Feeding

HCV may be found in human breast milk, but breast feeding does not promote HCV transmission except in cases of cracked, damaged, or bleeding nipples. Breast feeding can safely be recommended for women with HCV, except in HIV/HCV co-infection or instances of cracked, damaged, or bleeding nipples.

SCREENING FOR HEPATITIS C VIRUS IN WOMEN

The 1945 to 1965 ("baby boomer") birth cohort accounts for 75% of all cases of HCV in the United States, a phenomenon believed to result from high prevalence of HCV risk behaviors and iatrogenic exposure through unscreened blood products.[7] Because up to 50% of patients with HCV report no traditional risk factors, the CDC recommends all individuals born between 1945 and 1965 undergo testing for HCV, regardless of sex or risk factor status.[7,8] Additionally, testing should be offered to women of any age with risk factors.

Screening for Hepatitis C Virus in Pregnant Women

The American College of Obstetrics and Gynecology recommends HCV testing in pregnant women with infection risk factors but does not endorse routine screening for all pregnant women.[9] In large studies drawn from the general US population, HCV antibody positivity occurs in 0.24% to 4.3% of pregnant women.[5,10,11] In one review including 9 international studies of pregnant women with HCV, most had clear risk factors such as history of intravenous drug use (range, 17%–79%) or blood transfusion (2.5%–19%).[12] Furthermore, cost effectiveness analysis does not favor the use of routine HCV screening in pregnancy, even under the assumption that vertical transmission could be prevented.[13]

Most of HCV in pregnancy represents chronic rather than acute infection. Acute HCV in pregnancy rarely causes adverse maternal or fetal outcomes, although several case reports describe instances of fulminant hepatitis.[14] Pregnant women with abnormal liver function and HCV infection risk factors, such as recent intravenous drug use, should be ruled out for acute HCV through quantitative HCV viral load testing even if their antibody test result is negative.

NATURAL HISTORY OF HEPATITIS C VIRUS IN WOMEN

Spontaneous clearance of HCV occurs shortly after infection some exposed persons. Cohort studies of HCV-exposed women find higher rates of spontaneous clearance among women compared with men. In a landmark study of 376 young Irish women who contracted HCV in 1977 to 1978 from contaminated anti-D immune globulin,

Kenny-Walsh[15] found that 45% had spontaneously cleared the virus after 17 years. In contrast, spontaneous clearance occurs in approximately 20% of the general (predominantly male) HCV-exposed population.

Women with HCV progress to cirrhosis more slowly than men. Kenny-Walsh[15] reported that half the chronically infected women in their cohort had biopsy evidence of liver fibrosis after 17 years, with 1.9% having definite or probable cirrhosis. A follow-up study of this cohort examined patients who had undergone a repeat liver biopsy at least 5 years later (n = 184).[16] Compared with the baseline biopsy, fibrosis regressed in 24% of women, progressed in 27%, and remained the same in 49%.[16] At 24 years postinfection, just 2.1% of the women showed evidence of cirrhosis on liver biopsy.[16] This study did not address the rate of progression to cirrhosis over longer time intervals, and the cohort was composed of women infected with HCV at a young age and with minimal alcohol intake. However, other studies specifically examining women show low rates of progression to cirrhosis.[17] Rigorous natural history studies including both men and women consistently find that female sex is protective against liver fibrosis, even after adjusting for age at infection and a tendency toward heavier alcohol consumption in men.[18]

Hepatitis C Virus and Pregnancy

In general, pregnancy does not appear to affect the natural history of maternal chronic HCV.[19] Most women with chronic HCV experience a temporary decline in transaminase levels during pregnancy, and viral load may fluctuate. No high-quality evidence suggests that pregnancy impacts viral clearance or degree of hepatic fibrosis on a long-term basis.

Prospective evidence suggests that chronic HCV does not negatively affect pregnancy outcomes, unless there is established cirrhosis. Among Irish women with iatrogenic HCV infection after their first pregnancy (n = 36), no increase in spontaneous abortion, preterm delivery, or obstetric complications in subsequent pregnancies was observed relative to matched controls.[20] One retrospective population-based study examining birth records from 506 HCV-infected women found an increased rate of low birth weight, small size for gestational age, use of intensive care, or assisted ventilation relative to drug-using and randomly selected HCV-negative women.[21]

Comorbid Alcohol Use and Hepatitis C Virus in Women

Alcohol intake is an important cofactor in the progression of HCV in both sexes, but the effect of alcohol is more pronounced in women than in men. Chen and colleagues[22] identified 3187 deaths from HCV in a national study of death records from 2000 to 2002. Among women who died of HCV-related causes, the mean age of death declined from 61.0 years with HCV alone to 49.1 years with HCV plus heavy alcohol use. In men, the mean age of death decreased from 55.1 years with HCV alone to 50.0 years with HCV plus heavy alcohol use. The cumulative probability of death before age 65 was much higher in the setting of heavy alcohol with HCV (0.91 for men, 0.88 for women) than in HCV alone (0.68 for men, 0.47 for women). Although women generally seem to have a lower risk of mortality from HCV than men, in the setting of heavy alcohol their mortality rate becomes similar.

PHARMACOLOGIC MANAGEMENT OF HEPATITIS C VIRUS IN WOMEN

The goal of HCV antiviral therapy is to achieve sustained virologic response or permanent clearance of the virus as assessed by negative HCV viral load 6 months or more after treatment completion. HCV treatment is a rapidly developing area, with numerous new drugs entering the marketplace. Choice of regimen now depends primarily on viral genotype, cirrhosis status, and history of prior treatment exposure.

Until the 2013 approval of the polymerase inhibitor, sofosbuvir, and the second-generation protease inhibitor, simeprevir, all HCV antiviral regimens were based on the injectable cytokine interferon. Interferon is typically combined with the nucleotide analogue ribavirin. In 2011, the first protease inhibitors, telaprevir and boceprevir, were approved by the US Food and Drug Administration. These medications increased the effectiveness of interferon and ribavirin but with significantly greater inconvenience, pill burden, side effects, and financial costs. The second generation of direct-acting antiviral medications, including sofosbuvir, simeprevir, and ledipasvir, have significantly improved treatment outcomes and side-effect profiles relative to earlier drugs. Currently approved HCV treatment regimens are the same for both women and men and are outlined in **Table 2**. Outcomes of treatment are similar between women and men.

Historically, side effects and contraindications to interferon-based therapy (**Table 3**) constituted a major treatment barrier for men and women alike. Selected side effects of interferon include flulike symptoms, bone marrow suppression including anemia and neutropenia, and depression. Ribavirin causes hemolytic anemia and rash. Contraindications to traditional therapy with interferon and ribavirin include decompensated cirrhosis, severe thrombocytopenia, uncontrolled depression, renal failure, pregnancy or risk for pregnancy, and numerous others. Several interferon contraindications, including autoimmune hepatitis and thyroid dysfunction, are more common in women and should be ruled out before starting interferon.

In the past, low treatment efficacy, burdensome regimens, and treatment duration up to 48 weeks presented significant obstacles to both initiation and completion of therapy. Interferon-based regimens are rapidly becoming obsolete in favor of newer, highly effective, and more tolerable regimens. In the near future, the possibility of virologic cure for the majority of HCV patients may be realized for the first time.

Determination of Hepatitis C Virus Antiviral Treatment Candidacy

Antiviral treatment should be considered for all HCV-infected women interested in therapy and able to comply with treatment requirements. HCV-infected women with compensated or mildly decompensated cirrhosis are at high risk for eventual progression to liver failure and should be strongly considered for antiviral therapy. Interferon-free regimens now exist for all genotypes and are the treatments of choice for most patients. As with men, pretreatment counseling to explain the risks, benefits, indications, and expected side effects is essential to successful completion of antiviral therapy.

Hepatitis C Virus Treatment Considerations in Premenopausal Women

Premenopausal women face special treatment considerations in relation to the teratogenic potential of HCV antivirals. Ribavirin is contraindicated in pregnancy because it interferes with embryo development and is embryotoxic or embryolethal in animal models.[23] Drug manufacturers recommend avoiding ribavirin during pregnancy and up to 6 months postexposure for both females and their male partners. Ribavirin registries are maintained that track pregnancies occurring after maternal or paternal exposure. Premenopausal women with HCV, and HCV-infected men with premenopausal partners, must be counseled about the teratogenicity of ribavirin before beginning therapy. Two forms of contraception are recommended during ribavirin treatment and up to 6 months thereafter in addition to regular pregnancy testing during therapy.

Table 2
Outcomes of selected clinical trials of HCV treatment regimens in women and men

Study	Regimen	Treatment Duration (wk)	Population	Sustained Virologic Response, % (n)	
				Women	Men
Poordad et al,[31] 2011	Pegylated interferon/ribavirin/boceprevir	48	Gt 1, treatment naïve	67 (145)	66 (221)
Bacon et al,[32] 2011	Pegylated interferon/ribavirin/boceprevir	36	Gt 1, treatment experienced	56 (64)	60 (98)
		48	Gt 1, treatment experienced	65 (49)	67 (112)
Jacobson et al,[33] 2011	Pegylated interferon/ribavirin/telaprevir	48	Gt 1, treatment naïve	75 (149)	74 (214)
Zeuzem et al,[34] 2011	Pegylated interferon/ribavirin/telaprevir	48	Gt 1, treatment experienced	64[a] (171)	
Lawitz et al,[35] 2013	Pegylated interferon/ribavirin/sofosbuvir	12	Gt 1, 4, treatment naïve	94 (118)	88 (209)
	Sofosbuvir/ribavirin	12	Gt 2, treatment naïve	79 (85)	61 (168)
Zeuzem et al,[36] 2014	Sofosbuvir/ribavirin	12	Gt 2	94 (33)	92 (40)
		24	Gt 3	94 (95)	80 (155)
Kumada et al,[37] 2014	Pegylated interferon/ribavirin/simeprevir	12	Gt 1, treatment naïve	94 (16)	87 (8)
		12	Gt 1, prior relapsers	100 (13)	100 (16)
		12	Gt 1, prior nonresponders	38 (13)	38 (13)
Lawitz et al,[38] 2014	Sofosbuvir/simeprevir $\pm$ ribavirin	12–24	Gt 1	98 (60)	89 (107)
Jacobson et al,[39] 2014	Pegylated interferon/ribavirin/simeprevir	12	Gt 1, treatment naïve	80 (116)	79 (148)
Manns et al,[40] 2014	Pegylated interferon/ribavirin/simeprevir	12	Gt 1, treatment naïve	85 (117)	79 (140)
Afdhal et al,[41] 2014	Ledipasvir/sofosbuvir	12	Gt 1, treatment naïve	100 (86)	99.2 (126)
Afdhal et al,[42] 2014	Ledipasvir/sofosbuvir	12	Gt 1, treatment experienced	94.3 (35)	93.2 (74)

Abbreviation: Gt, genotype.
[a] Results not reported by sex.
Data from Refs.[30–42]

The first-generation protease inhibitors, telaprevir and boceprevir, introduced an additional layer of risk for unintended pregnancy because of drug interactions with hormonal contraceptives. Due to cytochrome p450-inducing effects, telaprevir and boceprevir lower the concentration of circulating estrogens, potentially reducing the efficacy of oral contraceptive pills. Women taking telaprevir or boceprevir must be counseled to use 2 nonhormonal forms of birth control to avoid pregnancy. Instead of oral contraceptives, acceptable alternatives include a male condom or female condom with spermicidal jelly (a combination of a male condom and a female condom is not suitable), diaphragm or cervical cap with spermicidal jelly, intrauterine device, or male or female sterilization. Newer HCV antivirals, including sofosbuvir and ledipasvir, have no pharmacokinetic interactions with hormonal oral contraceptives and may be safely co-administered.[24]

Hepatitis C Virus Treatment Considerations During Pregnancy and Breast Feeding

Safe HCV treatment options during pregnancy are limited and of limited efficacy (see **Table 3**). Therefore, treatment for acute HCV in pregnancy is rarely indicated. HCV antiviral medications are not currently approved for use in breast feeding women.

NONPHARMACOLOGIC MANAGEMENT STRATEGIES FOR HEPATITIS C VIRUS

Women who opt not to undergo HCV treatment or who have contraindications to treatment should be monitored at least annually for clinical or laboratory signs of cirrhosis. All patients with HCV should be counseled on harm reduction strategies including alcohol abstinence, hepatitis A and B vaccination, and transmission prevention. Treatment candidacy should be reassessed on an ongoing basis to identify patients whose eligibility and interest in treatment may have changed.

PSYCHOSOCIAL CONSIDERATIONS FOR WOMEN WITH HEPATITIS C VIRUS INFECTION

HCV is frequently linked to injection drug use in the public and medical consciousness, often creating a climate of stigma for individuals with HCV.[25] Qualitative studies focusing on women with HCV describe intense feelings of social stigma and shame.[26,27] Virtually all the women in one qualitative study by Grundy and Beeching[27] described fears of transmitting HCV to sexual partners and especially to their children (either vertically or through routine childcare activities), even when the women could verbalize the small absolute risk of such transmission. Grundy and Beeching[27] reported that women frequently avoided disclosing their HCV status to others, and some even perceived medical care for HCV as stigmatizing.

The subjective experience of HCV varies widely, particularly between women who are actively using injection drugs compared with those who quit using or who don't have traditional HCV risk factors.[26] Qualitative research suggests that many women with a history of injection drug use may regard HCV infection as an expected and inevitable consequence of that behavior. For individuals with HCV diagnosed many years after ceasing injection drug use, it may serve as a negative reminder of a previous identity from which the woman had hoped to separate herself. Women who are actively injecting drugs may not see HCV as immediately relevant in the context of their larger concerns about personal safety, addiction, substance use disorders treatment, and other immediate issues. In contrast, among women without classic HCV risk factors, the diagnosis can be personally devastating and disruptive to their individual identity.[26]

Although the subjective disease experience of women with HCV may vary, it has the potential to impact intimate and family relationships and influence their health care

Table 3
Side effects of HCV antiviral medications and safety during pregnancy and breast feeding

Drug	Common Side Effects	Pregnancy Category[a]	Breast Feeding Safety	Additional Concerns for Women
Pegylated interferon-alfa[43]	Flu-like symptoms, fatigue, marrow suppression, depression, insomnia, irritability, retinopathy, weight loss, nausea, diarrhea	C	Unknown	Potential abortifacient; may disrupt normal menstrual cycle or cause amenorrhea
Ribavirin[44]	Hemolytic anemia, rash	X; call pregnancy registry if exposed while pregnant	Unknown	May cause birth defects and fetal death; not to be initiated until negative pregnancy test and 2 forms of birth control; concern for female partners of male patients undergoing HCV treatment; continue birth control for 6 mo after completion of treatment
Telaprevir[45]	Anemia, rash, pruritis, hemorrhoids, diarrhea, dysgeusia, fatigue, vomiting, anorectal pain	B	Unknown; Manufacturer recommends discontinuing treatment or taking into account the importance of therapy	May interfere with hormonal contraceptives
Boceprevir[46]	Anemia, hypersensitivity reactions, dysgeusia, dry mouth, vomiting, diarrhea, nausea, neutropenia, thrombocytopenia	B	Unknown; Manufacturer recommends discontinuing treatment or considering the importance of therapy	May interfere with hormonal contraceptives; may affect estrogen in hormone replacement therapy

Sofosbuvir[47]	Nausea, pancytopenia, depression	B	Unknown; Manufacturer recommends discontinuing treatment or considering the importance of therapy	No data regarding use with hormonal contraceptives
Simeprevir[48]	Photosensitivity, rash, nausea, pruritis	C	Unknown; Manufacturer recommends discontinuing treatment or considering the importance of therapy	No data regarding use with hormonal contraceptives
Ledipasvir/sofosbuvir[49]	Fatigue, headache, nausea, diarrhea, insomnia	B	Unknown; Manufacturer recommends weighing benefits of breastfeeding vs potential adverse effects on breastfed child	No clinically significant drug interactions with oral contraceptives

[a] Category A: adequate and well-controlled (AWC) studies in pregnant women failed to show risk to the fetus in the first trimester of pregnancy (and there is no evidence of a risk in later trimesters). Category B: animal reproduction studies failed to show a risk to the fetus, and there are no AWC studies in pregnant women or animals that show an adverse effect; but AWC studies in pregnant women fail to demonstrate risk to the fetus during the first trimester of pregnancy (and there is no evidence of risk in later trimesters). Category C: animal reproduction studies show adverse effect on the fetus, there are no AWC studies in humans, and the benefits from the use of the drug in pregnant women may be acceptable despite its potential risks; or animal studies have not been conducted and there are no AWC studies in humans. Category D: positive evidence of human fetal risk based on adverse reaction data from investigational or marketing experience in humans, but potential benefits from use of the drug in pregnant women may be acceptable despite potential risks. Category X: studies in animals or humans show fetal abnormalities, or there is positive evidence of fetal risk based on reports from investigational or marketing experience, or both, and the risk of the use of the drug in a pregnant woman clearly outweighs any possible benefit.[50]

Data from Refs.[43–49]

interactions. Providers caring for women with HCV should consider proactively reassuring them that the virus is generally not transmissible to household members, including children, and that sexual transmission between monogamous partners is extremely rare.

FUTURE CONSIDERATIONS

HCV continues to be an important cause of liver-related morbidity and mortality as the high-prevalence "baby boomer" cohort transitions through the clinical phases of chronic infection and cirrhosis. New HCV antiviral regimens based on direct-acting antiviral agents without interferon have greatly expanded the pool of patients eligible for treatment and have dramatically improved treatment outcomes. Premenopausal women with HCV should be counseled regarding the risk of vertical transmission and risks surrounding HCV treatment during pregnancy and breast feeding. As newer treatments promise even greater efficacy, the challenge for health care providers is to identify women in need of HCV testing and to understand the rapidly developing array of HCV treatments.

REFERENCES

1. Denniston MM, Jiles RB, Drobeniuc J, et al. Chronic hepatitis C virus infection in the United States, National Health and Nutrition Examination Survey 2003 to 2010. Ann Intern Med 2014;160(5):293–300.
2. Davis GL, Albright JE, Cook SF, et al. Projecting future complications of chronic hepatitis C in the United States. Liver Transpl 2003;9(4):331–8.
3. Terrault NA, Dodge JL, Murphy EL, et al. Sexual transmission of hepatitis C virus among monogamous heterosexual couples: the HCV partners study. Hepatology 2013;57(3):881–9.
4. Roberts EA, Yeung L. Maternal-infant transmission of hepatitis C virus infection. Hepatology 2002;36(5 Suppl 1):S106–13.
5. Mast EE, Hwang LY, Seto DS, et al. Risk factors for perinatal transmission of hepatitis C virus (HCV) and the natural history of HCV infection acquired in infancy. J Infect Dis 2005;192(11):1880–9.
6. Ghamar Chehreh ME, Tabatabaei SV, Khazanehdari S, et al. Effect of cesarean section on the risk of perinatal transmission of hepatitis C virus from HCV-RNA+/HIV- mothers: a meta-analysis. Arch Gynecol Obstet 2011;283(2):255–60.
7. Smith BD, Morgan RL, Beckett GA, et al. Recommendations for the identification of chronic hepatitis C virus infection among persons born during 1945-1965. MMWR Recomm Rep 2012;61(RR-4):1–32.
8. Rein DB, Smith BD, Wittenborn JS, et al. The cost-effectiveness of birth-cohort screening for hepatitis C antibody in U.S. primary care settings. Ann Intern Med 2012;156(4):263–70.
9. American College of Obstetricians and Gynecologists. ACOG Practice Bulletin No. 86: viral hepatitis in pregnancy. Obstet Gynecol 2007;110(4):941–56.
10. Bohman VR, Stettler RW, Little BB, et al. Seroprevalence and risk factors for hepatitis C virus antibody in pregnant women. Obstet Gynecol 1992;80(4):609–13.
11. Silverman NS, Jenkin BK, Wu C, et al. Hepatitis C virus in pregnancy: seroprevalence and risk factors for infection. Am J Obstet Gynecol 1993;169(3):583–7.
12. Floreani A. Hepatitis C and pregnancy. World J Gastroenterol 2013;19(40):6714–20.
13. Plunkett BA, Grobman WA. Routine hepatitis C virus screening in pregnancy: a cost-effectiveness analysis. Am J Obstet Gynecol 2005;192(4):1153–61.

14. Sookoian S. Liver disease during pregnancy: acute viral hepatitis. Ann Hepatol 2006;5(3):231–6.
15. Kenny-Walsh E. Clinical outcomes after hepatitis C infection from contaminated anti-D immune globulin. Irish Hepatology Research Group. N Engl J Med 1999; 340(16):1228–33.
16. Levine RA, Sanderson SO, Ploutz-Snyder R, et al. Assessment of fibrosis progression in untreated irish women with chronic hepatitis C contracted from immunoglobulin anti-D. Clin Gastroenterol Hepatol 2006;4(10):1271–7.
17. Muller R. The natural history of hepatitis C: clinical experiences. J Hepatol 1996; 24(Suppl 2):52–4.
18. Poynard T, Bedossa P, Opolon P. Natural history of liver fibrosis progression in patients with chronic hepatitis C. The OBSVIRC, METAVIR, CLINIVIR, and DOSVIRC groups. Lancet 1997;349(9055):825–32.
19. Prasad MR, Honegger JR. Hepatitis C virus in pregnancy. Am J Perinatol 2013; 30(2):149–59.
20. Jabeen T, Cannon B, Hogan J, et al. Pregnancy and pregnancy outcome in hepatitis C type 1b. QJM 2000;93(9):597–601.
21. Pergam SA, Wang CC, Gardella CM, et al. Pregnancy complications associated with hepatitis C: data from a 2003-2005 Washington state birth cohort. Am J Obstet Gynecol 2008;199(1):38.e1–9.
22. Chen CM, Yoon YH, Yi HY, et al. Alcohol and hepatitis C mortality among males and females in the United States: a life table analysis. Alcohol Clin Exp Res 2007; 31(2):285–92.
23. Database R. Agent Name: Ribavirin. Available at: http://reprotox.us. Accessed July 16, 2014.
24. German P, Moorehead L, Pang P, et al. Lack of a clinically important pharmacokinetic interaction between sofosbuvir or ledipasvir and hormonal oral contraceptives norgestimate/ethinyl estradiol in HCV-Uninfected female subjects. J Clin Pharmacol 2014;54(11):1290–8.
25. Zickmund S, Ho EY, Masuda M, et al. "They treated me like a leper". Stigmatization and the quality of life of patients with hepatitis C. J Gen Intern Med 2003; 18(10):835–44.
26. Olsen A, Banwell C, Dance P. Reinforced biographies among women living with hepatitis C. Qual Health Res 2013;23(4):531–40.
27. Grundy G, Beeching N. Understanding social stigma in women with hepatitis C. Nurs Stand 2004;19(4):35–9.
28. Strader DB, Wright T, Thomas DL, et al. Diagnosis, management, and treatment of hepatitis C. Hepatology 2004;39(4):1147–71.
29. Recommendations for prevention and control of hepatitis C virus (HCV) infection and HCV-related chronic disease. Centers for Disease Control and Prevention. MMWR Recomm Rep 1998;47(RR-19):1–39.
30. Fried MW, Shiffman ML, Reddy KR, et al. Peginterferon alfa-2a plus ribavirin for chronic hepatitis C virus infection. N Engl J Med 2002;347(13):975–82.
31. Poordad F, McCone J Jr, Bacon BR, et al. Boceprevir for untreated chronic HCV genotype 1 infection. N Engl J Med 2011;364(13):1195–206.
32. Bacon BR, Gordon SC, Lawitz E, et al. Boceprevir for previously treated chronic HCV genotype 1 infection. N Engl J Med 2011;364(13):1207–17.
33. Jacobson IM, McHutchison JG, Dusheiko G, et al. Telaprevir for previously untreated chronic hepatitis C virus infection. N Engl J Med 2011;364(25):2405–16.
34. Zeuzem S, Andreone P, Pol S, et al. Telaprevir for retreatment of HCV infection. N Engl J Med 2011;364(25):2417–28.

35. Lawitz E, Mangia A, Wyles D, et al. Sofosbuvir for previously untreated chronic hepatitis C infection. N Engl J Med 2013;368(20):1878–87.
36. Zeuzem S, Dusheiko GM, Salupere R, et al. Sofosbuvir and ribavirin in HCV genotypes 2 and 3. N Engl J Med 2014;370(21):1993–2001.
37. Kumada H, Hayashi N, Izumi N, et al. Simeprevir (TMC435) once daily with peginterferon-alpha-2b and ribavirin in patients with genotype 1 hepatitis C virus infection: The CONCERTO-4 study. Hepatol Res 2014.
38. Lawitz E, Sulkowski MS, Ghalib R, et al. Simeprevir plus sofosbuvir, with or without ribavirin, to treat chronic infection with hepatitis C virus genotype 1 in non-responders to pegylated interferon and ribavirin and treatment-naive patients: the COSMOS randomised study. Lancet 2014;384(9956):1756–65.
39. Jacobson IM, Dore GJ, Foster GR, et al. Simeprevir with pegylated interferon alfa 2a plus ribavirin in treatment-naive patients with chronic hepatitis C virus genotype 1 infection (QUEST-1): a phase 3, randomised, double-blind, placebo-controlled trial. Lancet 2014;384(9941):403–13.
40. Manns M, Marcellin P, Poordad F, et al. Simeprevir with pegylated interferon alfa 2a or 2b plus ribavirin in treatment-naive patients with chronic hepatitis C virus genotype 1 infection (QUEST-2): a randomised, double-blind, placebo-controlled phase 3 trial. Lancet 2014;384(9941):414–26.
41. Afdhal N, Zeuzem S, Kwo P, et al. Ledipasvir and sofosbuvir for untreated HCV genotype 1 infection. N Engl J Med 2014;370(20):1889–98.
42. Afdhal N, Reddy KR, Nelson DR, et al. Ledipasvir and sofosbuvir for previously treated HCV genotype 1 infection. N Engl J Med 2014;370(16):1483–93.
43. PEGASYS (peginterferon alfa-2a) [package insert]. Genentech USA, Inc; 2013. Available at: http://www.gene.com/download/pdf/pegasys_prescribing.pdf.
44. COPEGUS (ribavirin) [package insert]. Genentech USA, Inc; 2013. Available at: http://www.gene.com/download/pdf/copegus_prescribing.pdf.
45. INCIVEK (telaprevir) [package insert]. Vertex Pharmaceuticals Incorporated; 2013. Available at: http://pi.vrtx.com/files/uspi_telaprevir.pdf.
46. VICTRELIS (boceprevir) [package insert]. Merck Sharp & Dohme Corp; 2013. Available at: http://www.merck.com/product/usa/pi_circulars/v/victrelis/victrelis_pi.pdf.
47. SOVALDI (sofosbuvir) [package insert]. Gilead Sciences, Inc; 2013. Available at: https://www.gilead.com/~/media/Files/pdfs/medicines/liver-disease/sovaldi/sovaldi_pi.pdf.
48. OLYSIO (simeprevir) [package insert]. Janssen Products, LP; 2013. Available at: https://www.olysio.com/shared/product/olysio/prescribing-information.pdf.
49. HARVONI (ledipasvir/sofosbuvir) [package insert]. Gilead Sciences, Inc; 2014. Available at: http://www.gilead.com/~/media/Files/pdfs/medicines/liver-disease/harvoni/harvoni_pi.pdf.
50. Ramoz LL, Patel-Shori NM. Recent changes in pregnancy and lactation labeling: retirement of risk categories. Pharmacotherapy 2014;34(4):389–95.

Osteoporosis

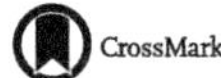

Screening, Prevention, and Management

Anna L. Golob, MD[a,*], Mary B. Laya, MD, MPH[b]

KEYWORDS

• Osteoporosis • Osteopenia • Fragility fractures • Prevention • Screening • Management

KEY POINTS

- Osteoporosis is underdiagnosed and undertreated despite evidence-based recommendations for screening and the availability of efficacious treatments.
- Bone mineral density (BMD) testing should be offered to all women age 65 and older and many younger postmenopausal women with elevated risk.
- The BMD rescreening interval for healthy nonosteoporotic women should take into account the baseline T-score.
- Clinically silent vertebral fractures found incidentally on imaging should prompt evaluation and treatment of osteoporosis.
- Patients with established osteoporosis or a 10-year risk of any major fracture of 20% or hip fracture of 3% should be treated with an osteoporosis-specific medication, lifestyle measures, and adequate calcium and vitamin D intake.

INTRODUCTION

Osteoporosis, a skeletal disorder of low bone density and disrupted bone architecture leading to fractures, is a common and costly condition among postmenopausal women. Nearly one-half of Caucasian women aged 50 years and older will experience an osteoporosis-related fracture in their lifetime.[1] In 2011, there were approximately 2 million osteoporotic fractures affecting US adults.[2] Current estimates suggest that 9.9 million Americans are affected by osteoporosis, and the prevalence is expected to increase as the population ages.[3]

Largely a silent disease before fracture, osteoporosis often goes undetected until a sentinel fracture event. The most common fracture sites are vertebrae (spine),

[a] Division of General Internal Medicine, Department of Medicine, VA Puget Sound Health Care System, University of Washington, 1660 South Columbian Way, Seattle, WA 98108, USA; [b] Division of General Internal Medicine, Department of Medicine, General Internal Medicine Center, UW Medical Centre, University of Washington, 4245 Roosevelt Way Northeast, Box 354765, Seattle, WA 98105, USA
* Corresponding author.
E-mail address: Anna.Golob@va.gov

Med Clin N Am 99 (2015) 587–606
http://dx.doi.org/10.1016/j.mcna.2015.01.010
0025-7125/15/$ – see front matter Published by Elsevier Inc.

proximal femur (hip), and distal forearm (wrist). Osteoporotic fractures often cause pain, deformity, and decreased mobility and can have a significant impact on a patient's quality of life. These fractures frequently result in a short- or long-term need for a higher level of care. In fact, about 20% of patients who suffer hip fractures require a long-term skilled nursing facility stay, and 60% of patients never regain their prefracture level of functional independence.[1] Osteoporotic fractures are also associated with an increased risk of mortality. A 2009 systematic review found an 8% to 36% excess mortality in adults the first year after hip fracture as compared with similar adults who did not have hip fracture.[4]

The economic toll of osteoporotic fractures is significant. In 2005, it was estimated that direct care expenditures for these fractures, including medical office visits, hospital admissions, and nursing home admissions, was $19 billion annually.[5] Given the aging population, this cost has been projected to rise to $25.3 billion by 2025.[5]

Despite evidence-based guidelines for screening and the availability of effective treatment, osteoporosis remains underdiagnosed and undertreated, especially in nonwhite women.[6] Given the high prevalence, morbidity, and excess mortality of osteoporotic fractures, which primarily affect postmenopausal women, we advise clinicians to counsel all women on preventative measures, regularly assess female patients for excess risk, screen when appropriate, and treat osteoporosis when it is diagnosed.

DEFINITIONS

Table 1 provides a lexicon of common terminology used in discussing osteoporosis.

PATHOPHYSIOLOGY

Bone is a dynamic, constantly remodeling tissue composed of specialized bone cells (osteoblasts, osteoclasts, and osteocytes) and a mineralized collagen matrix. Osteoblasts build new bone by secreting collagen fibers upon which calcium and phosphate crystallize. Osteoclasts break down bone tissue by secreting acid and enzymes to resorb the mineralized collagen fibers. Osteocytes secrete growth factors that

Table 1
Definitions of common terms

Term	Definition
Fragility fracture	A fracture occurring in the absence of major trauma, such as a fall from standing height, coughing, or sneezing. Usually involves the spine, ribs, hip, pelvis, wrist, or humerus
T-score	The number of standard deviations a patient's BMD is above or below the mean BMD of a young adult reference population
Z-score	The number of standard deviations a patient's BMD is above or below the mean BMD of an age-matched adult reference population
Osteoporosis	Low bone mass, microarchitectural deterioration of bone tissue and decreased bone strength associated with increased fracture risk. Diagnosed as BMD T-score on DXA at the hip or lumbar spine that is less than or equal to −2.5 *or* the presence of a fragility fracture regardless of BMD.
Osteopenia	BMD T-score on DXA at the hip or lumbar spine that is between −1.0 and −2.5.

Abbreviations: BMD, bone mineral density; DXA, dual-energy x-ray absorptiometry.

regulate osteoblast and osteoclast activity and hence bone formation. Multiple hormones, cytokines, growth factors, and other molecules act to influence the activity of osteoblasts and osteoclasts, including parathyroid hormone, calcitonin, calcitriol, human growth hormone, insulin-like growth factor I, glucocorticoids, thyroid hormones, and sex hormones.

Bone balance is determined by the relative activity of osteoblasts and osteoclasts. Most women achieve peak bone density by 18 to 25 years of age.[7] After peak bone density is achieved, bone continues to be remodeled throughout a person's lifetime to respond to new stresses and replace older, weakened bone. Age-related bone density loss begins shortly after peak bone density is attained owing to an imbalance of bone formation and bone resorption in the remodeling process. After menopause, the rate of bone remodeling increases, which accelerates bone loss owing to this inherent imbalance. Osteoporosis and other conditions of low bone density arise owing to an excess activity of osteoclasts that compounds age-related bone density loss (**Fig. 1**).

RISK FACTORS

Advancing age, female gender, and estrogen deficiency are widely recognized risk factors for osteoporosis; however, there are many other exposures that increase risk for bone density loss. These factors include behavioral factors, such as excess alcohol use, smoking, inadequate physical activity level, and inadequate calcium and vitamin D intake, as well as demographic factors such as white or Asian race, low body weight, and tall stature (**Table 2**). Several medical disorders can cause secondary osteoporosis, including hypogonadal conditions, rheumatoid arthritis, hyperparathyroidism, and many others (**Box 1**). Low bone density is also a recognized adverse effect of several classes of medications (**Box 2**). Glucocorticoids in particular are associated with a significant risk of bone loss and increased fracture risk. In fact, decreased bone density occurs with daily doses as low as 2.5 to 7.5 mg of prednisone or equivalent and is most rapid during the first few months of use.[8]

It is important to consider each woman's level of exposure to these risk factors when deciding when to initiate screening for osteoporosis (see section on screening).

In addition, because nearly all osteoporotic hip fractures and many vertebral compression fractures occur in the setting of falls, it is also important to consider a patient's risk factors for falls. These factors include environmental factors such as trip

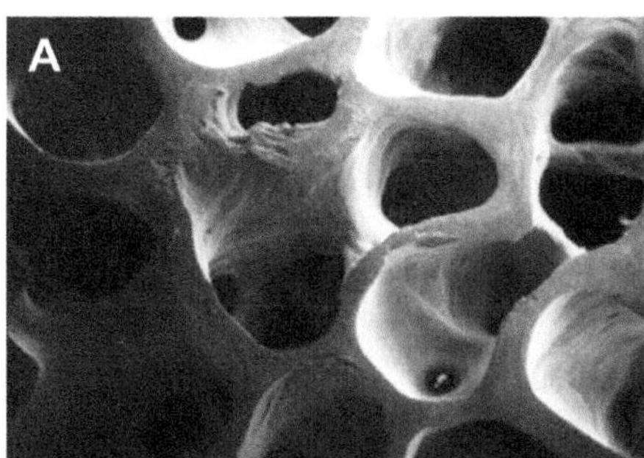

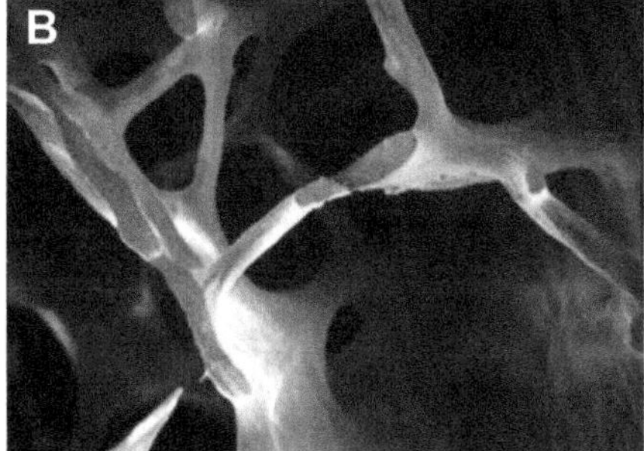

Fig. 1. Micrographs of normal and osteoporotic bone. (*A*) Normal bone. (*B*) Osteoporotic bone. (*From* Dempster DW, Shane E, Horbert W, et al. A simple method for correlative light and scanning electron microscopy of human iliac crest bone biopsies: qualitative observations in normal and osteoporotic subjects. J Bone Miner Res 1986;1(1):15–21; with permission.)

Table 2
Primary risk factors for osteoporosis

Demographic Factors	Behavioral Factors
Advancing age	Current smoking
Female gender	Excess alcohol use (>2 standard drinks per day)
White or Asian race	Inadequate weight bearing exercise
Low body weight (<127 lbs)	Inadequate calcium intake
Taller height	Inadequate vitamin D intake
Family history	

hazards in the home, patient neuromuscular factors such as impaired balance, reduced proprioception and deconditioning, and medical conditions such as orthostatic hypotension and vitamin D insufficiency (**Table 3**).

SCREENING

All women aged 65 and older should be screened for osteoporosis with bone mineral density (BMD) testing with dual-energy x-ray absorptiometry (DXA). This recommendation is universally endorsed by major society guidelines based on evidence of cost effectiveness in this age group (**Table 4**).[9,10]

Box 1
Secondary causes of osteoporosis

Hypogonadal conditions, including:

- Premature menopause
- Exercise oligomenorrhea
- Eating disorders

Hyperparathyroidism

Hyperthyroidism

Type 1 diabetes

Rheumatoid arthritis and other connective tissue diseases

Malabsorption syndromes, including:

- Celiac disease
- Bariatric surgery
- Pancreatic disorders

Chronic liver disease

Chronic kidney disease

Chronic obstructive pulmonary disease

Hematologic disorders, including:

- Multiple myeloma
- Hemoglobinopathies
- Hematologic malignancies

Box 2
Medications that cause or contribute to osteoporosis

Aluminum (in antacids)

Anticoagulants (heparin)

Anticonvulsants

Aromatase inhibitors

Barbiturates

Chemotherapy drugs

Cyclosporine

Depo-medroxyprogesterone

Glucocorticoids

Gonadotropin-releasing hormone agonists

Lithium

Methotrexate

Parenteral nutrition

Proton pump inhibitors

Selective serotonin reuptake inhibitors

Tacrolimus

Tamoxifen (premenopausal use)

Thiazolidinediones

Thyroid hormone (in excess)

Adapted from National Osteoporosis Foundation. Clinician's guide to prevention and treatment of osteoporosis. Washington, DC: National Osteoporosis Foundation; 2014. p. 12.

Table 3
Fall risk factors

Environmental Factors	Neuromuscular Factors	Medical Factors
Loose throw rugs	Poor balance/gait instability	Advanced age
Low level lighting	Low or impaired vision	Cardiovascular diseases including arrhythmia, congestive heart failure
Slippery surfaces	Reduced proprioception	Dehydration/orthostatic hypotension/vascular insufficiency
Obstacles on the floor	Impaired ability to transfer and mobilize	Vitamin D insufficiency (serum 25-OH-vitamin D <30 ng/mL)
Loose throw rugs	General deconditioning	Medications causing sedation
Lack of use of assistive devices	Neuromuscular, neurodegenerative, and joint diseases such as cerebrovascular accident, Parkinson's, arthritis	Dementia/cognitive impairment Urge urinary incontinence/overactive bladder

Adapted from National Osteoporosis Foundation. Clinician's guide to prevention and treatment of osteoporosis. Washington, DC: National Osteoporosis Foundation; 2014. p. 12.

Table 4
Major guideline recommendations for osteoporosis screening

National Osteoporosis Foundation (NOF) 2014	United States Preventive Services Task Force (USPSTF) 2011
All women aged ≥65	All women aged ≥65 (Grade B)
Younger postmenopausal women with clinical risk factors for fracture	Women aged <65 y whose 10-y fracture risk is equal to or greater than that of a 65 y old white woman without additional risk factors[a] (Grade B)
Women who have a fracture after age 50	—
Women with conditions that can cause secondary osteoporosis	—

[a] Per the FRAX fracture risk assessment tool, the 10-year fracture risk in a 65-year-old white woman without additional risk factors is 9.3%.

For women aged 50 to 64, there is no universal consensus regarding when to begin BMD screening. The United States Preventative Services Task Force 2011 osteoporosis screening guideline recommends that clinicians utilize a "validated prediction tool" to identify higher risk asymptomatic younger women (aged 50–64).[11] Specifically, they advise screening younger women whose 10-year risk of any major osteoporotic fracture is equivalent to that of a 65-year-old white woman without additional risk factors, that is, 9.3% or higher.[11]

Several risk factor-based assessment tools have been validated to help identify asymptomatic younger women who are at greater risk to have osteoporosis and who would therefore benefit most from screening while avoiding unnecessary testing.[12] One frequently utilized risk assessment calculator is the web-based World Health Organization "Fracture Risk Assessment Tool" (FRAX). Originally developed as a treatment decision tool, the FRAX tool uses clinical risk factors with or without femoral neck BMD to estimate 10-year probability of hip and major osteoporotic fractures (hip, clinical vertebral, humerus, or wrist).

Clinicians may also use other validated risk assessment tools such as the Osteoporosis Self-assessment Tool.[13] The Osteoporosis Self-assessment Tool uses a mathematical formula, (weight in kg − age)/5, to generate a risk score: the lower the score, the higher the risk for osteoporosis. A score of less than 2 was 88% to 95% sensitive and 37% to 52% specific for identifying osteoporosis (T score ≤−2.5) among postmenopausal women.[14] Some authors have found that older tools such as the Osteoporosis Self-assessment Tool are more sensitive than FRAX in identifying younger women with osteoporosis.[14] They suggest that clinicians consider using a lower cutoff point of 10-year major osteoporotic fracture risk greater than 4.1% to improve the sensitivity of the FRAX tool. Of note, none of these screening strategies for women less than 65 years of age have been prospectively evaluated for cost effectiveness.

Given that BMD decreases with advancing age among all women, it is advisable to consider rescreening women who did not meet criteria for osteoporosis on initial evaluation. There are no consensus guidelines regarding the most appropriate interval for rescreening. However, some experts advise rescreening individuals based on the severity of bone density loss on baseline DXA and demonstrated rates of bone density loss from large population-based observational studies.[15,16] **Table 5** provides suggested rescreening intervals using this approach. Clinicians may consider shortening the interval between screenings for woman with a low body mass index or who begin taking agents that increase resorption (eg, corticosteroids, aromatase inhibitors).

Table 5
Bone mineral density rescreening intervals in postmenopausal women

Category	T Score Range	Rescreening Interval (y)
Normal or mild osteopenia	>−1.5	7–15
Moderate osteopenia	−1.50 to −1.99	5
Advanced osteopenia	−2.00 to −2.49	1

CLINICAL SYNDROMES OF COMMON OSTEOPOROTIC FRACTURES

Hip Fractures

Osteoporotic hip fracture should be suspected in women aged older than 50 who present with new groin pain or pain with hip motion or weight-bearing after a fall from ground level height or greater.[2] In some cases, the affected leg may be shortened or rotated, depending on the fracture characteristics and degree of displacement. When hip fracture is considered, it is important to obtain plain radiographs of the affected hip including an anterioposterior image of the hip with maximal internal rotation, a lateral hip image, and an anterioposterior pelvis image to compare the unaffected side. Of note, hip fractures are radiographically occult in 3% to 6% of cases. Therefore, if the initial radiographs are normal but there is still a high clinical suspicion of fracture, further imaging such as a bone scan, CT, or MRI should be obtained.[17]

Initial care for a patient diagnosed with a hip fracture includes pain management and orthopedic surgery referral. Most hip fractures are treated surgically unless the patient is severely debilitated. Complications from hip fractures include pain, decreased mobility, leg length discrepancy, deep venous thrombosis, requirement for increased level of care, and increased risk of mortality (**Fig. 2**).

Vertebral Compression Fractures

Vertebral compression fractures are often asymptomatic and found incidentally on spine imaging obtained for other reasons.[18] These “morphometric” fractures are as important as symptomatic fractures in predicting future risk of fracture, found to be 19.3% in the first year after fracture.[19] When symptomatic, vertebral compression fractures usually present with acute onset back pain after a low mechanism insult, such as a ground level fall or lifting a heavy object, or, in the setting of severe osteoporosis, a very low mechanism insult such as sneezing, coughing, or even turning in

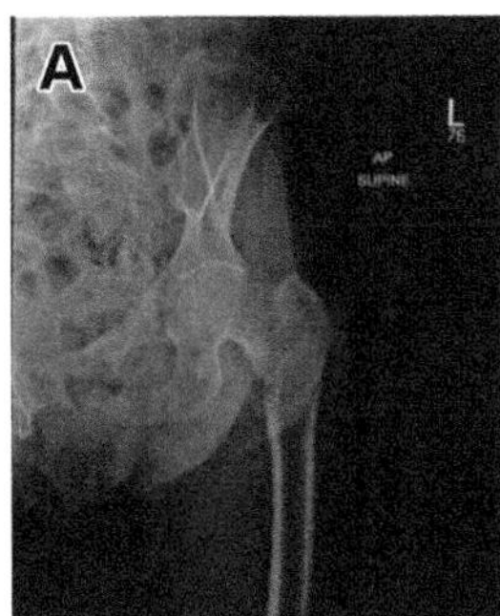

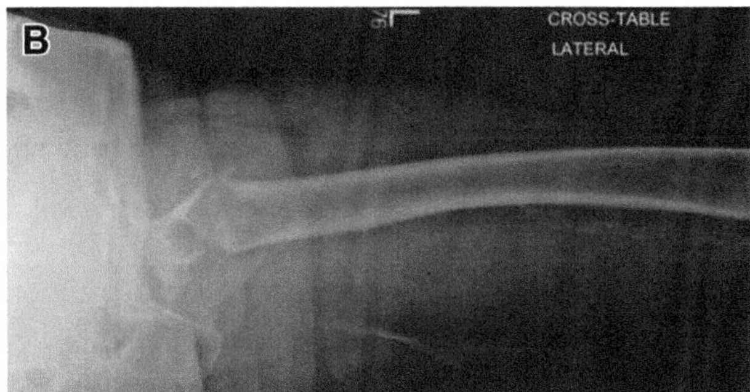

Fig. 2. Radiograph of hip fracture. Anteroposterior (*A*) and lateral (*B*) radiographs of the left hip, showing a hip fracture in a 94-year-old woman with a history of osteoporosis. (*From* Varacallo MA, Fox EJ. Osteoporosis and its complications. Med Clin North Am 2014;98(4):817–31; with permission.)

bed. The back pain typically increases with postural changes, may radiate around the truck as a "girdle of pain," and improves with lying flat on the back. There is often acute tenderness to palpation at the affected vertebrae.[20] Compression fractures usually do not cause neurologic deficits because they most often involve the anterior half of the vertebral body.[20] However, occasionally the fracture involves the entire vertebral body and may cause retropulsion of bone fragments into the vertebral canal, resulting in radicular pain and neurologic deficits.

Radiographs (and advanced imaging as needed) should always be obtained in patients older than age 50 with back pain after trauma, when accompanied by neurologic deficits, or when pain persists for longer than 4 to 6 weeks. Clinicians should also consider obtaining plain spine radiographs in all women older than 50 with new back pain even in the absence of trauma or neurologic symptoms to evaluate for compression fracture. In patients under the age of 50 who sustain a vertebral compression fracture in the absence of trauma, or in patients older than 50 with unusual fracture appearance or a history of malignancy, metastatic disease (pathologic compression fracture) should also be considered.

The treatment of vertebral compression fractures is usually nonsurgical, and includes pain management, external orthoses for stabilization, and physical therapy. Surgical management is indicated in patients with neurologic compromise, severe spine deformity, or intractable pain failing conservative therapy.[20] Complications of vertebral compression fractures include chronic back pain, spine deformity owing to progressive loss of vertebral body height leading to excessive thoracic kyphosis and lumbar lordosis, and respiratory compromise owing to alterations in thoracic cavity pressure (**Fig. 3**, **Table 6**).

DIAGNOSTIC EVALUATION

Osteoporosis is diagnosed in the presence of any of the following conditions provided other bone conditions that mimic osteoporosis (eg, osteomalacia) have been excluded:

- Screening DXA study T-score of −2.5 or less.
- Clinical fragility fracture regardless of bone density.
- Incidentally found (asymptomatic) vertebral compression fracture.

All patients should undergo a diagnostic workup to[21]:

- Evaluate the causes and contributory factors leading to low bone density;
- Exclude diseases that mimic osteoporosis;
- Assess the risk of subsequent fractures; and
- Select the most appropriate treatment.

This evaluation should include a focused history and physical examination, laboratory tests, and imaging.

History

A focused history should be obtained to determine possible exposures to the risk factors in **Boxes 1** and **2** and **Table 2**, and should include:

- Lifestyle factors such as dietary/supplemental calcium and vitamin D intake, smoking, alcohol use, activity level, fall history;
- Personal and family history of fractures;
- Comorbid medical conditions that cause secondary osteoporosis (from **Box 1**, eg, rheumatoid arthritis, hypogonadism from any cause, hyperthyroidism); and

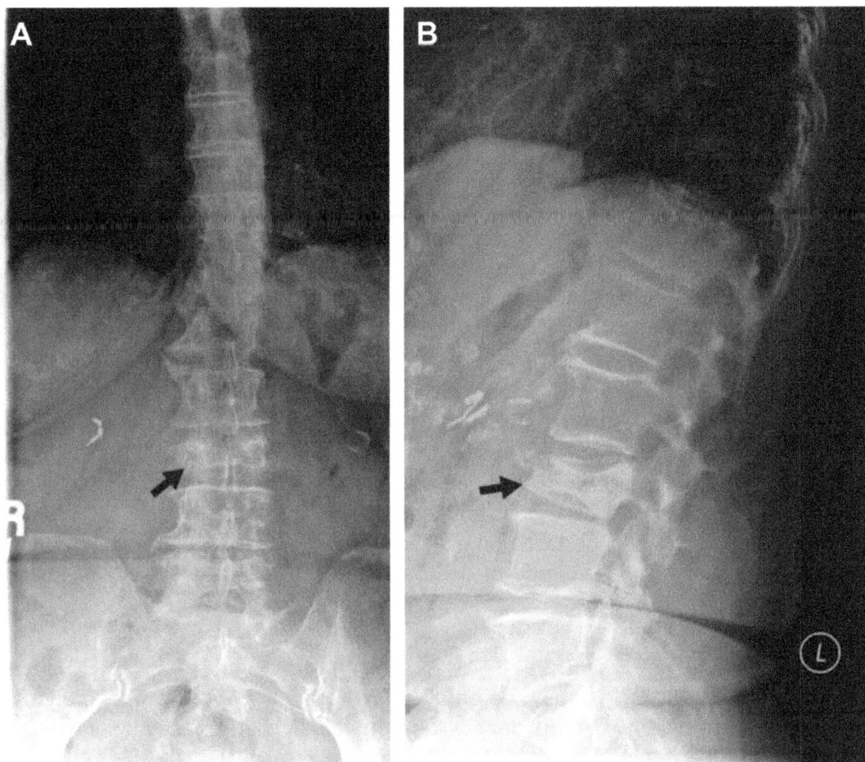

Fig. 3. Radiograph of vertebral compression fracture. Anteroposterior (*A*) and lateral (*B*) radiographs of the lumbar spine showing an L3 vertebral compression fracture in an 86-year-old woman with a history of osteoporosis. Arrows are pointing to the fractured L3 vertebral body. (*From* Varacallo MA, Fox EJ. Osteoporosis and its complications. Med Clin North Am 2014;98(4):817–31; with permission.)

Table 6
Common symptoms and complications of hip and vertebral compression fractures

	Symptoms	Complications
Hip fracture	Groin pain after fall Leg length discrepancy after fall Abnormal hip rotation after fall Inability to bear weight after fall	Chronic groin/hip pain Leg length discrepancy Decreased mobility Deep venous thrombosis Increased level of care requirement Increased risk of mortality
Vertebral compression fracture	None (often asymptomatic) Acute localized back pain after fall/lifting/forceful sneeze or cough (low mechanism insult) Tenderness to palpation of the affected level Decreased spinal mobility Acute back pain with radiculopathy after low mechanism insult (rare) Neurologic deficits such as numbness/weakness after low mechanism insult (rare)	Chronic back pain Spine deformity including thoracic kyphosis and lumbar lordosis Decreased respiratory capacity Deep venous thrombosis

- Medication use (past and present), particularly corticosteroids, antiepileptics, chemotherapy, and hormonal medications, as well as others listed in **Box 2**.

Physical Examination

The focused physical examination should evaluate for[22]:

- Physical manifestations of osteoporotic complications (eg, thoracic kyphosis, height loss);
- Signs of comorbid medical conditions that cause secondary osteoporosis; and
- Fall risk assessment (gait stability, muscle strength and balance).

Laboratory Testing

Certain tests should be obtained in all patients with osteoporosis to evaluate for common causes of secondary bone density loss. Others tests should be ordered only in select patients based on the clinical scenario (eg, patients whose BMD is more than 2 standard deviations below the age-matched mean or Z score <−2.0) and perceived likelihood of abnormal findings, for example, those in whom a specific secondary cause of osteoporosis is suspected. **Table 7** lists the advised tests.

Imaging

- BMD testing with DXA should be obtained in all patients at the time of diagnosis to determine severity of bone density loss and to establish a baseline for which to compare the effects of treatment.
- Consider radiographs (or advanced imaging such as CT bone scan, MRI, etc) if any concern for undiagnosed or subtle hip or vertebral compression fractures (eg, unexplained chronic back pain, height loss of >2 inches from maximum adult height, etc).

MANAGEMENT

Once the diagnosis of osteoporosis has been made and a workup for underlying causes initiated, we advise specific osteoporosis treatment with the goal to prevent future fractures. Unfortunately, studies indicate that many patients diagnosed with osteoporosis are undertreated despite the presence of a fragility fracture or abnormal DXA result.[23–25] Some barriers to initiating treatment include lack of knowledge and awareness by both patient and provider, perception by the provider (eg, orthopedic surgeon, primary care provider, emergency room provider) that osteoporosis diagnosis and treatment is not their responsibility, low rates of referral to osteoporosis clinics or specialists, costs of therapy, side effects of therapy, and multiple medical comorbidities.[23,24]

However, it is well-established that patients who suffer an osteoporotic fracture are at increased risk (between 2- and 5-fold depending, on the site of initial fracture) to suffer subsequent fractures.[20,26] At the same time, effective treatments as outlined herein are available to decrease this risk.[23] Thus, prompt evaluation and treatment of osteoporosis is indicated to prevent further fracture-related morbidity and mortality. **Box 3** provides indications for prescribing osteoporotic-specific medications. Treatment for osteoporosis includes both pharmacologic agents (**Table 8**) and nonpharmacologic therapies including behavioral modifications as outlined.

Table 7
Laboratory evaluation for diagnostic workup of osteoporosis in women

	Test Name	Evaluates for
Essential tests	Complete blood count	Hematologic cancer, anemia
	Serum calcium	Hyperparathyroidism or other disorder of calcium homeostasis
	Serum phosphate	Osteomalacia or other disorder of phosphate homeostasis
	Serum creatinine	Kidney disease (may cause secondary hyperparathyroidism)
	Serum thyroid stimulating hormone	Thyroid disorders
	Serum liver transaminases	Chronic liver disease
	Serum alkaline phosphatase	If high: chronic liver disease or Paget's disease of bone If low: hypophosphatemia
	Serum 25-OH vitamin D	Vitamin D insufficiency
Optional tests according to clinical scenario	Serum parathyroid hormone (in patients with elevated serum calcium)	Hyperparathyroidism
	24-h urinary calcium	If low (<50–100 mg/24 h): calcium malabsorption If high (>250 mg/24 h in women): excessive calcium absorption or renal calcium leak
	Serum and urine protein electrophoresis, kappa and lambda light chains	Multiple myeloma
	Serum celiac antibodies when malabsorption is suspected	Celiac disease (small bowel biopsy required to confirm diagnosis)
	24-h urinary free cortisol or dexamethasone suppression test when hypercortisolism is suspected	Cushing syndrome
	Serum tryptase	Systemic mastocytosis
	Serum rheumatoid factor and anti-citrullinated peptide antibodies	Rheumatoid arthritis

Adapted from Lewiecki EM. In the clinic: osteoporosis. Ann Intern Med 2011;155(1):ITC1-1–15.

Box 3
Indications to prescribe osteoporotic specific medications

Osteoporotic fracture of the vertebra (symptomatic or asymptomatic) or hip

T score of ≤−2.5 at the femoral neck, total hip, or lumbar spine on DXA

T score between −1.0 and −2.5 and United States adapted WHO (FRAX) 10-year hip fracture risk ≥3% or 10-year major osteoporotic fracture risk ≥20% (primary prevention)

Abbreviations: DXA, dual energy x-ray absorptiometry; FRAX, Fracture Risk Assessment Tool; WHO, World Health Organization.

Adapted from National Osteoporosis Foundation. Clinician's guide to prevention and treatment of osteoporosis. Washington, DC: National Osteoporosis Foundation; 2014; and Watts NB, Bilezikian JP, Camacho PM, et al. American Association of Clinical Endocrinologists medical guidelines for clinical practice for the diagnosis and treatment of postmenopausal osteoporosis: executive summary of recommendations. Endocr Pract 2010;16:1016–19.

Table 8
Pharmacologic treatments for osteoporosis

Drug Category	Drug Names/Dose	Mechanism of Action	Benefits	Side Effects	Notes
Bisphosphonates	Alendronate 10 mg PO daily or 70 mg PO weekly Ibandronate 150 mg PO monthly or 3 mg IV every 3 mo Risedronate 5 mg PO daily, 35 mg PO weekly, 150 mg PO monthly Zoledronic acid 5 mg IV yearly	Decrease bone resorption by attenuating osteoclast activity	All bisphosphonates have been shown to increase bone density and decrease both vertebral and nonvertebral fractures by 25%–70% except for ibandronate, which only has evidence for vertebral fracture risk reduction[27–29]	Esophageal irritation Osteonecrosis of the jaw (very rare when used for long-term osteoporosis treatment[30] Low trauma atypical femur fractures (very rare, associated with long term use >5 y[31])	Oral bisphosphonates should be taken on an empty stomach with lots of water Patients should remain upright for 30–60 min after ingestion; Do not use if creatinine clearance is ≤35 mL/min
Parathyroid hormone antagonist	Calcitonin 200 U (1 spray) intranasal daily	Decrease bone resorption by attenuating osteoclast activity	Slight increase in bone density Decrease risk of vertebral fractures only (30% risk reduction)[32]	Rhinitis, irritation of nasal mucosa Possible increased risk of malignancies[33]	Not considered a first-line agent for fracture risk reduction May help to decrease pain in acute or subacute vertebral compression fracture
Estrogen	Conjugated estrogens (+progesterone if intact uterus); dosing varies	Suppressive effects on osteoclasts; decreases bone resorption	Increase bone mass Decrease risk of vertebral and nonvertebral osteoporotic fractures by 23%–34%[34]	Deep venous thrombosis and pulmonary embolism Cardiovascular disease (in women >10 y postmenopause) Stroke Invasive breast cancer (only seen in combined estrogen/progesterone group)	Not first line for treatment of osteoporosis owing to risks

Estrogen agonist/ antagonists (formerly called "SERMs")	Raloxifene 60 mg PO daily	Acts as estrogen agonist on bone tissue thus suppressive effects on osteoclasts Acts as estrogen antagonist in uterine and breast tissue	Increases bone mass Decreases vertebral compression fractures by 30%–55%[35] Reduces risk for invasive breast cancer	Deep venous thrombosis and pulmonary embolism Hot flashes Leg cramps	Consider in women with a history of breast cancer who have osteoporosis Does not reduce risk for nonvertebral fractures
Parathyroid hormone (1–34)	Teriparatide 20 μg daily SQ injection	Stimulates bone formation	Increases bone mass Decreases vertebral (65%) and nonvertebral fracture risk (53%)[36]	Leg cramps Nausea Dizziness Possible increased risk of osteosarcoma	Avoid in patients with an increased risk of osteosarcoma (history of Paget's disease; bony radiation; skeletal metastases, etc) Lifetime duration of use should not exceed 18–24 mo When stopped, should be replaced by other antiresorptive osteoporosis treatment, such as bisphosphonate
RANK ligand inhibitor	Denosumab 60 mg SQ every 6 mo (administered by health care professional)	Decreases bone resorption by attenuating osteoclast formation, activity, and survival	Increases bone mass Decreases risk of vertebral fractures by 68%, hip fractures by 40% and other nonvertebral fractures by 20%[37]	Hypocalcemia Increased risk of cellulitis Osteonecrosis of the jaw (very rare) Atypical femur fractures (very rare)	No restrictions in dosing according to renal function

Abbreviations: PO, per os; SQ, subcutaneously.

Pharmacologic Treatment

Osteoporotic-specific medications

When choosing which osteoporosis medication to utilize, it is important to consider:

- Demonstrated benefit (eg, does the medication reduce all fracture types or only vertebral fractures)
- Ease of administration
- Side effect profile
- Cost
- Patient-specific indications
  - Personal or family history of breast cancer may make raloxifene a more favorable agent
- Contraindications
  - Advanced chronic kidney disease precludes bisphosphonates
  - History of bone cancer or bone radiation precludes teriperatide

We advise clinicians to involve patients actively and use a shared decision making approach to help guide medication choice. Regarding duration of treatment, in general osteoporosis-specific medications seem to have decreased efficacy and increased concern for adverse effects (eg, insufficiency fractures with long-term use of bisphosphonates) when used longer than 5 years. Therefore, the recommended approach is that these medications should be used for an initial treatment period of 5 years (except teriparatide, which should be used for 2 years or less), at which time the patient should be reevaluated with history, physical examination, and repeat BMD testing.

If the patient seems to be at relatively low risk for recurrent fractures (stable or improved bone density, no interval fractures, no new high-risk exposures such as glucocorticoids), then it is reasonable to stop therapy and monitor closely. Of note, the reduction in fracture risk associated with bisphosphonate use does extend for several years after therapy is stopped; this is not the case for all other osteoporosis medications, whose benefits end when therapy is stopped. If instead the patient seems to be at high risk for recurrent fractures (history of fractures while on therapy, decreased interval bone density, new high-risk exposure), then it is advisable to consider extending the duration of bisphosphonate use or switch to another agent.[38] Primary care clinicians may also consider consultation with an osteoporosis treatment expert regarding treatment duration.

Calcium and vitamin D

In addition to disease-specific medications, clinical guidelines recommend that patients with osteoporosis receive adequate calcium and vitamin D.[22,39–41] There has been some recent debate in the medical literature about possible adverse effects of supplemental calcium, including kidney stones and cardiovascular disease.[42,43] However, current consensus is that, for patients with established osteoporosis who are at the highest risk for future fracture events, the benefits of adequate calcium intake outweigh the possible risks. Current clinical guidelines from the National Osteoporosis Foundation and Institute of Medicine recommend that women age 51 and older, especially those with osteoporosis, take in 1200 mg of calcium each day.[39,41] Ideally, this should be achieved through diet, which seems to carry less risk of cardiovascular events,[43,44] but supplements should be used if dietary intake is inadequate.

For vitamin D intake, the Institute of Medicine recommends that women aged 70 years and younger take in 600 IU daily and those 71 and older take in 800 IU daily.[41] The National Osteoporosis Foundation recommends a higher dose, 800 to 1000 IU of vitamin D daily for all adults aged 50 and older.[39] They also advise checking a serum 25-OH vitamin D level in women at risk for deficiency, such as those with malabsorption, chronic renal insufficiency, other chronic illnesses, taking antiepileptics, housebound, institutionalized, limited sun exposure, or very dark skin. For these patients, the National Osteoporosis Foundation advises a target serum 25-OH vitamin D level of 30 ng/mL or greater whereas the Institute of Medicine recommends a target of greater than 20 ng/mL. Patients with a serum 25-OH Vitamin D level of 20 ng/mL or less will likely require an initial bolus regimen of ergocalciferol (vitamin D_2) 50,000 IU by mouth weekly for 8 to 12 weeks to achieve goal vitamin D level, followed by maintenance dosing of cholecalciferol (vitamin D_3) 800 to 2000 IU daily.[39] Per the Institute of Medicine, the safe upper limit of daily vitamin D intake is 4000 IU. We advise against exceeding serum 25-OH vitamin D concentrations of 50 ng/mL owing to concern for hypercalcemia and other adverse effects.

Nonpharmacologic Treatments

It is important to counsel patients diagnosed with osteoporosis regarding specific lifestyle and behavioral recommendations to decrease their risk of future fractures, including:

- Participation in regular weight-bearing and muscle strengthening exercise, targeting 30 minutes on most days of the week.
- Cessation of tobacco use.
- Decrease alcohol intake if excessive (limit one drink daily for women).
- Fall risk reduction[45,46]:
  - Physical therapy for balance/gait training/strength training;
  - Appropriate use of assistive mobility devices such as canes or walkers;
  - Home and environmental modifications, such as removal of rugs and cords, and improved lighting, use of glasses, and proper footwear.
  - Consider physical therapy and occupational therapy consultations for home safety evaluation.

MONITORING

Patients undergoing treatment for osteoporosis should be evaluated regularly to ensure appropriate calcium and vitamin D intake, adherence to lifestyle modifications, medication adherence and tolerance, and fracture occurrence or new exposures that increase risk for fractures. There is no universal consensus regarding the appropriate frequency to repeat DXA tests. The National Osteoporosis Foundation practice guidelines advise obtaining surveillance bone density tests approximately every 2 years or when the outcome will affect management, including after 3 to 5 years of medication use to guide further medication management decisions.[39] Clinicians may consider other monitoring tools, such as biochemical markers of bone turnover and sequential vertebral imaging, in select patients based on risk profile and consultant recommendations.

PREVENTION

Patients who do not meet diagnostic criteria for osteoporosis, that is, a T-score greater than −2.5, but who are at high risk—for example, presence of osteopenia, chronic use of glucocorticoids, or family history of osteoporosis—should be advised regarding strategies to reduce their risk.

Table 9
Institute of Medicine recommended daily allowance for calcium intake

Population Group	Recommended Daily Allowance (mg)
Children 1–3 y	700
Children 4–8 y	1000
Preteens and teens 9–18 y	1300
Adults 19–50 y	1000
Adults ≥51	1200

Nonpharmacologic Interventions to Prevent Osteoporosis or Osteoporotic Fractures

These interventions parallel the lifestyle and behavioral recommendations advised for patients diagnosed with osteoporosis; please see "Nonpharmacologic treatments" in the Management section.

Calcium and Vitamin D

Most organizations, including the Institute of Medicine, American Association of Clinical Endocrinologists, and the National Osteoporosis Foundation, advise adequate calcium intake across the life spectrum (**Tables 9** and **10**). However, the US Preventative Services Task Force concluded in 2013 that there was insufficient evidence to assess the benefits and harms of calcium and vitamin D supplementation for the primary prevention of fracture in community-dwelling postmenopausal women.[47] This is because the medical literature shows some discrepancy in the effectiveness of calcium and vitamin D supplementation in reducing fracture risk among community-dwelling versus institutionalized individuals for primary prevention.[42,48] Current literature supports the conclusion that the patients who most benefit from higher calcium and vitamin D supplementation for primary prevention are those at highest risk to be deficient, particularly institutionalized adults or others with poor food access or malabsorption.

Another recent area of debate in the medical literature is a possible adverse cardiovascular risk associated with calcium supplementation (not dietary calcium). Thus far, this risk has been demonstrated primarily through secondary analyses of previous trials that did not have cardiovascular disease as a prespecified endpoint.[43] Of note, a large, retrospective analysis of the Nurse's Health Cohort did not show an adverse cardiovascular risk effect with calcium supplement use.[44] Further randomized studies with cardiovascular disease as a pre-specified outcome are needed to evaluate this risk further.

Overall, for primary prevention, we advise that clinicians counsel patients on the importance of adequate calcium and vitamin D for general bone health, emphasizing that calcium intake is safest if achieved through diet, and consider supplementation

Table 10
Institute of Medicine recommended daily allowance for vitamin D intake

Population Group	Daily (IU)
Birth to 11 mo	400
Age 1 to 70	600
Age 70 and over	800
Homebound/institutionalized elderly	800

Box 4
Indications to consider osteoporosis medications for the prevention of osteoporotic fractures

T score between −1.0 and −2.5 and U.S. adapted WHO 10-year hip fracture risk ≥3% or 10-year risk for any major osteoporotic fracture ≥20%

High risk premenopausal and postmenopausal women who are receiving chronic glucocorticoids >5–7.5 mg/d prednisone or equivalent for anticipated duration ≥3 months[a]

Abbreviation: WHO, World Health Organization.

[a] See the 2010 American College of Rheumatology guidelines for a detailed recommendation.[49]

primarily in women who clearly have inadequate dietary intake, malabsorption, or in those who are institutionalized.

Pharmacologic Interventions to Prevent Osteoporosis

The use of osteoporosis-specific medications is recommended to reduce the risk of developing osteoporosis (see **Box 3**) in some high risk women, including those with a 10-year risk of hip fracture of greater than 3% or any major osteoporotic fracture of greater than 20%, or who use glucocorticoids chronically (**Box 4**).[39,49] Bisphosphonates and raloxifene are the most commonly utilized medications for prevention of osteoporosis in high-risk postmenopausal women.

REFERENCES

1. Office of the Surgeon General (US). Bone health and osteoporosis: a report of the surgeon general. Rockville (MD): Office of the Surgeon General (US); 2004.
2. Bukuta SV, Sieber FE, Tyler KW, et al. A guide to improving the care of patients with fragility fractures. Geriatr Orthop Surg Rehabil 2011;2:5–39.
3. Wright NC, Looker A, Saag K, et al. The recent prevalence of osteoporosis and low bone mass based on bone mineral density at the femoral neck or lumbar spine in the United States. J Bone Miner Res 2014;29:2520–6.
4. Abrahamsen B, van Staa T, Ariely R, et al. Excess mortality following hip fracture: a systematic epidemiological review. Osteoporos Int 2009;20(10):1633–50.
5. Burge R, Dawson-Hughes B, Solomon DH, et al. Incidence and economic burden of osteoporosis-related fractures in the United States, 2005–2025. J Bone Miner Res 2007;22(3):465–75.
6. Cunningham TD, Di Pace BS, Ullal J. Osteoporosis treatment disparities: a 6-year aggregate analysis from national survey data. Osteoporos Int 2014;25(9):2199–208.
7. Khosla S, Riggs BL. Pathophysiology of age-related bone loss and osteoporosis. Endocrinol Metab Clin North Am 2005;34:1015–30.
8. Van Staa TP, Leufkens HG, Cooper C. The epidemiology of corticosteroid induced osteoporosis: a meta-analysis. Osteoporos Int 2002;13:777.
9. Tosteson AN, Burge RT, Marshall DA, et al. Therapies for treatment of osteoporosis in US women: cost-effectiveness and budget impact considerations. Am J Manag Care 2008;14(9):605–15.
10. Nelson HD, Haney EM, Dana T, et al. Screening for osteoporosis: an update for the U.S. Preventive Services Task Force. Ann Intern Med 2010;153:99–111.
11. U.S. Preventive Services Task Force. Screening for osteoporosis: U.S. preventative services task force recommendation statement. Ann Intern Med 2011;154:356–64.

12. Rubin KH, Abrahamsen B, Friis-Holmberg T, et al. Comparison of different screening tools (FRAX®, OST, ORAI, OSIRIS, SCORE and age alone) to identify women with increased risk of fracture. A population-based prospective study. Bone 2013;56(1):16–22. Available at: http://www.ncbi.nlm.nih.gov/pubmed/23669650.
13. Richy F, Gourlay M, Ross PD, et al. Validation and comparative evaluation of the osteoporosis self-assessment tool (OST) in a Caucasian population from Belgium. QJM 2004;97(1):39–46.
14. Crandall CJ, Larson J, Gourlay ML, et al. Osteoporosis screening in postmenopausal women 50 to 64 years old: comparison of US preventive services task force strategy and two traditional strategies in the women's health initiative. J Bone Miner Res 2014;29(7):1661–6.
15. Gourlay ML, Fine JP, Preisser JS, et al. Bone density testing interval and transition to osteoporosis in older women. N Engl J Med 2012;366:225–33.
16. Frost SA, Nguyen ND, Center JR, et al. Timing of repeat BMD measurements: development of an absolute risk-based prognostic model. J Bone Miner Res 2009;24:1800–7.
17. Frihagen F, Nordsletten L, Tariq R, et al. MRI diagnosis of occult hip fractures. Acta Orthop 2005;76:524.
18. Picazo DR, Villaescusa JR, Martinez EP, et al. Late collapse osteoporotic vertebral fracture in an elderly patient with neurologic compromise. Eur Spine J 2014;23:2696–702.
19. Lindsay R, Silverman SI, Cooper C, et al. Risk of new vertebral fracture in the year following a fracture. JAMA 2001;285:320–3.
20. Alexandru D, So W. Evaluation and management of vertebral compression fractures. Perm J 2012;16:46–51.
21. Compston J, Bowring C, Cooper C, et al. Diagnosis and management of osteoporosis in postmenopausal women and older men in the UK: National Osteoporosis Guideline Group (NOGG) update 2013. Maturitas 2013;75(4):392–6.
22. Lewiecki EM. In the clinic: osteoporosis. Ann Intern Med 2011;155(1). ITC1-1–ITC1-15.
23. Bogoch ER, Elliot-Gibson V, Beaton DE, et al. Effective initiation of osteoporosis diagnosis and treatment for patients with a fragility fracture in an orthopedic environment. J Bone Joint Surg Am 2006;88:25–34.
24. Marsh D, Akesson K, Beaton DE, et al, IOF CSA Fracture Working Group. Coordinator-based systems for secondary prevention of fragility fracture patients. Osteoporos Int 2011;22:2051–65.
25. Dell R, Green D. Is osteoporosis disease management cost effective? Curr Osteoporos Rep 2010;8:49–55.
26. Colon-Emeric C, Kuchibhatla M, Pieper C, et al. The contribution of hip fracture to risk of subsequent fractures: data from two longitudinal studies. Osteoporos Int 2003;11:879–83.
27. Black DM, Cummings SR, Karpf DB, et al. Randomised trial of effect of alendronate on risk fracture in women with existing vertebral fractures. Fracture Intervention Trial Research Study Group. Lancet 1996;348(9041):1535–41.
28. Cranney A, Wells G, Willan A, et al. Meta-analysis of alendronate for the treatment of post-menopausal women. Endocr Rev 2002;23:508–16.
29. Cranney A, Tugwell P, Adachi J, et al. Meta-analysis of risedronate for the treatment of postmenopausal osteoporosis. Endocr Rev 2002;23:517–23.
30. Khosla S, Burr D, Cauley J, et al, American Society for Bone and Mineral Research. Bisphosphonate associated osteonecrosis of the jaw: report of a

task force of the American Society for Bone and Mineral Research. J Bone Miner Res 2007;22(10):1470–91.
31. Shane E, Burr D, Abrahmsen B, et al, American Society for Bone and Mineral Research. Atypical subtrochanteric and diaphyseal femoral fractures: second report of a task force of the American Society for Bone and Mineral Research. J Bone Miner Res 2014;29(1):1–23.
32. Chesnut CH 3rd, Silverman S, Andriano K, et al. A randomized trial of nasal spray salmon calcitonin in postmenopausal women with established osteoporosis: the prevent recurrence of osteoporotic fractures study. PROOF Study Group. Am J Med 2000;109(4):267–76.
33. Overman RA, Borse M, Gourlay ML. Salmon calcitonin use and associated cancer risk. Ann Pharmacother 2013;47(12):1675–84.
34. Cauley JA, Robbins J, Chen Z, et al. Effects of estrogen plus progesterone on risk of fracture and bone mineral density: the Women's Health Initiative randomized trial. JAMA 2003;290:1729–38.
35. Cranney A, Tugwell P, Zytaruk N, et al. Meta-analysis of raloxifene for the prevention and treatment of postmenopausal osteoporosis. Endocr Rev 2002;23:524–8.
36. Neer RM, Arnaud CD, Zanchetta JR, et al. Effect of parathyroid hormone (1,34) on fractures and bone mineral density in postmenopausal women with osteoporosis. N Engl J Med 2001;344:1434–41.
37. Cummings SR, San Martin J, McClung MR, et al. Denosumab for the prevention of fractures in postmenopausal women with osteoporosis. N Engl J Med 2009; 361:756–65.
38. Black DM, Bauer DC, Schwartz AV, et al. Continuing bisphosphonate treatment for osteoporosis-for whom and for how long? N Engl J Med 2012;366(22):2051–3.
39. National Osteoporosis Foundation. Clinician's guide to prevention and treatment of osteoporosis. Washington, DC: National Osteoporosis Foundation; 2014.
40. Watts NB, Bilezikian JP, Camacho PM, et al. American Association of Clinical Endocrinologists Medical Guidelines for Clinical Practice for the diagnosis and treatment of postmenopausal osteoporosis: executive summary of recommendations. Endocr Pract 2010;16:1016–9.
41. Institute of Medicine (US) Committee to Review Dietary Reference Intakes for Vitamin D and Calcium, Ross AC, Taylor CL, et al, editors. Dietary reference intakes for calcium and vitamin D. Washington, DC: National Academies Press (US); 2011. Available at: http://www.ncbi.nlm.nih.gov/books/NBK56070/.
42. Jackson RD, LaCroix AZ, Gass M, et al. The Women's Health Initiative trial of calcium plus vitamin D supplementation on risk for fractures. N Engl J Med 2006; 354:669–83.
43. Bolland MJ, Grey A, Avenell A, et al. Calcium supplements with or without vitamin D and risk of cardiovascular events: re-analysis of the WHI limited access dataset and meta-analysis. BMJ 2011;342:d2040.
44. Paik JM, Curhan GC, Sun Q, et al. Calcium supplement intake and risk of cardiovascular disease in women. Osteoporos Int 2014;25(8):2047–56.
45. Sattin RW. Falls among older persons: a public health perspective. Annu Rev Public Health 1992;13:489–508.
46. Gillespie LD, Robertson MC, Gillespie WJ, et al. Interventions for preventing falls in older people living in the community. Cochrane Database Syst Rev 2012;(9):CD007146.
47. Moyer VA, U.S. Preventive Services Task Force. Vitamin D and calcium supplementation to prevent fractures in adults: a U.S. Preventive Services Task Force recommendation statement. Ann Intern Med 2013;158:691–6.

48. Chung M, Lee J, Terasawa T, et al. Vitamin D with or without calcium supplementation for the prevention of cancer and fractures: an updated meta-analysis for the USPSTF. Ann Intern Med 2011;155:827–38.
49. Grossman JM, Gordon R, Ranganath VK, et al. American College of Rheumatology 2010 recommendations for the prevention and treatment of glucocorticoid-induced osteoporosis. Arthritis Care Res (Hoboken) 2010;62:1515.

Female Sexual Dysfunction

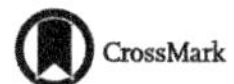

Jennifer J. Wright, MD[a,b,*], Kim M. O'Connor, MD[a,b]

KEYWORDS

- Female sexual dysfunction • Hypoactive sexual desire disorder
- Testosterone therapy • SSRI-induced sexual dysfunction • Atrophic vaginitis

KEY POINTS

- Ask patients about their sexual health and explore their concerns: broad categories of female sexual dysfunction include decreased desire, difficulty with arousal, delayed or absent orgasm, and pain with intercourse.
- Evidence supports the use of topical testosterone to treat hypoactive sexual desire disorder; although the magnitude of the benefit was small, there is a lack of long-term safety data, the studied testosterone replacement preparations are not available in the United States, and it is not approved by the Food and Drug Administration.
- Selective serotonin reuptake inhibitor–induced female sexual dysfunction can be treated with addition of bupropion or use of sildenafil.
- Topical estrogen is the most effective treatment for atrophic vaginitis, which is a common cause of pain with intercourse.

INTRODUCTION

The topic of female sexual health and dysfunction is a challenging one for health care providers. Discomfort with the topic, inadequate training, and insufficient clinical time with patients to discuss in-depth sexual histories and limited treatment options hinder providers' desire to address this issue. Academically, before the 1950s, this topic was rarely discussed. In the 1950s, Kinsey[1] introduced landmark literature addressing the sexual lives of women and their sexual practices in the United States. In the 1960s, Masters and Johnson[2] introduced a model of the female sexual response cycle, defined as the linear progression of 4 distinct physiologic phases, including excitement, plateau, orgasm, and resolution (**Fig. 1**). In the late 1970s, Kaplan[3] modified

Conflict of Interest Disclosures: We have no conflicts of interest to report including no financial conflicts of interest.

Role in Authorship: All authors had access to the data and had a role in writing the article.

[a] Division of General Internal Medicine, Harborview Medical Center, The University of Washington, Box 359780, 325 Ninth Ave Campus, Seattle, WA 98104, USA; [b] Department of Medicine, General Internal Medicine Center, University of Washington General Internal Medicine Clinic, Box 354760, 4245 Roosevelt Way Northeast, Seattle, WA 98105, USA

* Corresponding author. Department of Medicine, General Internal Medicine Center, University of Washington General Internal Medicine Clinic, Box 354760, 4245 Roosevelt Way Northeast, Seattle, WA 98105.

E-mail address: sonic@u.washington.edu

Med Clin N Am 99 (2015) 607–628
http://dx.doi.org/10.1016/j.mcna.2015.01.011 **medical.theclinics.com**
0025-7125/15/$ – see front matter

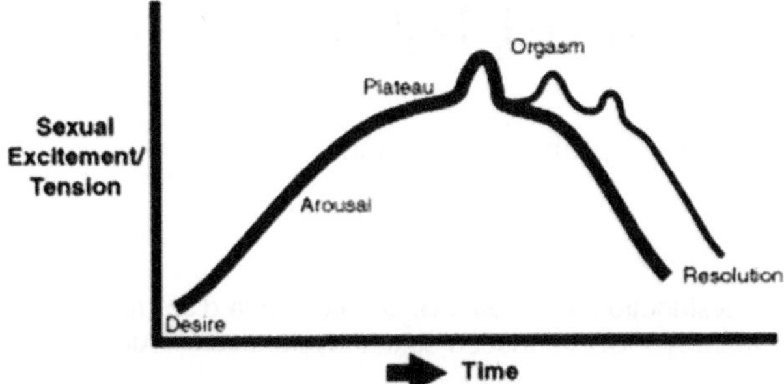

Fig. 1. Traditional sexual response cycle. (*From* Basson R. Female sexual response: the role of drugs in the management of sexual dysfunction. Obstet Gynecol 2001;98(2):351; with permission.)

this to a 3-phase model, including desire, arousal, and orgasm. In both of these genitally focused models, orgasm was considered essential for sexual fulfillment and the importance of intimacy and the emotional aspects of sexuality were not addressed. Basson[4] significantly modified this linear model of female sexual response. She proposed a cyclical model incorporating intimacy, relationship satisfaction, and sexual stimuli. In Basson's model,[4] the stages of female sexual functioning occur in a nonlinear fashion and orgasm is not essential for sexual fulfillment (**Fig. 2**).

It is important to realize that the Diagnostic and Statistical Manual of Mental Disorders-IV-text revision (DSM-IV-TR) criteria for female sexual dysfunction is based on the traditional linear model, which we have learned may not represent the most accurate pattern of sexual functioning for most women.[5] However, many women still believe normal sexual functioning to be the traditional desire-arousal-orgasm process. As a provider, some brief education about alternative theories and the importance of intimacy and emotionality and not just orgasm can go far in decreasing women's distress about their sexual health.

Not surprisingly, numerous biopsychosocial factors impact sexual function. Multiple medical and mental health conditions and medications can impact sexual health.

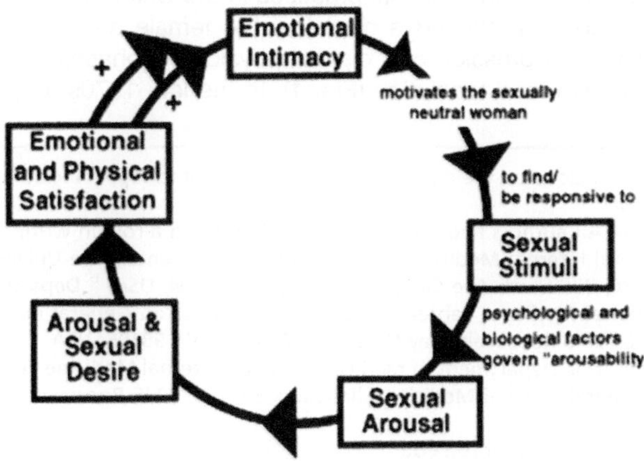

Fig. 2. Cyclical sexual response cycle. (*From* Basson R. Female sexual response: the role of drugs in the management of sexual dysfunction. Obstet Gynecol 2001;98(2):351; with permission.)

Family and cultural beliefs, early sexual experiences, partner relationship, and external stressors also play a strong role. Exploring these issues with patients may reveal modifiable obstacles to sexual fulfillment through better disease management, medication changes, mental health treatment, and discussion around personal and cultural beliefs or counseling.

As providers, we should bring up the topic of sexual health because only approximately 18% of women with sexual concerns will spontaneously volunteer information about sexual dysfunction to their doctor.[6] Simple screening questions could include the following: "*Sexuality is such an important part of our overall health. I would like to ask you some questions about that now. Is that okay with you?" "Are you currently sexually active?" "With men, women, or both?" "Do you have any concerns about your sexual health?*" Based on her responses, clinicians should further tailor their questioning around areas of concern. In 2000, the Female Sexual Function Index (FSFI) was developed for use in research. It is a brief, 19-item, multidimensional self-report instrument that assesses key dimensions of desire, arousal, lubrication, orgasm, satisfaction, and pain. Although it is validated for use in research, it is not yet used in clinical practice. However, the questions are quite useful and may be helpful to clinicians in obtaining a more comprehensive sexual history. How to interpret FSFI scores in the clinical setting has yet to be determined, but the individual responses to each question may be very informative when evaluating a sexual complaint.[7,8]

To meet criteria for a diagnosis of female sexual dysfunction, symptoms must be recurrent or persistent and they must cause significant personal distress. Sexual complaints are common and occur in approximately 40% of US women with 12% to 22% of those reporting personal distress related to their sexual issue.[9] The next step is determining whether it is a primary or lifelong issue, or a secondarily acquired problem. Understanding whether their problem is more generalized or situational is also important.

The classification of female sexual dysfunction (FSD), based on the DSM-IV-TR criteria, falls under the 4 categories of desire, arousal, orgasm, and pain.[5] The most common disorders are related to desire. Desire disorders include hypoactive sexual desire disorder (HSDD) and sexual aversion disorder. HSDD, which is described as decreased libido, is by far the most common issue for women, whereas sexual aversion disorder is quite rare. The prevalence rates for arousal, orgasm, and pain complaints are similar. Based on a 2006 review of published literature on prevalence studies of FSD, in women with sexual complaints, the average prevalence of women who experienced desire difficulties was 64%, arousal difficulties 31%, orgasm difficulties 35%, and sexual pain 26%.[10]

As mentioned before, there are new theories about the female sexual response cycle that are moving away from the linear model with distinct phases of arousal. The DSM-5, published in May 2013, aimed to incorporate these new philosophies and made some subtle changes to their diagnostic criteria. In the new criteria, female hypoactive desire disorder and female arousal dysfunction were merged into a single syndrome called sexual interest/arousal disorder. The diagnosis of sexual aversion disorder was deleted from the DSM-5 based on the fact that the diagnosis had limited empirical support and shared more similarities with phobias and anxiety disorders rather than sexual disorders. Also, the previously separate categories of dyspareunia and vaginismus are now called genito-pelvic pain/penetration disorder. Female orgasmic disorder remains in place. Different from the DSM-IV criteria, diagnosis of sexual dysfunction requires a minimum duration of 6 months of symptoms and symptoms must occur 75% to 100% of the time for all diagnoses except substance-induced and medication-induced sexual dysfunction. Also, the disorder must cause "clinically significant distress in the individual" and not just "interpersonal difficulty."[11,12] A number of other subtle changes were added that can be reviewed in the DSM-5 handbook or cited articles.[5,11,12] Please refer to **Table 1** for summary.

For the purpose of this article, we focus on the 4 categories of desire, arousal, orgasm, and pain so as to help delineate history taking and treatment options for each component. As one can imagine, despite having criteria that defines sexual dysfunctions in relation to the phases of the sexual response cycle, in clinical practice it is uncommon to see a disorder that is limited to a single phase.[5] Although there are many controversies around these diagnostic criteria and whether sexual difficulties are being overclassified as true "disorders," it is still at least helpful to have a generalized approach to history taking, diagnosis, and treatment. This approach will help women with these issues regardless of whether they should be defined as disorders or not.

Case:

A 34-year-old female, Mrs Jones, presents to your clinic for several issues. She is 6 months post-partum and she reports fatigue, difficulty with losing the weight she gained with pregnancy, and notes that her husband thinks they are not having sex very often. She has a history of depression and insomnia. Her medications include norethindrone 0.35 mg daily, citalopram 20 mg daily, and diphenhydramine 25 mg at bedtime as needed for insomnia.

DESIRE DISORDERS

In the DSM-IV, the desire disorders consist of HSDD and sexual aversion disorder. The patient's history for both these conditions will be very similar, apart from one major difference. The patient with HSDD will not report anxiety or aversion to sex, whereas the patient with sexual aversion disorder will report severe anxiety or aversion to sex. They will be similar in their reports of having absent or diminished interest in sex, infrequent sexual activity, decreased receptivity to sex, and infrequent or absent initiation of sexual activity.

Case:

Additional patient history: Mrs Jones feels that she is not currently interested in sex, she attributes this to feeling tired and unattractive, but the lack of interest bothers her: she previously had a good sexual relationship with her husband and she would like to again.

Table 1
Categories for female sexual dysfunction

DSM-IV Categories	DSM-5 Categories
Desire disorders • Hypoactive sexual desire disorder • Sexual aversion disorder	Desire/arousal disorders • Merged desire and arousal into one category • Deleted sexual aversion disorder
Arousal disorders	
Orgasm disorder	Female orgasm disorder
Pain • Dyspareunia: Pelvic pain with intercourse • Vaginismus: Pelvic floor muscle spasm leading to pain with penetration	Genito-pelvic pain/penetration disorder • Merged dyspareunia and vaginismus

Abbreviation: DSM, Diagnostic and Statistical Manual of Mental Disorders.

Potential causes for the desire disorders are similar; however, a history of sexual abuse or trauma is more common in women with sexual aversion disorder compared with those with HSDD. Relationship issues and religious or cultural beliefs can certainly influence libido. Sleep deprivation, stress, depression, or treatments with antidepressants or antipsychotics are common contributors. Pregnancy, breast-feeding, or a postmenopausal state can be associated with decreased libido. Any number of chronic medical conditions, including hypothyroidism, may contribute as well.

Many women will ask whether their form of contraception may be contributing. The data on this are conflicting. Most of the available data are on combined oral contraceptives (COCs), and most often they are libido neutral. A comprehensive review article on the subject was published in 2012.[13] In some cases, libido may be decreased from COCs due to antiandrogenic effects and a decrease in lubrication. In other studies, libido may increase due to decreased fear of pregnancy and improvement in certain gynecologic conditions, such as dysmenorrhea, menorrhagia, or endometriosis. The data for the NuvaRing (etonogestrel/ethinyl estradiol vaginal ring), the combined contraceptive patch (norelgestromin/ethinyl estradiol patch), and Depo-Provera (medroxyprogesterone acetate injection) appear similar. There are minimal data on the progesterone-only "mini pill" (norethindrone). One study of the Mirena (levonorgestrel) intrauterine device showed an increase in desire, whereas Implanon (etonogestrel) subdermal implant showed a decrease in libido in 2.5% of patients.[14,15]

Laboratory evaluation for FSD is rarely indicated unless there is a suspicion for a specific medical condition contributing to the patient's complaint. There are no data to support checking testosterone levels for FSD unless you are concerned about a hyperandrogenic medical condition. Endogenous serum androgen levels do not appear to be an independent predictor of sexual function in women.[16]

Simple interventions that may help your patient include discussions about stress reduction and education about average frequency of sex. Unfortunately, the media has given us an unrealistic view of typical sexual practices. Helping your patients understand that there are a wide variety of practices and frequency of sexual activity may help alleviate concern. Based on the results of a survey performed in the United States in 2009, you can provide the patient with information regarding the average frequency of sexual activity in women: for women older than 25 years, the most common frequency of vaginal intercourse reported was "a few times per month to weekly"; overall, in women in their 40s, 30.5% reported intercourse a few times a month to weekly, 17.5% reported intercourse 2 to 3 times a week, and 3.5% reported intercourse 4 or more times a week. Overall, the frequency of intercourse decreased with age and intercourse is more frequent in partnered women than single women.[17]

Case:

Mrs Jones feels better knowing that it is not uncommon for her to feel diminished libido considering the multiple issues affecting her on a daily basis. However, she still asks about testosterone therapy. She heard about it from a friend of hers.

Many women will ask their providers about whether testosterone therapy is an option. The benefit of testosterone therapy in postmenopausal women with HSDD is supported by several randomized controlled trials. See **Table 2** for a summary of important trials, including the patient population studies, testosterone preparation, and risks and benefits.[18–21]

Review of the literature is of benefit for several reasons. There is a good evidence base regarding a benefit of testosterone therapy in the treatment of HSDD, but the

Table 2
Summary of major randomized, placebo-controlled studies of testosterone therapy for hypoactive sexual desire disorder

Study	Patient Population	Testosterone Preparation	Results	Testosterone Side Effects
Davis SR, Moreau M, Kroll R, et al. Testosterone for low libido in postmenopausal women not taking estrogen.[18]	814 postmenopausal women not on hormone replacement therapy	Transdermal testosterone patches, 150 μg/d or 300 μg/d	300-μg/d patch resulted in an increase of 2.1 satisfying sexual episodes/4 wk; the placebo group had increase of 0.7 episodes/4 wk. No significant increase with the 150-μg/d dose of testosterone.	Hair growth, but very few women withdrew from the study because of this. More frequent vaginal bleeding, attributed to endometrial atrophy. No significant increase in acne, alopecia, or voice deepening. Three cases of breast cancer, all in the testosterone-treatment group.
Panay N, Al-Azzawi F, Bouchard C, et al. Testosterone treatment of HSDD in naturally menopausal women: the ADORE study.[19]	272 postmenopausal women with nonsurgical menopause, many of whom were also being treated with estrogen replacement	Transdermal testosterone patches, 300-μg/d	Testosterone therapy resulted in an increase of 1.69 satisfying sexual episodes/4 wk, compared with an increase of 0.53 episodes/4 wk in the placebo group.	Hair growth and acne, neither severe enough to lead to withdrawal from the trial. No major adverse effects were noted.

Braunstein GD, Sundwall DA, Katz M, et al. Safety and efficacy of a testosterone patch for the treatment of hypoactive sexual desire disorder in surgically menopausal women: a randomized, placebo-controlled trial.[20]	447 postmenopausal women who underwent surgical menopause, all on oral estrogen replacement	Transdermal testosterone patch, 150 μg/d, 300 μg/d or 450 μg/d	300 μg/d patch resulted in an increase of 0.58 satisfying sexual episodes a week. No significant increase on 150 μg/d or 450 μg/d dose of testosterone.	No major adverse effects.
Davis S, Papalia MA, Norman RJ, et al. Safety and efficacy of a testosterone metered-dose transdermal spray for treating decreased sexual satisfaction in premenopausal women: a randomized trial.[21]	261 premenopausal women with low circulating testosterone levels	Transdermal testosterone spray, 56 μL, 90 μL or 180 μL	90 μL/d dose resulted in an increase of 2.48 satisfying sexual episodes/ 4 wk compared with an increase of 0.8 episodes/ 4 wk on placebo.	Increased hair growth, primarily at the application site, and an increase in severity of acne. No other significant adverse events.

Data from Refs.[18–21]

magnitude of this benefit is small. It is thought that an increase of ≥1 satisfying sexual episodes per 4 weeks is meaningful to patients, but when weighed against potential risks, this needs to be carefully considered.[22] It also should be noted that long-term safety data are nonexistent. Finally, availability of the studied testosterone replacement preparations is limited. In the United States, there are no testosterone preparations approved for use in women. There is no 300-μg per day transdermal testosterone patch available; the patches designed for men are much higher doses than those studied for use in women. There are ongoing trials of a low-dose testosterone gel, brand name LibiGel, designed for use in women. The trial under way is being completed to assess long-term safety data in response to requests by the Food and Drug Administration (FDA) for cardiovascular and breast cancer safety data before potential approval of testosterone therapy for treatment of postmenopausal women with HSDD.[23] It also should be noted that efficacy of this preparation has not yet been demonstrated in the literature.

Use of products designed for use in men would clearly be off-label and should be done with caution. As noted, the concentration of testosterone in these preparations is much higher, and therefore the dose would need to be carefully adjusted. Transdermal patches designed for men cannot be cut; therefore, options primarily include injections and gels.

Case:

Mrs Jones is on an antidepressant. Is there anything to help with HSDD in this population?

Selective serotonin reuptake inhibitors (SSRIs) can negatively affect any component of the sexual response cycle, including desire, arousal, and/or orgasm, with estimates of 30% to 70% of patients on SSRIs reporting some degree of sexual dysfunction.[24] Delay of orgasm and lack of orgasm are the most commonly reported side effects. Sexual dysfunction is a potential side effect for all drugs within the SSRI class of antidepressants. In addition, sexual side effects are frequently reported with venlafaxine, a serotonin-norepinephrine reuptake inhibitor (SNRI). Evidence regarding the severity of sexual side effects with mirtazapine is mixed, in some studies comparable to SNRIs, in others much less severe.[25,26] Notably, bupropion, an antidepressant that is thought to primarily act on the dopamine and noradrenergic receptors, is not commonly associated with high rates of sexual side effects.

There are several potential strategies to manage sexual dysfunction in the setting of antidepressant use; see **Box 1** for a concise summary. First, it is important to investigate the onset of a patient's sexual dysfunction. Depression itself may lead to sexual dysfunction, and treatment with an SSRI may actually be helpful, although this may take weeks of therapy. It is also possible that the symptom will resolve spontaneously;

Box 1
Strategies for managing FSD in the setting of depression and SSRI therapy

- Continue SSRI, add bupropion sustained release 150 mg twice a day
- Continue SSRI, prescribe sildenafil 50–100 mg as needed before sexual activity
- Reduce dose of SSRI if possible
- Switch antidepressant classes from SSRI to bupropion

Abbreviations: FSD, female sexual dysfunction; SSRI, selective serotonin reuptake inhibitor.

similar to other common SSRI side effects, such as nausea, it has been estimated that 10% of the time sexual side effects will resolve as the body adapts to the medication.[25]

Several studies have found a reduction in SSRI-related sexual side effects with the addition of bupropion. In a Cochrane Database Systematic Review, Taylor and colleagues[27] performed a review of management of SSRI-induced sexual dysfunction. They identified 5 high-quality randomized trials, including a total of 579 participants, regarding addition of bupropion to an SSRI for management of sexual side effects. One of these studies was exclusively of women; the other studies included predominately women. They found improvement in sexual rating scores with use of bupropion sustained release 150 mg twice daily, but no statistically significant improvement with bupropion sustained release 150 mg once daily. Based on the limited data available in the studies, there was no evidence of a worsening of control of patients' underlying mental illness with augmentation.

The use of sildenafil for management of SSRI-induced FSD may be considered as well. In a randomized, double-blinded, placebo-controlled trial of 49 premenopausal women with SSRI-induced sexual dysfunction, patients treated with sildenafil 50 to 100 mg as needed before sexual activity had an improved global sexual function score, the study's primary outcome measure.[28] Improvement in sexual function based on other scales, used as secondary outcome measures, was not consistently seen with sildenafil compared with placebo.

Other strategies can be considered, although they are less evidence-based. One option is a reduction in dose of a patient's SSRI or SNRI, in hopes of reducing sexual side effects. A switch in antidepressants could be made, from an SSRI to bupropion. Or a "drug holiday" could be considered. There is one small observational study regarding this in which 30 patients were instructed to hold their SSRI antidepressant, fluoxetine, sertraline, or paroxetine, on Friday and Saturday for a month.[29] There was a reported improvement in sexual function for the patients taking a "holiday" from sertraline and paroxetine; there was no improvement in patients on fluoxetine. There was no worsening in depression scores. These strategies would all carry the risk of worsening control of a patient's depression and should be undertaken with caution if the patient's symptoms are well controlled on their current drug regimen.

There is some evidence to support the use of bupropion for treatment of HSDD even in the absence of depression or SSRI therapy. There have been 2 studies completed regarding this question.[30,31] Studies were of premenopausal women with HSDD who did not have depression. Different doses were used in each study, bupropion sustained release 150 mg daily and 300 to 400 mg daily; both studies found benefit compared with placebo. Bupropion improved all domains of sexual function. In the study by Safarinejad and colleagues,[31] common side effects of bupropion included headache, insomnia, dry mouth, and nausea, although overall these symptoms were well tolerated, only leading to withdrawal of 3 of the 112 participants in the study group.

Case:

Mrs Jones returns to your clinic a month later. She is concerned that when she and her husband have been sexually active over the past several weeks it has been uncomfortable, noting that she has poor vaginal lubrication.

AROUSAL DISORDERS

Arousal disorder is defined as the recurrent inability to attain or maintain sufficient sexual arousal despite adequate stimulation. Once again, numerous psychosocial issues and mental health conditions can influence arousal, as can medications, such as SSRIs, tricyclic antidepressants, antihistamines, anticholinergics, certain antihypertensives (alpha-blockers, beta-blockers, calcium channel blockers, diuretics), and illicit substances. Pelvic neurogenic or vascular impairments due to local nerve damage from pelvic surgeries or spinal cord injuries, peripheral nerve disorders from conditions such as diabetes and multiple sclerosis, and vascular impairment from diabetes, hypertension, hyperlipidemia, and smoking can affect arousal.

Educating patients on the importance of adequate stimulation and the use of lubricants and vaginal moisturizers can be helpful. There are a variety of lubricant products on the market available without a prescription. Broad categories include water-based, silicon-based, and oil-based lubricants. The water-based formulations are most commonly used; examples include Astroglide, K-Y Jelly, and Slippery Stuff. They are unlikely to cause skin irritation or stain bedding but may dry up more quickly than the silicone-based products. Silicone-based products are more expensive and more likely to stain bedding; examples include Pjur and ID Millenium. Many women will report using oil-based lubricants, such as baby oil, which can irritate the vaginal tissues and should not be used with latex condoms as they can reduce the effectiveness of the contraception and the prevention of sexually transmitted illnesses. Natural oils, including olive oil or avocado oil, are less irritating, although still should be avoided if the patient is using condoms with her partner.

Teaching patients about self-stimulation with vibrators or medical devices such as the Eros Clitoral Therapy device can be effective. The Eros Clitoral Therapy device is an FDA-approved hand-held vacuum used to increase blood flow to the clitoris and surrounding vaginal tissues. Whereas vibrators do not require a prescription and come in a variety of prices, the Eros Therapy device does require a prescription and costs approximately $179 as listed on the Eros Therapy Web site, eros-therapy.com.

Zestra is a natural oil-based topical therapy marketed as an "arousal oil." It contains a combination of natural oils, including borage seed and evening primrose oils, and extracts and vitamins. In a randomized controlled study comparing efficacy of Zestra to placebo, a soybean oil–based product, in 178 patients with FSD, including arousal, desire and orgasmic disorders, there was a significant improvement in arousal and desire with the Zestra product, with a nonstatistically significant improvement in global satisfaction as well.[32] This product was associated with mild-to-moderate genital burning in approximately 15% of subjects in the study.

Case:

Her husband is using Viagra. She wonders if that will help her too.

As reviewed previously, there have been encouraging data regarding the use of sildenafil in the treatment of SSRI-induced FSD.[28] However, the evidence supporting the use of sildenafil in women who have female sexual arousal disorder has not been consistent. A study performed in premenopausal and postmenopausal women found no benefit with sildenafil doses ranging from 10 to 100 mg, although other, smaller studies have found some benefit.[33–35] At this time, sildenafil would not be a recommended therapy.

Case:

Mrs Jones returns to clinic again, several months later. Several issues have improved; she feels that her interest in sexual activity has returned to a level she is happy with, and with adequate stimulation she has normal vaginal lubrication. Today she is concerned about a decrease in the frequency of orgasms; she feels that she more frequently had orgasms before her pregnancy.

ORGASM DISORDERS

Female orgasmic disorder can be primary or secondary. A patient who has never had an orgasm would be described as having primary orgasmic disorder. There may be a history of sexual abuse, and if so, psychotherapy may be useful in treatment. But in some cases it is idiopathic, in which case there are no recommended treatments. Patients with secondary orgasmic disorder have achieved orgasm in the past but have a distressing change in their ability to achieve orgasm at the time of presentation. There are many possible etiologies, including psychosocial causes such as relationship conflict, religion or cultural beliefs, and body image issues. Neurologic and vascular disease can lead to orgasm disorders; examples include spinal cord injury, diabetes, and multiple sclerosis. A class of medications frequently associated with anorgasmia and delayed orgasm is SSRIs. Management of secondary female orgasm disorder involves normalizing the patient's experience, educating the patient on possible ways to achieve orgasm, consideration of counseling, and possible change of antidepressant if the patient is taking an SSRI, as described previously.

A model of assessment and treatment that could be used by the primary care provider is the PLISSIT model. PLISSIT stands for *P*ermission, *Li*mited Information, *S*pecific *S*uggestions, *I*ntensive *T*herapy. Permission stands for the discussion with the patient around normalization of sexual behaviors. Limited Information could include information about behaviors that may increase arousal, including foreplay and a discussion of medical conditions or medications that could be contributing to the problem. Specific Suggestions could include use of lubricants, vaginal estrogen, and position changes. Intensive Therapy would be referral to a specialist, such as a sex therapist or couples counselor, if appropriate. "Sex therapy" is psychotherapy aimed at treating sexual dysfunction. The organization American Association of Sexuality Educators, Counselors, and Therapists offers certification. The focus of sex therapy can be variable based on the patient's needs. It frequently focuses on reducing anxiety in sexual situations, based on the assumption that anticipation and performance anxiety often contribute to sexual dysfunction, in addition to discussion of sexual skills. Sexual exercises are frequently assigned; these may include sensate focus, in which the focus of intimate physical interactions is on sensations and not orgasm. This therapy has not been well studied, and there is great heterogeneity in both specific treatments and results.[36]

Case:

Mrs Jones returns to clinic 2 years later. She had her second child 4 months ago. Despite reviewing all the recommendations you made to her previously she is again having pain with intercourse. Even with adequate stimulation she feels that she doesn't have adequate vaginal lubrication and is having significant pain with insertion. She is currently breast-feeding and is back on the norethindrone "mini pill."

PAIN DISORDERS

In the DSM-5 criteria, the categories of dyspareunia and vaginismus were merged under a new category called genito-pelvic pain/penetration disorder (GPPD). The primary reason for this change was because these 2 disorders could not be reliably differentiated. The presence of "vaginal muscle spasm," which is part of the diagnostic criteria for vaginismus, has not been supported by empirical evidence and the fear of pain or the fear of penetration is common in the clinical descriptions of vaginismus.[12] Because there is tremendous overlap between dyspareunia and vaginismus, the term "genito-pelvic pain/penetration disorder" is all encompassing. For the diagnosis of GPPD, one of the following should occur persistently or recurrently: difficulty in vaginal penetration, marked vulvovaginal or pelvic pain during penetration or attempt at penetration, fear or anxiety about pain in anticipation of, during, or after penetration, and tightening of pelvic floor muscles during attempted penetration.[12] Sexual pain may be localized to the vulva, vestibule, vagina, pelvis, or at multiple sites simultaneously. Currently research in pelvic pain syndromes is lacking in women for whom insertive vaginal intercourse may not be part of their typical sexual practices. Future revisions to the DSM criteria will hopefully incorporate more information about nonpenetrative sexual activities and women without partners.[11]

To diagnose GPPD, other causes of pelvic pain must be ruled out. Etiologies for genito-pelvic pain are numerous. From the perspective of a health care provider, it may be easier to think of broader categories such as "irritative," "anatomic," and "infectious" causes; see **Table 3**. Regarding infectious causes, evaluate for sexually transmitted illnesses, candidiasis, and pelvic inflammatory disease when appropriate. Under the category of "anatomic," one might elicit a history or physical examination finding of previous pelvic surgery, episiotomy, fibroids, uterine or bladder prolapse, gynecologic malignancy, or endometriosis, to name a few. In this article, we focus on "irritative" causes, which include diminished lubrication, atrophic vaginitis, vulvar dermatoses, and vulvodynia.

Atrophic vaginitis is most common in menopausal women. Hypoestrogenic states also can occur in the postpartum period, during lactation, and in premenopausal women with the administration of antiestrogenic drugs, such as tamoxifen, aromatase inhibitors, and medroxyprogesterone that may cause vaginal atrophy. Typical physical examination findings for vaginal atrophy include loss of labial or vulvar fullness, minimal vaginal moisture, pallor of urethra or vagina, narrow introitus, and loss of vaginal rugae (**Fig. 3**). Placing a piece of pH paper on the vaginal wall until it is moistened can test vaginal pH. The pH of an estrogenized vagina ranges from 3.5 to 5.0. A vaginal pH of 4.5 or greater in the absence of infection or recent semen in the vaginal vault can be an indicator of vaginal atrophy due to estrogen deficiency.

Table 3
Causes of pelvic pain

Categories	Examples
Irritative	Vaginal dryness Atrophic vaginitis Vulvar dermatoses Vulvodynia/vestibulitis
Anatomic	Endometriosis Fibroids Uterine or bladder prolapse Scarring related to previous pelvic surgery, episiotomy Gynecologic malignancy
Infectious	Sexually transmitted infections (gonorrhea, chlamydia) Vulvovaginal candidiasis Pelvic inflammatory disease

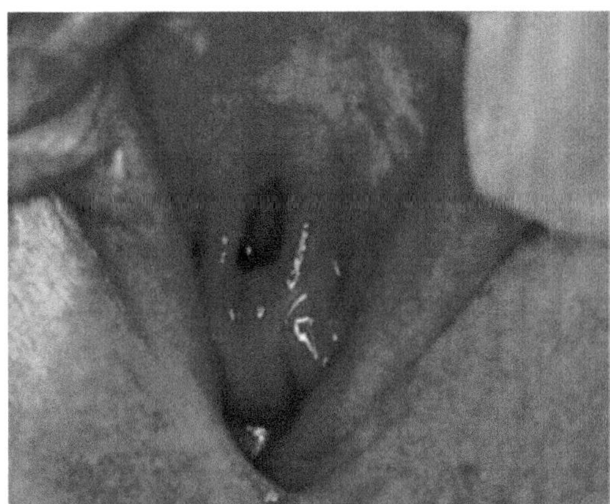

Fig. 3. Atrophic vulva. Slightly enlarged clitoris owing to loss of estrogen, with a pale, thin vulvar vestibule. (*From* Apgar BS, Brotzman GL, Spitzer M. Colposcopy, principles and practice, an integrated textbook and atlas. Philadelphia: WB Saunders; 2002; with permission.)

Women with atrophic vaginitis should be encouraged to use vaginal moisturizers and lubricants. The different lubricant products available are outlined previously in the section on arousal disorders. Over-the-counter vaginal moisturizers used on a regular basis with intercourse rather than as needed can help manage symptoms of atrophic vaginitis. Replens is an example of a vaginal moisturizer, with results of 2 small studies showing equal efficacy as topical estrogen, although the authors' clinical experience would suggest it is less effective.[37] Vaginal estrogen is also an option for many women. Unless there is clinical indication for systemic estrogen therapy, the recommendation is to use low-dose vaginal estrogen for atrophic vaginitis, as it appears more effective with less risk of side effects. This is based on a meta-analysis of 58 studies demonstrating higher patient satisfaction with vaginal versus oral estrogen therapy for the relief of urogenital atrophy symptoms.[38] Low-dose vaginal estrogen options include estradiol (Vagifem) 10-μg tablets, estradiol ring (Estring), conjugated estrogen cream (Premarin) 0.625 mg/g (low dose ≤0.3 mg), or estradiol cream (Estrace) 100 μg/g (low dose ≤50 μg). Remember that the high-dose estradiol ring of 50 to 100 μg/d (Femring) is not a low-dose option and is equal to systemic estrogen therapy. For the tablets and creams, treatment is usually initiated nightly for 2 weeks, then twice weekly for maintenance. The low-dose estradiol ring in placed intravaginally for 3 months and then replaced with a new ring. Symptoms may improve within the first few weeks of starting therapy but it may take up to 4 to 6 weeks for complete restoration of the urogenital tissue. See **Table 4** for summary of therapies for atrophic vaginitis.

There is minimal systemic absorption with these vaginal preparations, but the highest absorption may occur with the creams. Circulating estradiol levels measured in women treated with the low-dose vaginal estradiol tablet and estradiol ring are similar to normal levels in menopausal women.[39] There are fewer data available on estradiol levels in women treated with the vaginal creams. Well-designed, long-term studies evaluating potential risks of low-dose vaginal estrogen are lacking. Therefore, it is still controversial whether these preparations are safe in the setting of a previous history of breast cancer, particularly hormone-receptor–positive breast cancer, or venous thromboembolism and whether progesterone therapy should be used in the setting of an intact uterus. We recommend conferring with a woman's oncologist before

Table 4
Therapies for atrophic vaginitis

Categories	Examples	Dosing	Comments
Over-the-counter vaginal lubricants	Water-based: Astroglide, K-Y Jelly, Slippery Stuff	As needed with intercourse	Dry up more quickly than other products
	Silicon-based: Pjur, ID Millenium	As needed with intercourse	More expensive than other products Potential to stain bedding
	Oil-based: synthetic (baby oil) or natural oils (olive, avocado)	As needed with intercourse	Reduce effectiveness of condoms Synthetics: Vaginal irritation
Over-the-counter vaginal moisturizers	Replens	Every 3 d	
Prescription topical estrogen therapy	Estradiol (Vagifem) 10-μg tablets Estradiol ring (Estring) Conjugated estrogen cream (Premarin) 0.625 mg/g (low dose ≤0.3 mg) Estradiol cream (Estrace) 100 μg/gram (low dose ≤50 μg)	Tablets and creams: treatment typically initiated nightly for 2 wk then twice weekly for maintenance The low-dose estradiol ring is placed intravaginally every 3 mo	Endometrial safety: Use of an opposing progestin unnecessary when using low-dose vaginal tablets and rings, less clear with the creams Patients with an h/o breast cancer: Risk likely very low, confer with a woman's oncologist before initiating treatment with vaginal estrogen
Prescription oral medications	Ospemifene (Osphena), a selective estrogen receptor modulator that acts as an estrogen agonist in the vagina	60 mg daily	FDA recommends use of opposing progestin. Potential risk of venous thromboembolism. Yet to be determined if safe in women with history of breast cancer and if protective in women at high risk for breast malignancy.

Abbreviations: FDA, Food and Drug Administration; h/o, history of.

initiating treatment with vaginal estrogen in patients with breast cancer. Based on limited data, it appears that use of vaginal estrogen in women on tamoxifen is safe.[40] Data are lacking about the effects of low-dose vaginal estrogen on endocrine therapy for breast cancer. At this point, we would recommend against use of vaginal estrogen in women taking aromatase inhibitors for treatment of breast cancer. The goal of aromatase inhibitor therapy is to maximally reduce systemic estrogen levels. There is a very small study demonstrating that the use of low-dose vaginal estrogen reversed the suppression of serum estradiol levels achieved by aromatase inhibitor therapy.[41]

Regarding endometrial safety, low-dose vaginal estrogen used for the treatment of atrophic vaginitis does not appear to cause proliferation of the endometrial epithelium regardless of vaginal preparation used.[39,42] The use of an opposing progestin is likely unnecessary when using low-dose vaginal tablets and rings, but it is less clear with the use of the creams. The conservative approach would be to use opposing progestin in women treated with vaginal estrogen creams. Progestin can be taken either daily or for 10 to 12 consecutive days per month. Typical progestin formulations include medroxyprogesterone 10 mg, norethindrone acetate 5 to 10 mg, or micronized progesterone 200 mg. Regardless of the type of vaginal estrogen used, any menopausal woman who develops vaginal bleeding should be evaluated for endometrial hyperplasia or cancer.

Ospemifene (Osphena) 60 mg/day is a newly FDA-approved oral tablet for the treatment of moderate to severe menopausal dyspareunia. This is a selective estrogen receptor modulator (SERM) that acts as an estrogen agonist in the vagina. Two randomized trials have shown that ospemifene 60 mg per day is more effective than placebo in the treatment of menopausal dyspareunia and vaginal dryness at 12 weeks.[43,44] To date, there are no studies comparing ospemifene to vaginal estrogen. Other SERMs on the market (tamoxifen and raloxifene) have not shown the same improvements in atrophic vaginitis symptoms. The most common side effect of ospemifene is hot flashes. Whether opposing progestin should be used in women with an intact uterus is still unclear. In a 1-year, long-term safety extension study of ospemifene for the treatment of atrophic vaginitis, neither ospemifene 30 mg or 60 mg daily resulted in significant endometrial changes.[45] Currently, the FDA recommends the use of opposing progestin; however, studies evaluating the protective effects of progestin are lacking. There is also a potential risk of venous thromboembolism; however, further data are needed. Additional studies also are needed to determine if ospemifene is safe in women with history of breast cancer and whether it has protective effects for women at high risk for breast malignancy.

Is it important to evaluate for evidence of vulvar dermatoses when women complain of dyspareunia. Lichen sclerosis is a chronic, progressive inflammatory skin condition of unknown etiology. It most commonly affects the labia minora and/or labia major, but can extend to the perineum and around the anus. Women will complain of pruritus and/or pain. Dyspareunia is often a late symptom due to introital stenosis, fissuring, or labial agglutination. Classic findings include white atrophic papules that may coalesce into ivory or pink plaques. Lichen sclerosis can also be hemorrhagic, purpuric, hyperkeratotic, bullous, eroded, or ulcerated. Fissuring perianally, around the clitoris and in the intralabial folds is common (**Figs. 4** and **5**). As the condition progresses, labial scarring may occur, which can lead to the loss of the vulvar architecture and narrowing of the introitus. Women with lichen sclerosis are at higher risk of developing squamous cell cancer of the vulva. Treatment usually involves the use of superpotent topical steroids to improve symptoms and prevent progression of the disease. It is not known whether topical steroids prevent the development of squamous cell cancer. Typical treatment includes the application of a thin film of clobetasol or halobetasol propionate 0.05% ointment nightly to the affected areas for 6 to 12 weeks and then 1 to 3 times per week for maintenance.

Another vulvar dermatosis that can lead to dyspareunia is vulvar lichen planus. This is a chronic, desquamative, erosive dermatitis that can result in severe destruction of the vulvar tissues and stenosis of the vaginal opening. Symptoms most often develop in women age 50 to 60 years and include severe pruritus or vulvar pain, soreness, or burning. Vulvar lichen planus can involve the labia minor and vestibule. The anus is

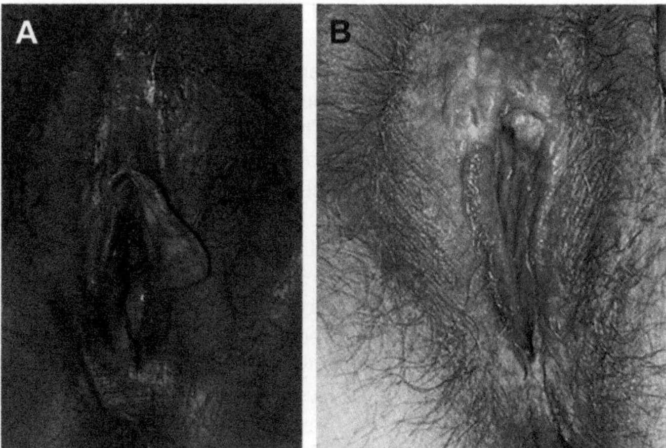

Fig. 4. (*A*) Vulvar lichen sclerosus. Pallor, atrophy (wrinkled aspect on the perineum) and perineal fissures. (*B*) Early changes in lichen sclerosus. White thickened areas of vulva caused by lichen sclerosus. (*From* Moyal-Barracco M, Wendling J. Vulvar dermatosis. Best Pract Res Clin Obstet Gynaecol 2014;28:949; with permission.)

rarely affected. Lesions can be isolated or diffuse. Vulvar lichen planus is described as glassy, brightly erythematous erosions with white striae or a serpentine white border along the margin (Wickham striae) (**Figs. 6–8**). A violaceous border is occasionally seen. Data regarding efficacy of treatments for vulvar lichen planus are limited; however, treatment often involves the use of super-potent topical steroids with daily

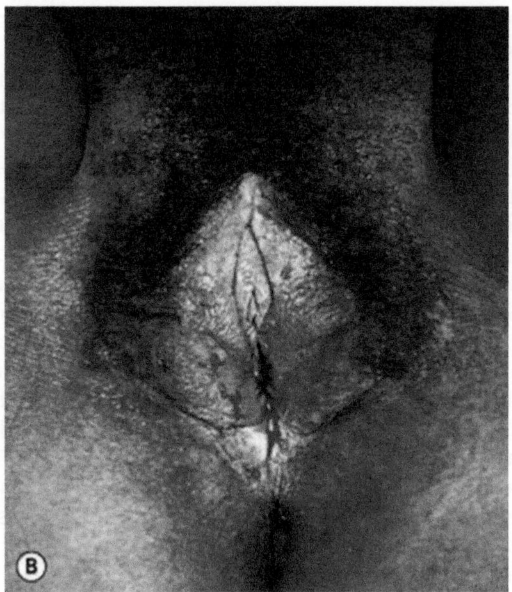

Fig. 5. More advanced vulvar lichen sclerosis. Hypertrophic plaques, edema, loss of normal architecture, introital narrowing, and perineal involvement. (*From* Moreland A, Kohl P. Genital and dermatologic examination. In: Morse SA, editor. Atlas of sexually transmitted diseases and AIDS. 4th edition. Philadelphia: Saunders; 2011. p. 1–23; with permission.)

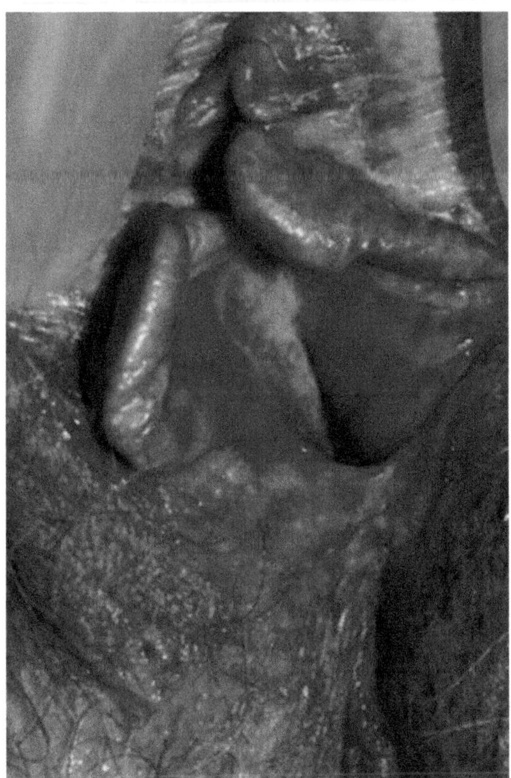

Fig. 6. Lichen planus of the vulva. White lacelike pattern and erythema. (*From* Laga AC, Lazar AJ, Haefner HK, et al. Noninfectious inflammatory disorders of the vulva. In: Crum CP, editor. Diagnostic gynecologic and obstetric pathology. 2nd edition. Philadelphia: Saunders; 2011. p. 21–48; with permission.)

treatment followed by maintenance therapy. Evaluation and management by a dermatologist is recommended.

Vulvar pain disorders also can include localized or generalized vulvodynia. Once other causes for pain are excluded, localized vulvodynia can be diagnosed using the Q-tip test, in which pain is "provoked" in the vestibule, interlabial sulci, introitus, or around the clitoris with light touch from a moistened Q-tip (**Fig. 9**). Pain may be prevented or reduced with the use of topical lidocaine 5% ointment or EMLA (lidocaine-prilocaine) cream applied to the painful areas 10 minutes before intercourse.

Generalized vulvodynia is defined as "unprovoked" stinging, burning, irritation, rawness, or pain anywhere on the vulva that is not explained by another condition. In generalized vulvodynia, physical examination is often normal or there may be areas of tenderness, hyperesthesia, or hypesthesia. The use of topical anesthetics before intercourse can be tried, otherwise numerous oral medications used for the treatment of chronic pain can be considered. Working closely with a gynecologist and possibly a pelvic floor physical therapist is recommended.

Once other conditions have been excluded, the treatment of GPPD is often multifactorial. Referral to a psychiatrist or psychotherapist may be necessary to deal with any potential psychological factors contributing to the pain. Pelvic floor physical therapists are able to instruct women in desensitization techniques, such as Kegel exercises and

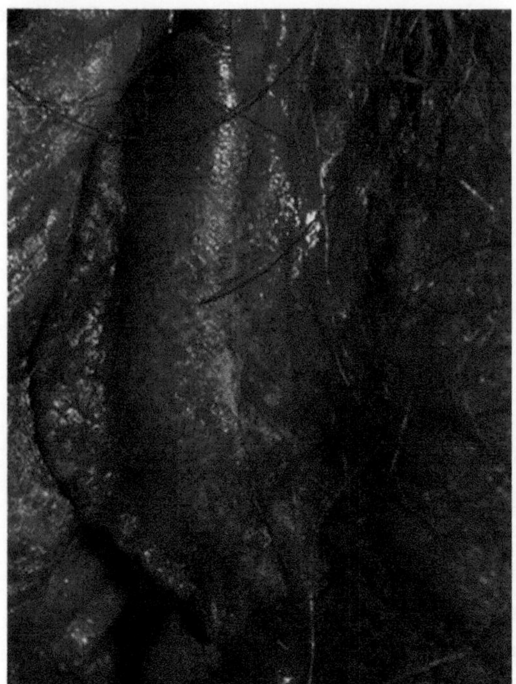

Fig. 7. Wickham striae. The most classic and only pathognomonic findings of vulvar lichen planus are the white, reticulate, lacy papules. Even these papules are most often accompanied by vulvar or vaginal erosions. (*From* Mirowski GW, Goddard A. Treatment of vulvovaginal lichen planus. Derm Clinics 2010;28(4):720; with permission.)

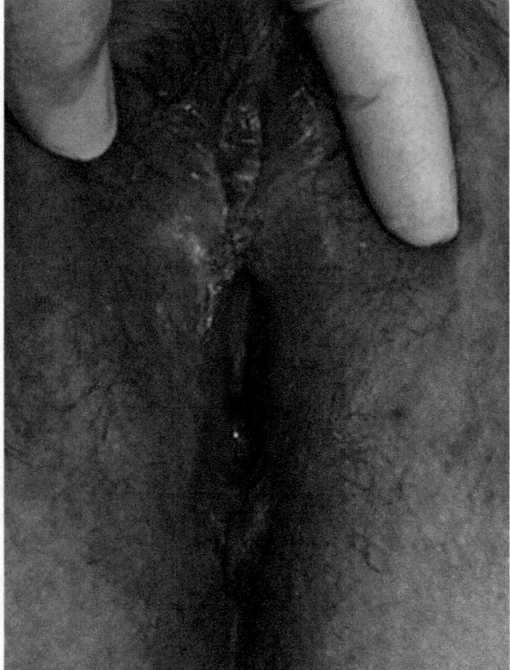

Fig. 8. Vulvar lichen planus. Most often manifested by vestibular erosions, loss of vulvar architecture caused by scarring, and surrounding white epithelium; patients experience both itching and pain. (*From* Stewart KM. Clinical care of vulvar pruritus, with emphasis on one common cause, lichen simplex chronicus. Derm Clinics 2010;28(4):673; with permission.)

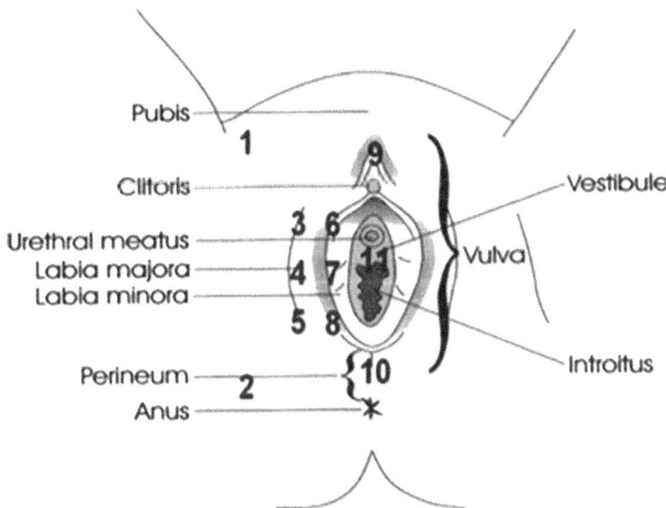

Fig. 9. Cotton swab testing for vulvodynia. Check clockwise: 1–2, inner thigh; 3–5, labia majora; 6–8, interlabial sulcus; 9, clitoris and hood; 10, perineum; 11, vestibule. (*From* Shah M, Hofstetter S. Vulvodynia. Obstet Gynecol Clin North Am 2014;41(3):456; with permission.)

vaginal dilator therapy with the goal of giving the woman control over her pelvic floor tonicity and relaxation. Numerous other treatments have been tried but lack well-designed studies. Working with a gynecologist or other women's health provider versed in the treatment of this condition is important.

SUMMARY

FSD is a term applied to a heterogeneous group of disorders. Providers and patients are frequently uncomfortable discussing sexual health, leading to neglect of this important issue in patients' well-being. When a patient has sexual concerns, these should be explored and if distressing to the patient, may represent an FSD "disorder." There are several broad categories of FSD to consider, including desire, arousal, orgasm, and pain disorders, although it should be acknowledged that frequently one patient may have symptoms of several of these types of sexual dysfunction. We hope to have offered the reader guidance in how to evaluate a patient with sexual concerns, how the history can lead to diagnosis and in turn treatment strategies for the patient. In the setting of HSDD, there is evidence to support the use of topical testosterone therapy, although the magnitude of the benefit was small, there is a lack of long-term safety data and the studied testosterone replacement preparations are not available in the United States. At this time, use of testosterone for HSDD in women is not FDA approved. For patients with SSRI-induced FSD, addition of bupropion or use of sildenafil may be helpful. Patient education regarding adequate stimulation and use of lubricants is likely one of the most effective means of treating arousal disorders. In the absence of SSRI therapy, treatment of secondary female orgasmic disorder also involves patient education and potentially more intensive "sex therapy." Pain with intercourse is common, especially in postmenopausal women. Treatment of atrophic vaginitis is most effectively accomplished with topical estrogen treatment. In the absence of other painful vaginal conditions, GPPD can be diagnosed. Treatments are not well studied, but may include pelvic floor physical therapy for desensitization exercises.

REFERENCES

1. Kinsey A. Sexual behavior in the human female. Philadelphia: W.B. Saunders Company; 1953.
2. Masters W, Johnson V. Human sexual response. Boston: Little, Brown and Company; 1966.
3. Kaplan H. Disorders of sexual desire and other new concepts and techniques in sex therapy. New York: Brunner/Hazel Publications; 1979.
4. Basson R. Human sex-response cycles. J Sex Marital Ther 2001;27(1):33–43.
5. American Psychiatric Association. Sexual dysfunctions. Diagnostic and statistical manual of mental disorders. 5th edition. Arlington (VA): American Psychiatric Publishing; 2013.
6. Nusbaum MR, Helton MR, Ray N. The changing nature of women's sexual health concerns through the midlife years. Maturitas 2004;49(4):283–91.
7. Wiegel M, Meston C, Rosen R. The female sexual function index (FSFI): cross-validation and development of clinical cutoff scores. J Sex Marital Ther 2005;31(1):1–20.
8. Rosen R, Brown C, Heiman J, et al. The Female Sexual Function Index (FSFI): a multidimensional self-report instrument for the assessment of female sexual function. J Sex Marital Ther 2000;26(2):191–208.
9. Shifren JL, Monz BU, Russo PA, et al. Sexual problems and distress in United States women: prevalence and correlates. Obstet Gynecol 2008;112(5):970–8.
10. Hayes RD, Bennett CM, Fairley CK, et al. What can prevalence studies tell us about female sexual difficulty and dysfunction? J Sex Med 2006;3(4):589–95.
11. Sungur MZ, Gunduz A. A comparison of DSM-IV-TR and DSM-5 definitions for sexual dysfunctions: critiques and challenges. J Sex Med 2014;11(2):364–73.
12. IsHak W, Tobia G. DSM-5 changes in diagnostic criteria of sexual dysfunctions. Reprod Sys Sexual Disorders 2013;2(2):122.
13. Burrows LJ, Basha M, Goldstein AT. The effects of hormonal contraceptives on female sexuality: a review. J Sex Med 2012;9(9):2213–23.
14. Gezginc K, Balci O, Karatayli R, et al. Contraceptive efficacy and side effects of Implanon. Eur J Contracept Reprod Health Care 2007;12(4):362–5.
15. Skrzypulec V, Drosdzol A. Evaluation of quality of life and sexual functioning of women using levonorgestrel-releasing intrauterine contraceptive system–Mirena. Coll Antropol 2008;32(4):1059–68.
16. Davis SR, Davison SL, Donath S, et al. Circulating androgen levels and self-reported sexual function in women. JAMA 2005;294(1):91–6.
17. Herbenick D, Reece M, Schick V, et al. Sexual behaviors, relationships, and perceived health status among adult women in the United States: results from a national probability sample. J Sex Med 2010;7(Suppl 5):277–90.
18. Davis SR, Moreau M, Kroll R, et al. Testosterone for low libido in postmenopausal women not taking estrogen. N Engl J Med 2008;359(19):2005–17.
19. Panay N, Al-Azzawi F, Bouchard C, et al. Testosterone treatment of HSDD in naturally menopausal women: the ADORE study. Climacteric 2010;13(2):121–31.
20. Braunstein GD, Sundwall DA, Katz M, et al. Safety and efficacy of a testosterone patch for the treatment of hypoactive sexual desire disorder in surgically menopausal women: a randomized, placebo-controlled trial. Arch Intern Med 2005;165(14):1582–9.
21. Davis S, Papalia MA, Norman RJ, et al. Safety and efficacy of a testosterone metered-dose transdermal spray for treating decreased sexual satisfaction in premenopausal women: a randomized trial. Ann Intern Med 2008;148(8):569–77.

22. Symonds T, Spino C, Sisson M, et al. Methods to determine the minimum important difference for a sexual event diary used by postmenopausal women with hypoactive sexual desire disorder. J Sex Med 2007;4(5):1328–35.
23. White WB, Grady D, Giudice LC, et al. A cardiovascular safety study of LibiGel (testosterone gel) in postmenopausal women with elevated cardiovascular risk and hypoactive sexual desire disorder. Am Heart J 2012;163(1):27–32.
24. Safarinejad MR. Reversal of SSRI-induced female sexual dysfunction by adjunctive bupropion in menstruating women: a double-blind, placebo-controlled and randomized study. J Psychopharmacol 2011;25(3):370–8.
25. Higgins A, Nash M, Lynch AM. Antidepressant-associated sexual dysfunction: impact, effects, and treatment. Drug Healthc Patient Saf 2010;2:141–50.
26. Anderson HD, Pace WD, Libby AM, et al. Rates of 5 common antidepressant side effects among new adult and adolescent cases of depression: a retrospective US claims study. Clin Ther 2012;34(1):113–23.
27. Taylor MJ, Rudkin L, Bullemor-Day P, et al. Strategies for managing sexual dysfunction induced by antidepressant medication. Cochrane Database Syst Rev 2013;(5):CD003382.
28. Nurnberg HG, Hensley PL, Heiman JR, et al. Sildenafil treatment of women with antidepressant-associated sexual dysfunction: a randomized controlled trial. JAMA 2008;300(4):395–404.
29. Rothschild AJ. Selective serotonin reuptake inhibitor-induced sexual dysfunction: efficacy of a drug holiday. Am J Psychiatry 1995;152(10):1514–6.
30. Segraves RT, Clayton A, Croft H, et al. Bupropion sustained release for the treatment of hypoactive sexual desire disorder in premenopausal women. J Clin Psychopharmacol 2004;24(3):339–42.
31. Safarinejad MR, Hosseini SY, Asgari MA, et al. A randomized, double-blind, placebo-controlled study of the efficacy and safety of bupropion for treating hypoactive sexual desire disorder in ovulating women. BJU Int 2010;106(6):832–9.
32. Ferguson DM, Hosmane B, Heiman JR. Randomized, placebo-controlled, double-blind, parallel design trial of the efficacy and safety of Zestra in women with mixed desire/interest/arousal/orgasm disorders. J Sex Marital Ther 2010;36(1):66–86.
33. Basson R, McInnes R, Smith MD, et al. Efficacy and safety of sildenafil citrate in women with sexual dysfunction associated with female sexual arousal disorder. J Womens Health Gend Based Med 2002;11(4):367–77.
34. Schoen C, Bachmann G. Sildenafil citrate for female sexual arousal disorder: a future possibility? Nat Rev Urol 2009;6(4):216–22.
35. Berman JR, Berman LA, Toler SM, et al. Safety and efficacy of sildenafil citrate for the treatment of female sexual arousal disorder: a double-blind, placebo controlled study. J Urol 2003;170(6 Pt 1):2333–8.
36. Pereira VM, Arias-Carrion O, Machado S, et al. Sex therapy for female sexual dysfunction. Int Arch Med 2013;6(1):37.
37. Sinha A, Ewies AA. Non-hormonal topical treatment of vulvovaginal atrophy: an up-to-date overview. Climacteric 2013;16(3):305–12.
38. Cardozo L, Bachmann G, McClish D, et al. Meta-analysis of estrogen therapy in the management of urogenital atrophy in postmenopausal women: second report of the Hormones and Urogenital Therapy Committee. Obstet Gynecol 1998;92(4 Pt 2):722–7.
39. Krychman ML. Vaginal estrogens for the treatment of dyspareunia. J Sex Med 2011;8(3):666–74.

40. Le Ray I, Dell'Aniello S, Bonnetain F, et al. Local estrogen therapy and risk of breast cancer recurrence among hormone-treated patients: a nested case-control study. Breast Cancer Res Treat 2012;135(2):603–9.
41. Kendall A, Dowsett M, Folkerd E, et al. Caution: vaginal estradiol appears to be contraindicated in postmenopausal women on adjuvant aromatase inhibitors. Ann Oncol 2006;17(4):584–7.
42. Santen RJ, Pinkerton JV, Conaway M, et al. Treatment of urogenital atrophy with low-dose estradiol: preliminary results. Menopause 2002;9(3):179–87.
43. Bachmann GA, Komi JO, Ospemifene Study Group. Ospemifene effectively treats vulvovaginal atrophy in postmenopausal women: results from a pivotal phase 3 study. Menopause 2010;17(3):480–6.
44. Portman DJ, Bachmann GA, Simon JA, et al. Ospemifene, a novel selective estrogen receptor modulator for treating dyspareunia associated with postmenopausal vulvar and vaginal atrophy. Menopause 2013;20(6):623–30.
45. Simon JA, Lin VH, Radovich C, et al. One-year long-term safety extension study of ospemifene for the treatment of vulvar and vaginal atrophy in postmenopausal women with a uterus. Menopause 2013;20(4):418–27.

Intimate Partner Violence

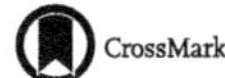

Prevalence, Health Consequences, and Intervention

Nancy Sugg, MD, MPH

KEYWORDS

• Intimate partner • Violence • Health • Intervention • Spouse abuse
• Domestic violence

KEY POINTS

- Intimate partner violence (IPV) affects women and men regardless of race, sexual orientation, or socioeconomic status.
- One in 3 women and 1 in 4 men experience some form of IPV in their lifetimes.
- Patients who experience IPV are more likely to present with health complaints that are not acute injuries, such as headache, gastrointestinal disorders, insomnia, or depression.
- The medical provider's role is to acknowledge the problem of IPV, assess safety, make appropriate referrals, and provide appropriate medical documentation.

DEFINITION

Intimate partner violence (IPV) can be defined in many ways and encompasses many different types of physical and emotional abuse.[1,2] The US Centers for Disease Control and Prevention (CDC) provides a basic definition: "Physical, sexual, or psychological harm by a current or former partner or spouse."[1]

Important caveats are that the violence can occur between couples of any sexual orientation and the relationship does not have to include sexual intimacy.

A variety of behavior can be classed in each of these broad categories. The behaviors may occur in isolation or as an ongoing pattern of abuse.

Physical Violence

Physical violence can range from slapping or shoving to severe physical violence such as a hit with a fist or an object, burning, beating, choking, or the use of a knife or gun.

Sexual Violence

Sexual violence can include noncontact sexual experiences such as coercing or forcing to participate in sexual photographs or videos, unwanted kissing or fondling,

Department of Medicine, Harborview's Pioneer Square Clinic, University of Washington, 206 3rd Avenue South, Seattle, WA 98104, USA
E-mail address: sugg@uw.edu

Med Clin N Am 99 (2015) 629–649
http://dx.doi.org/10.1016/j.mcna.2015.01.012 medical.theclinics.com
0025-7125/15/$ – see front matter

sexual contact when the victim is unable to consent because of drug or alcohol use, and attempted or completed rape.

Psychological Aggression

Psychological aggression can involve name calling and derogatory statements or use of intense anger as a means of control. Threatening behaviors can range from threats to pets or property to threats of suicide or death threats. Forced or coerced social isolation, restriction of ability to freely come and go, control or coercion of finances, and deprivation or control of food or medical care are all in this category.

Stalking

Stalking includes behaviors or tactics such as unwanted contact by phone, texting, or e-mail; being followed; or entering a home uninvited, which results in fear for safety.

Control of Reproductive and Safe Sex Choices

This category can involve manipulation or control of birth control, refusal to use a condom or failure to disclose a sexually transmitted disease (STD), or attempting to impregnate or attempting to get pregnant without the partner's consent.

Patterns of IPV

The terms "perpetrator" and "victim" are used in this article but are inherently poor terms. The term "victim" diminishes the reality of the strength and resilience of people who are dealing with the effects of IPV in their lives. It also carries the connotation of being helpless and without power, which is not a useful message for patients experiencing IPV.

In addition, the terms "victim" and "perpetrator" do not take into account various patterns of IPV in which the abuse and violence is bidirectional. Johnson and Ferraro[3] categorize IPV into 4 patterns.

Situational couple violence (SCV) is violence that does not arise from a pattern of control but is in response to a specific stress, frustration, or argument. The investigators found that this type of violence was more likely to be mutual, less likely to be severe violence, and less likely to escalate over time and become chronic.

Intimate terrorism is a pattern of violence and abuse that is motivated by the desire to control the partner. As opposed to SCV, intimate terrorism is less likely to be mutual, and more likely to escalate and involve serious injury.

Violent resistance describes violence used by the primary victim to defend against violence or controlling behavior of a partner, and is most often used by women against a partner in response to intimate terrorism.

Mutual violent control (MVC) defines situations in which the violence and abusive behavior are bidirectional and motivated by each partner attempting to control the other.[3–5] There are data to suggest that, among adolescent and young adults in heterosexual relationships, reciprocal violence such as SCV and MVC may be the most dangerous in terms of injury.[6]

PREVALENCE IN THE GENERAL POPULATION

The CDC-sponsored National Intimate Partner and Sexual Violence Survey (NISVS), is one of the largest national surveys examining the prevalence, characteristics, and impact of IPV on women and men in the United States.[7] The study found the following:

- More than 1 in 3 women (35.6%) and 1 in 4 men (28.5%) have experienced rape, physical violence, and/or stalking by an intimate partner in their lifetimes.

- When women experience rape, physical violence, or stalking they are 3 times as likely to be injured compared with men (41.6% vs 13.9% respectively).
- Women are nearly twice as likely to experience severe physical violence (eg, being hit with fist, kicked, choked, beaten, burned, or the use of a knife or gun) compared with men (24.3% vs 13.8% respectively).
- Nearly 1 in 10 women in the United States have been raped by an intimate partner.

These prevalence rates are likely to be an underestimate of the actual rates. The denominator includes participants who responded "do not know" or refused to answer. It is also likely that, because of safety concerns or ongoing emotional stress from current or past violence, some participants were not willing to disclose abuse. The survey also did not capture populations that speak languages other than English or Spanish, those that live in institutions (prisons, nursing homes), or those who are homeless.

Gender

There is no typical battered woman. Certain factors such as young age, female gender, and having a lower income are associated with higher rates of violence, but IPV affects all socioeconomic and demographic groups. As noted earlier, although women are more likely to be injured in violent relationships, men are also victims of violence. The prevalence rate among men is significant and the NISVS study found that nearly two-thirds of men affected by IPV did not receive the services needed.

Age

The NISVS found that among both men and women more than 18 years of age, the highest risk of IPV occurs between the ages of 18 and 24 years. However, 1.4% of men and women more than 55 years of age experienced IPV in the past year, which represents more than 1 million people per year in this older age group. Adolescence (ie, ages 11–18 years) is also a high-risk time for violence. This age group is more likely to experience violence from intimate partners as well as other family members or care givers. The CDC Youth Risk Behavior Surveillance Survey found that 10% of adolescents had experienced physical violence in a dating relationship in the past year, with female adolescents having higher rates than male adolescents (13% and 7.4% respectively).[8] Other studies have found rates of ever experiencing physical or sexual violence to be between 20% and 40% among female adolescents.[9,10] More disturbing is the NISVS finding that, among adults who have experienced rape, physical violence, or stalking by an intimate partner, 22.4% of women and 15% of men had their first experience of IPV between the ages of 11 and 17 years.

Race

Multiracial women experience a significantly higher lifetime prevalence of IPV (53.8%) and Asian-Pacific Islanders experience a significantly lower rate (19.6%) compared with white women (34.6%).[7] Among men experiencing rape, physical violence, or stalking, Native American or Alaska Native men experience significantly higher rates compared with Hispanic men (45.3%vs 26.6%). Across all racial groups the prevalence of IPV is high. The lower prevalence found among Asian-Pacific Islander women still represents 1 in 5 women experiencing IPV during their lifetimes. Place of birth also influences rates of IPV. Breiding and colleagues[7] found that men and women born in the United States are significantly more likely to experience IPV compared with those born outside the United States.

Sexual Orientation

Although much of the medical literature regarding IPV mirrors public perception that IPV is mainly an issue for heterosexual couples, recent studies have shown high rates among lesbian, gay, bisexual, and transgendered (LGBT) couples. The NISVS found the highest prevalence of lifetime physical violence, rape, and stalking to be among bisexual women (61.1%) compared with lesbian (43.8%) or heterosexual (35%) women.[11] Bisexual women experiencing IPV were significantly more likely to experience severe violence and most (89.5%) report having only male perpetrators. Similarly, bisexual men had the highest prevalence of IPV (37.3%), although this is not statistically different from gay (26%) or heterosexual (29%) men. There was no significant difference in rates of severe physical violence between gay and heterosexual men, with bisexual men having numbers too small to report. Note that most (78.5%) bisexual men reported only having a female perpetrator of violence.

A systematic review of studies involving IPV among men who have sex with men (MSM) found rates of physical violence ranging from 13% to 38% from a variety of socioeconomic groups and study locations (human immunodeficiency virus [HIV] clinics, gay pride events, state and national random digit dialing).[12] The investigators noted that all forms of IPV occur among MSM at rates similar to or higher than those reported for women. Transgendered individuals have similarly high rates of lifetime physical abuse (34.6%) and may have difficulty accessing IPV services and shelters that are mostly oriented toward heterosexual women.[13]

Socioeconomic Status

Income status can also not be used to determine risk for IPV. Although rape, physical violence, and stalking by an intimate partner in the previous 12 months was significantly more likely to be reported among individuals with incomes less than $25,000 per year, 2% to 4% of men and women with incomes more than $75,000 also reported IPV. This percentage translates to more than 2 million men and women in the higher socioeconomic group experiencing IPV every year. Beyond just using income as a marker of socioeconomic status, food and housing insecurity also measures an important social determinant of health. Women and men who lived with food and housing insecurity were significantly more likely to report IPV in the last 12 months.[7]

PREVALENCE IN HEALTH CARE SETTINGS

It is challenging to compare prevalence rates between different health care settings because a variety of different approaches are used in measuring IPV. The type or types of behaviors studied vary (ie, physical violence only versus various combinations of physical, psychological, or sexual aggression). The definitions of each behavior type vary: for sexual aggression, some investigators only study attempted or completed rape, whereas others include all forms of unwanted sexual experiences. Studies have differed in using direct questions or validated tools. Means of data collection vary, including direct face-to-face surveys, written questionnaires, computerized questionnaires, or random digit dialing telephone surveys. The recall times studied include the past 30 days, the past 6 months, the past 12 months, current relationship, most recent relationship, adult life, or lifetime. Eligibility criteria have varied by age, gender, or sexual orientation. Acutely ill or cognitively impaired patients were often not included in studies. Participation was often limited to English or English and Spanish speaking only.

Primary Care

Over the past 2 decades several studies in family and internal medicine clinics have attempted to determine the prevalence of current or lifetime IPV in populations seen at their clinics. In a systematic review of medical clinics, Sprague and colleagues[14] tabulated the results from a variety of primary care and subspecialty studies in the United States and internationally. In the United States, among patients in family medicine clinics, lifetime IPV rate (physical, sexual, and emotional) ranged from 45% to 66%. The prevalence rate in the current relationship ranged from 13% to 21%.

Specialty Care

Even among patients attending specialty care clinics, high rates of IPV are identified. Orthopedic surgery is considered a specialty likely to have a high rate of patients injured in IPV assaults. A study in 2 Canadian orthopedic fracture clinics confirms this assumption, with an overall (physical, sexual, emotional) IPV rate of 32% in the past 12 months for women attending the clinic, with 2.5% of women reporting their current injury to be IPV related.[15]

Emergency Department

Studies in emergency departments (EDs) find high rates of lifetime IPV, ranging from 30% to 60%, and 1-year prevalence ranging from 12% to 20%.[16–20] Among women seen in the ED, approximately 2% are there for acute trauma related to IPV and 11.7% are there for IPV trauma or other IPV-related medical conditions.[19,20] Among female patients with trauma admitted to a level 1 trauma center, 46.3% experienced severe IPV in their lifetimes and 26% in the past year.[21]

Obstetrics/Reproductive Health

The prevalence of violence against women during pregnancy ranges from 0.9% to 20.1%, with most studies being in the 4% to 8% range.[22] The higher rates were often associated with asking more than once during the pregnancy with face-to-face interviews and with asking during the third trimester and not just as an intake at the beginning of the pregnancy. Higher rates of prenatal violence (16%) have been reported among pregnant adolescents.[23]

Prevalence rates in family planning clinics are also high. In one study of women aged 14 to 26 years who attended a family planning clinic and had a current partner, 43% reported physical abuse.[24] Of those who reported physical abuse, 36% reported more than 1 episode of severe abuse.

HEALTH CONSEQUENCES OF INTIMATE PARTNER VIOLENCE

Medical Consequences

Medical providers often envision lacerations and contusions when they think about IPV. However, women and men who experience IPV are far more likely to present with health complaints that are not acute injuries. Experiencing physical or psychological abuse is associated with significantly higher self-report of poor health.[25,26] The sequelae of IPV often persist long after the violence has ended[27,28] and although it would be logical to assume that most sequelae are directly related to physical violence, Coker and colleagues[25] found that higher scores for psychological IPV were more strongly associated with negative health outcomes than physical IPV scores.

Chronic pain

As expected, chronic pain issues are common among both men and women who experience any form of IPV. Abdominal pain, pelvic pain, headache including migraine, neck pain, and chronic low back pain have all been associated with IPV.[27–29] Wuest and colleagues'[27] study of Canadian women who were survivors of IPV found that

35% experienced high levels of disability chronic pain and that, on average, had 3 separate locations of pain. Along these same lines, Breiding and colleagues[30] found significantly more activity limitations and use of disability equipment among men and women who experience IPV violence.

Gastrointestinal disorders

Gastrointestinal disorders are also common, including peptic ulcer disease, irritable bowel syndrome, gastroesophageal reflux, indigestion, diarrhea, and constipation.[29] It is postulated that both psychological and physiologic mechanisms related to chronic stress are responsible for increases in gastrointestinal symptoms in abused women.[31] These increased gastrointestinal symptoms often lead to increased imaging and invasive diagnostics. Of concern is the finding that patients seen in a gastroenterology clinic with irritable bowl syndrome, dyspepsia, or chronic abdominal pain and a history of childhood or adult abuse were significantly more likely to have lifetime surgeries compared with nonabused patients.[32]

Multiple physical symptoms

Women who experience IPV often have more physical symptoms than nonabused women.[29] A wide range of symptoms, including insomnia, fatigue, fainting, shortness of breath, loss of appetite, vaginal discharge, vaginal bleeding, painful intercourse, and urinary symptoms, have also been associated with current IPV.[26,29,33] Even increased risk of influenza and upper respiratory infections, possibly related to poor immune function caused by stress, have been noted with IPV.[28] However, no discrete set of symptoms has been consistently identified that would inform providers to screen based solely on symptoms.

Chronic disease

Less obvious is the increased association of IPV with chronic diseases. Breiding and colleagues[30] found that both women and men with experience of IPV had increase risk of asthma and stroke. However, only women had a higher risk of high blood pressure, high cholesterol, heart attack, and heart disease associated with IPV.

For many reasons, medical management of all chronic diseases is more challenging for patients experiencing IPV. The chronic stress of violence acutely exacerbates conditions such as hypertension and asthma. Chronic and acute stress are known to activate autonomic, neuroendocrine, immune/inflammatory, and cardiovascular systems, increasing the likelihood of developing and exacerbating cardiovascular disease.[34] Furthermore, men and women who experience IPV are more likely to engage in risky behaviors, such as smoking, that are associated with poorer outcomes for patients with chronic diseases.[30] In addition, perpetrators can use control of medication or access to care as a form of abuse. One study found that nearly 1 in 5 women with a history of IPV in the past year had a partner who prevented them from going to a doctor or interfered with their health care.[35] Conversely, of women who reported interference with their health care, more than half reported IPV in the past year.

Increased Health Risk Behavior

Sexually transmitted diseases/human immunodeficiency virus

Multiple studies have shown a significant association between STD and IPV.[28,33,36] Among women attending an STD clinic, 11% had experienced IPV within the last year and 24% within their lifetime[37], rates similar to those found in other clinical settings. The study also found that abused women were twice as likely to have a history of STD compared with never-abused women. As the study investigators point out, multiple different mechanisms may be responsible, including coercive behavior from the perpetrator impairing the victim's ability to practice safe sex; or impaired decision making on the part of the victim caused by psychological trauma, posttraumatic stress disorder (PTSD), or substance use. IPV was significantly associated with the victim having used alcohol at the last sexual encounter and with the partner not being monogamous.

HIV shares some of the same risk behaviors as other STDs but also includes behaviors such as intravenous (IV) drug use and sex with partners at high risk for HIV. Among predominantly minority women seeking care at an urban hospital, those who had ever experienced IPV were 3 times as likely to have had multiple sexual partners and 2 to 4 times as likely to intermittently or never use condoms. Of increasing concern is that women who were experiencing IPV in their current relationship were 4 times as likely to have a partner with a known HIV risk factor (IV drug user, recent STD symptoms or diagnosis, recent sex with another man or woman, or known to be HIV positive).[38] The large multistate Behavioral Risk Factor Surveillance System found that men and women with lifetime IPV experience were more than twice as likely to have HIV risk factors including having used IV drugs, history of an STD, ever having given or received money or sex for drugs, or having had anal sex without a condom in the past year. Using data from the National Epidemiologic Survey on Alcohol and Related Conditions, Sareen and colleagues[39] found a significant association between HIV infection and IPV, with an odds ratio of 3.4. Based on these data it is estimated that 12% of the cases of HIV infection among women are attributable to IPV.

Alcohol and substance abuse

Multiple studies have documented the increased risk of alcohol and substance abuse among persons experiencing IPV.[25,29,33] Bonomi and colleagues[33] found that women experiencing current abuse were nearly 6 times as likely to have a substance abuse diagnosis. Conversely, patients who are diagnosed with alcohol or substance abuse issues are at higher risk of IPV.[40–42] Among women who attended a methadone maintenance clinic, nearly half had experienced IPV in the past month and nearly 20% experienced severe physical or sexual violence or severe injury by an intimate partner in the past 6 months.[41] Similarly, Waller and colleagues[42] found that women who drank heavily, infrequently, or frequently (but not occasionally) were 2 to 3 times more likely to experience IPV. One theory is that victims of IPV abuse alcohol or illegal substances as a coping mechanism for the IPV.[28] Another possibility is that women who are alcohol or drug dependent are more likely to be in relationships with men who are alcohol or drug dependent, and the strong association between male substance use and IPV perpetration is well documented.[40,43] Regardless of which came first or the multiple complex causalities, if a provider diagnoses alcohol or substance abuse, it is important to screen for IPV, and vice versa. In addition, it needs to be recognized that IPV and substance abuse are 2 distinct health risks and both need to be addressed separately. Just because a person stops drinking does not mean that the IPV risk will necessarily decrease, and, similarly, ending a violent relationship does not always mean that the alcohol abuse will resolve.

Mental Health Consequences

Depression

The recurrent emotional abuse, threats, and physical violence experienced by victims of IPV result in an increased risk of depression and anxiety.[25,28,29,33] Depressed mood, poor sleep, inability to concentrate, and feelings of hopelessness are often experienced by patients in abusive relationships. A meta-analysis by Devries and colleagues[44] found evidence that women with preexisting depression were more likely to experience IPV. Not only do depressive symptoms negatively affect quality of life but they also may hinder people's ability to protect themselves.

Posttraumatic stress disorder

PTSD is also frequently diagnosed among women who experience IPV, with rates ranging from 31% to 84.4%.[45] More severe or frequent physical violence, sexual violence, or use of a weapon have been related to the development and increased symptoms of PTSD, but there is also evidence that psychological abuse may be an even stronger predictor of PTSD.[45,46] The intrusive thoughts or nightmares, hyperarousal state, avoidant behavior, and negative and sometimes distorted thoughts and beliefs can occur for years after the abuse has ended. Neuroendocrine and immune function abnormalities associated with PTSD lead to increased insulin resistance and increased central obesity, thereby increasing the risk of obesity, diabetes, and cardiovascular disease.[47] PTSD is often associated with substance abuse and other poor health habits.[45] Furthermore, depression and PTSD are highly likely to co-occur.[46]

Suicide

Suicide attempts are strongly associated with IPV. A study of formerly abused women experiencing chronic pain found that 31% had attempted suicide at some point in their lifetimes[27] and a study of urban women found that abused women were nearly 8 times more likely to attempt suicide than nonabused women.[48] In the latter study, women who were abused and HIV positive were nearly 13 times more likely to attempt suicide compared with nonabused, HIV-negative women.[48] Among male veterans receiving Veterans Health Administration services, nearly 30% of men with a history of IPV had attempted suicide, which was twice the rate of men without a history of IPV.[49] Only 1 of the 53 men who screened positive for IPV reported perpetration without victimization. Data on completed suicides and IPV are scarce but one report from the New Mexico Office of the Medical Investigator found that IPV was documented in 5% of female suicide deaths.[50] The National Violent Death Reporting System found that, in 2010, intimate partner problems were a precipitating factor for 32% of male and 27% of female suicides.[51] The report further found that 1% of female and 0.3% of male suicide victims had experienced interpersonal violence and 4% of male and 1.4% of female suicide victims had perpetrated interpersonal violence in the month before the suicide. However, the terms "intimate partner problems" and "interpersonal violence" may not be synonymous with IPV. However, given the high rates of depression and PTSD, persons experiencing IPV are at higher risk of suicide attempts and completed suicides.

As with substance abuse, the strong association of mental health issues with IPV makes screening for both imperative. If depression or PTSD is diagnosed or a patient has attempted suicide, screening for IPV must be part of the assessment. If a patient is experiencing IPV, then screening for depression, PTSD symptoms, and suicidal ideation must also be part of the evaluation.

Pregnancy

As noted earlier, the prevalence of IPV during pregnancy is significant. For some women, preexisting abuse continues despite the pregnancy. For others the abuse abates during this time. For some, their first experience of abuse occurs with the pregnancy. Identification of IPV during pregnancy is crucial because the consequences of violence affect not only the health of the mother but also the baby.

A strong association exists between IPV and unintended pregnancies.[52] Unintended pregnancies can include mistimed pregnancies that would be wanted if they occurred at a different time, and unwanted pregnancies that would not be wanted at any time.

Goodwin and colleagues[53] found that women with unintended pregnancies that resulted in a live birth were 2.5 times as likely to experience physical abuse around the time of pregnancy as women with intended pregnancies, and this increased risk remained strongest for older, more educated women of higher socioeconomic status when controlling for maternal characteristics. Conversely, Pallitto and colleagues[52] found that women who had been physically or sexually abused had a 41% higher risk of an unintended pregnancy in the past 5 years. Multiple factors may account for the increase in mistimed and unwanted pregnancies. Miller and colleagues[54] found that, among young adult women seeking care in a family planning clinic, 35% reporting IPV also reported reproductive control by their partner. Reproductive control included pregnancy coercion and birth control sabotage. Pregnancy coercion included behavior such as attempts to force or pressure the victim into becoming pregnant and threats to leave the relationship or threats to harm the victim if they did not agree to become pregnant. Birth control sabotage included sabotaging or refusing to use condoms or preventing access to birth control pills. Other factors have also been cited to account for the overlap of IPV and unintended pregnancies, including the role that stress around an unintended pregnancy might play in increasing violence between partners. In addition, women who experience sexual violence and rape are at increased risk of unintended pregnancies. In addition to unintended pregnancies, Hathaway and colleagues[55] found that women described pressured or forced abortions or forced sterilizations as an additional means of reproductive control by an abusive partner.

Determining adverse pregnancy outcomes related specifically to IPV is challenging. Patient characteristics such as young age and low income are risk factors for both IPV and poor pregnancy outcomes. Known risk behaviors for poor pregnancy outcomes such as smoking and substance abuse are also risk behaviors found in pregnant women who experience IPV.[56] Women who experience IPV are nearly twice as likely to delay entry into prenatal care (entering care in the second or third trimester) but after controlling for maternal characteristics this association only remains for older, more affluent women.[57]

The overlap of risk factors between IPV and pregnancy outcomes and the heterogeneity of study methods used in various studies makes teasing out the specific role of IPV difficult. Low birth weight, premature and very premature births, antepartum hemorrhage, and perinatal deaths are some of the adverse pregnancy outcomes documented in the literature as being associated with IPV during pregnancy.[58–61] However, other studies have failed to show an association of abuse with low birth weight or the association was no longer significant after adjusting for confounding factors such as smoking, alcohol, maternal weight gain, or maternal health.[52] A meta-analysis of 8 studies did find abused women who experienced physical, sexual, or emotional abuse to be at increased risk of giving birth to a low birth weight baby by an odds ratio of 1.4%.[62]

The mechanisms by which adverse pregnancy outcomes can occur include direct trauma resulting in antepartum hemorrhage or perinatal death; stress leading to poor weight gain by the mother; or risk behaviors including alcohol, smoking, and substance abuse, for which abused women are known to be at higher risk. Prematurity and low birth rates often result in long-term sequelae for the children, including cognitive impairment, motor and language delays, as well as behavioral and psychological problems.[56] Thus the physical and psychological consequences of IPV can extend directly to the children.

Adolescent Health

Given the high rate of IPV among adolescents and very young adults, their health risks and health consequences require specific attention. Silverman and colleagues[10] found that among female students in grades 9 to 12, those experiencing physical and/or sexual violence or both were significantly more likely to use alcohol, tobacco, and cocaine; to use laxatives, diet pills, or to intentionally vomit; to have early sexual intercourse and multiple partners; and to have suicidal ideation and suicide attempts. Female students who experience both physical and sexual violence were 4 times as likely to ever have been pregnant and 8 times as likely to attempt suicide. A study of adolescent and young women attending a family planning clinic found that those with very recent IPV were nearly twice as likely to have unprotected vaginal sex and more than twice as likely to have unprotected anal sex.[63] The study found that physically or sexually abused young women were 4 times as likely to fear asking to use a condom and 11 times more likely to fear refusing sex. Furthermore, female adolescents experiencing recent teen dating violence were more than 3 times as likely to use IV drugs or have a partner who used IV drugs compared with those not currently experiencing teen dating violence.[63] Teens experiencing dating violence are at high risk of STD (including HIV), teen pregnancy, and substance abuse.

Teen girls who report poor health are more likely to have experience dating violence.[9] The adverse effects of teen dating violence extend into early adulthood. A study of men and women who reported psychological or physical violence by a dating partner in their adolescence found that, in follow-up 5 years later, women reported increased heavy episodic drinking and depression, whereas men reported increased antisocial behavior and marijuana use.[64] Both men and women reported increased suicidal ideation and adult IPV victimization.

Injury

Physical injury from IPV can include scratches, bruises, contusions, lacerations, fractured teeth, bone fractures, joint dislocations, strains, sprains, abdominal and pelvic injuries, head injuries, and strangulation-related injuries. A meta-analysis of ED studies found that head, neck, or facial injuries were significantly associated with IPV in women who presented to the ED, whereas extremity injuries were less likely to involve IPV.[65] In an earlier study by Muelleman and colleagues,[66] in addition to head, neck, and facial injuries, thorax and abdominal injuries were also significantly more common among abused women. Although the study was able to identify 12 specific injury types that occurred more frequently in abused women, the positive predictive value was low. Other studies have also noted that women injured by IPV were more likely to have multiple injuries compared with women who experienced accidental injuries.[65] Among injured women, excluding motor vehicle accidents, multiple injuries mainly involving the head, neck, and trunk should increase the suspicion for IPV.

The good news regarding injury is that over the past 2 decades the US Department of Justice has found that the rate of serious IPV has declined by 72% for women and 64% for men.[67] However, among those who have injuries, 13% of women and 5% of men have severe injury such as internal injury, unconsciousness, or broken bones. In addition, only 18% of women and 11% of men sought medical treatment of their injuries.

Kothari and Rhodes[68] found that, among female victims of IPV identified in a police database, 64% received care in an ED in the year before the assault. The median number of ED visits over the course of 3 years was 4 for this same group. For most visits (71%), the victims were being seen for non–injury-related complaints. This finding again emphasizes that by only screening patients who present with injuries a large number of people who are at risk for IPV-related health consequences are missed.

Homicide

Homicide is the ultimate injury inflicted on a victim by an intimate partner. Based on information reported to the US Federal Bureau of Investigation, 14% of all homicides in the United States are committed by an intimate partner.[69] Women account for 70% of victims killed by an intimate partner. Put another way, when women are murdered, 45% of the time they are killed by a spouse, ex-spouse, boyfriend, or girlfriend. In comparison, 5% of male homicide victims are killed by an intimate partner. However, there is positive progress even in these grim statistics. Although 14% of all homicides are committed by an intimate partner, this represents a 29% reduction between 1993 and 2007. During this time period, female intimate partner homicides decreased by 35% and male intimate partner homicides decreased by 46%.

Of special note are the homicide-suicide incidents that occur, in which the perpetrator of the homicide then commits suicide. In one study of homicide-suicide incidents, most of the homicide victims were female (75%) and in nearly 60% of all homicide-suicide incidents, the victim is a current or former intimate partner of the perpetrator.[70] Furthermore, the study found that 31% of men who killed their intimate partner went on to commit suicide within 24 hours compared with 6% of women.[70] Another study of medical examiner records found that in cases of intimate partner homicide-suicide, 95% were female homicides followed by male suicides. Of the women who were murdered, 11% were pregnant or within 1 year postpartum.[71]

The homicide rates presented earlier do not fully take into account all the lives lost because of IPV because most homicide rates only focus on the intimate partner couple. The rates do not reflect the deaths of others at the hands of the perpetrator. A study using data from the National Violent Death Reporting System found that in IPV-related homicide incidents, 80% of the homicide victims are the intimate partner, but 20% are corollary homicide victims.[72] These victims included family members, new intimate partners, friends, neighbors, acquaintances, police officers, and sometimes strangers, and 38% of the family member homicide victims were aged 11 years or younger.

SCREENING

Many professional organizations, including the American Medical Association, the American College of Obstetrics and Gynecology, the American Nurses Association, the Joint Commission on the Accreditation of Hospitals and Health Care Organizations, and the Institute of Medicine (IOM) have all recommended routine screening for IPV. The IOM recommendations were adopted by the Department of Health and Human Services and are now incorporated into their Women's Preventive Service Guidelines to be covered under the Affordable Care Act.[73] Although screening is supported by many medical organizations, there is little consensus on best methods, tools, or intervals for screening. There is also lack of consensus regarding routine (universal) screening of all patients versus selective screening (case finding) of patients who have higher-risk symptoms (somatization or chronic pain), belong to a high-risk group (adolescent girls, unintended pregnancies), or have known risk factors (mental illness, substance abuse).

Despite the acceptance of the importance of screening by many large medical organizations there is still controversy regarding the efficacy of screening. In 2010 the US Preventive Services Task Force (USPSTF) recommended routine screening of all women of childbearing age[74]; however, a Cochrane Review determined that there was insufficient evidence for routine screening in health care settings.[75] The Cochrane Review found that routine screening did increase identification of abused women in antenatal settings but not other health care settings, and found no evidence that screening significantly improved health outcomes such as recurrence of violence, quality of life, PTSD, or substance abuse. The USPSTF recommendations for routine screening of women in childbearing years were based on research showing several screening tools having high diagnostic accuracy and on intervention trials that showed lower rates of recurrent abuse experiences.

Whether screening is done routinely or for case finding, it is important to create an environment in which patients are comfortable in discussing IPV. Placing posters in the waiting room and brochures in the bathroom gives the message that IPV is an important health issue and indicates a willingness on the part of providers to discuss it. If an intake health questionnaire is used, having a question about IPV communicates to patients that this is a standard question asked of all patients, provides permission for patients to discuss the issue, and reminds providers to ask as part of a general history. It is also of paramount importance to interview the patient alone. Finding nonthreatening ways to have the partner or older children (age >2 years) leave the room can be challenging but is the only safe and effective way to have a discussion about IPV and other highly confidential health issues.

Screening can occur by many different methods: self-report either in writing or via computer or face-to-face verbal questioning. The method used to screen varies by the patient populations; younger patients may opt for computers, non–English-speaking or low-literacy patients may require face-to-face questioning, and older patients may find written questions to be a less threatening means of screening. Ideally all 3 methods of screening would be available to patients to maximize the case finding and increase patients' comfort levels. However, financial resources and the clinic flow may dictate choosing only 1.

When asking face to face about IPV, it often helps to open with a generalized statement such as:

Many people experience problems at home or in their relationships that can affect their health, so I have started to ask all my patients about any issues at home.

Assure the patient of confidentiality unless it becomes clear that a child is in danger or abused. Use nonjudgmental language, avoiding words that can be misinterpreted (like "abused" or "battered woman"), and then ask directly about behavior:

Have you ever had problems with anyone hitting you or hurting you or threatening you?

There are also a variety of screening tools that have been developed. Again, these can be adapted to self-report via computer or writing or used in a face-to-face screening. An excellent review and critique of the most common tools was done by Rabin and colleagues,[76] who described the complexity of developing a tool when no gold standard exists and the tool must be both comprehensive (covering physical, emotional, and sexual abuse) and concise to make it acceptable to busy medical practices (**Table 1**).

INTERVENTION

Whether by universal screening, symptom-based, or risk factor–based screening, or spontaneous self-report by a patient, medical providers will be faced with patients who are experiencing IPV. When a patient reveals IPV, nonresponse by a medical professional can be devastating. Medical providers must be prepared to engage patients around the issue of IPV and provide assessment and referral.

Much of what is known about effective intervention comes from studies involving women seeking family planning, obstetric, perinatal, or primary care who received

Table 1
Screening tools

Name	Description	Sensitivity (%)/Specificity (%)
HITS[77]	Developed for use in primary care. Four-item tool captures emotional and physical abuse in current relationship but not past sexual abuse	Women: sensitivity, 86; specificity, 99[74] Men: sensitivity, 88; specificity, 97[78]
OVAT[79]	Developed for EDs. Four-item tool measures severe physical violence, emotional abuse, and threats with weapons over past month	Sensitivity: 86 Specificity: 83
PVS[80]	Developed for EDs. Three-item tool measuring past physical violence with any perpetrator and safety with current or former partners	Sensitivity: 35–71[76] Specificity: 80–94[76]
AAS[81]	Developed for prenatal clinics. Five-item tool	Sensitivity: 93–94[76] Specificity: 55–99[76]
WAST[82]	Tested in primary and emergency care settings. Eight-item tool covering physical, emotional, and sexual abuse	Sensitivity: 47[76] Specificity: 96[76]

Abbreviations: AAS, Abuse Assessment Screen; HITS, Hurt, Insulted, Threatened, or Screamed; OVAT, Ongoing Violence Assessment Tool; PVS, Partner Violence Screen; WAST, Woman Abuse Screening Tool.

counseling by social workers, nurses, or community mentors.[83] Many of these studies showed a reduction in IPV and improved birth outcomes but some studies failed to show a significant difference.

However, there are currently no randomized controlled trials to help inform medical providers regarding their role in intervention in the context of a clinical visit. Unique methodological, safety, and ethical issues prevent the important longitudinal studies of effective intervention from readily fitting the classic randomized control trial model. However, best practices, as informed by IPV advocates, IPV survivors, researchers, and medical providers, include acknowledging the problem, assessing safety, referring to appropriate resources, and documenting appropriately in the medical record.

Acknowledge the Problem

Providers must respectfully but effectively convey to their patients that they consider IPV to be a serious health issue. Directly relating the effect that the IPV is currently having on a patient's health is often useful: "Your frequent asthma exacerbations may be related to the stress of what you are experiencing at home." Discussing the linkages between depression or substance use issues and IPV may help patients begin to see connections with their health. Taking an injury prevention stance and discussing the risk of future, potentially worse injuries can be appropriate. Whatever the approach, the message that patients must hear is that this is a serious health issue and their medical providers are concerned.

Assess Safety

Before the patient leaves the office, a safety assessment is critical. The assessment informs the type of resources that the patient needs; for instance, are they safe to go home or do they need to access a domestic violence shelter? The assessment provides the additional benefit of educating the patient about making a safety plan. In addition, it can be used as a tool to assess whether the patient is in significant danger of serious or fatal injury.

The safety assessment can be done by the medical provider, nurse, social worker, or by providing the patient with a private area in which they can call the local domestic violence organization if one is available. Although others in the clinical area can do the assessment, it is important for providers to have a general knowledge of assessing safety. Patients do not always want to talk with the social worker, may be under time constraints, or the nurse or social worker may be unavailable.

Important safety questions to address:

- Do you feel safe to go home?
  - If not, can you stay with a friend or family member safely?
  - Otherwise, refer to a domestic violence shelter
- Do you have a plan if the violence recurs?
  - Can you plan an escape route out of each room of your house, avoiding the bathroom because of lack of egress and the kitchen because of the availability of knives and other objects?
  - Do you have access to money and transportation?
  - Can you make copies of important documents (birth certificates, passports, green cards, marriage license) and put them in a safe place in case you need to leave suddenly?
  - Do you have a plan with your children about what to do if violence starts?
  - Do you know how to call 911 (this is especially important to problem solve if the patient is non–English speaking)?
- Do you believe your partner is capable of killing you?

The last question, if answered positively, could indicate a situation in which the victim may be in greater danger. A danger assessment tool was developed by Campbell and colleagues[84] to assess the likelihood of future severe injury or death and was refined down to 5 questions to increase its utility in a busy clinical environment such as an ED.[85] If 3 of the following 5 questions are answered positively, it is predictive that the patient is at risk of severe injury or death with 83% sensitivity:

1. Has the physical violence increased in frequency or severity over the past 6 months?
2. Has he ever used a weapon or threatened you with a weapon?
3. Do you believe he is capable of killing you?
4. Have you ever been beaten by him while you were pregnant?
5. Is he violently and constantly jealous of you?

If the patient has multiple risk factors for serious injury, the medical provider must frankly discuss the situation with the patient and encourage a strong safety plan. Ultimately it is the patient's decision regarding the next steps to take but, as with any health risk, patients need to be fully informed when making their decisions.

It is not always feasible to do the safety planning during the clinic visit but patients can be educated regarding safety and provided with basic information for formulating a plan. Many small, wallet-sized cards are available that have a detailed safety plan, but patients must decide whether having the card found on them might increase their danger. Importantly, the medical provider must listen to the patients to learn what the patients have tried in the past and are currently doing to keep themselves and their families safe. Supporting the patients and emphasizing their strength and resilience goes further than authoritatively laying out a plan that may not be workable.

Referral

Every medical clinic and ED would ideally have specific staff members who are well trained in addressing IPV with patients. However, this is not the reality for many practice sites. For those lucky enough to be well resourced, a warm hand-off from provider to the staff member goes a long way in helping patients engage in care. For those clinics without on-site resources, the organization Futures Without Violence has developed an excellent guide for helping health care settings develop a protocol for responding to IPV. The National Consensus Guidelines on Identifying and Responding to Domestic Victimization in Health Care Settings can be downloaded from their Web site at www.futureswithoutviolence.org/.[86]

Knowledge of the local IPV resources is imperative. The small investment of time required to become familiar with community resources and how to quickly and effectively access them saves enormous time and frustration at the moment when referrals are needed. Having the local domestic violence agency or shelter present at a staff meeting makes collaboration and communication easier. Patients also sense that they are being referred to a known resource in which the provider has confidence.

Referral to couples therapy may seem appropriate, but should only be done in selective cases with extreme caution. Couples therapy can only be done safely and effectively if both partners feel safe, both come committed to developing an abuse-free relationship, and if the therapist is experienced with issues regarding IPV. Both partners must be equally empowered for counseling to be helpful, which is a situation that does not exist if one person uses violence to control their partner.

At a minimum, have the numbers to the 24-hour crisis line, the local domestic violence agency, the state domestic violence hotline, and/or the National Domestic Violence Hotline (1-800-799-7233) readily available.

The National Domestic Violence Hotline assist patients in finding resources in their area. Their Web site, www.thehotline.org/, also has a chat room for patients to ask questions of an advocate. However, patients should be alerted that computer use can be monitored by an abuser and it is not possible to wipe out all traces of a search. Other options are to use a computer at a public library or community center to protect themselves. The National Domestic Violence Hotline has linkages to all the state domestic violence coalitions, national organizations, and resources specific to teens and LGBT individuals. They are also a valuable resource to obtain IPV brochures and posters. Again, brochures can be informative, but make sure that they do not increase the danger for patients who have them on their persons.

Other Web sites for resources and education:

American Congress of Obstetrics and Gynecology: www.acog.org/
The National Coalition against Domestic Violence: www.ncadv.org/
The National Resource Center on Domestic Violence: www.nrcdv.org/
National Network to End Domestic Violence: www.nnedv.org/
Futures without Violence: www.futureswithoutviolence.org/.

Documentation

Good documentation is vital for many reasons. Documentation helps coordinate care between multidisciplinary providers, including primary care, ED, inpatient, and mental health providers as well as chemical dependency counselors and social workers. It provides legal protection for providers when it is clear that IPV was addressed appropriately. Prosecutors also rely on the documentation in court to bring perpetrators to justice and victims depend on accurate documentation for custody and other legal issues.

If patients are willing to divulge the identity of their assailants, record the name and the relationship of the assailant to the victim (eg, "Patient said to have been stabbed by boyfriend, John Doe …"). This statement does not mean that the provider is accusing John Doe or that the provider has knowledge that the event occurred as stated, only that this is an accurate recording of what the patient stated while in the process of receiving medical care.

If injuries are involved, specify the mechanism of injury (eg, "hit with bat" or "strangled with hands"). Describe all injuries, old and new. Use a body map or, with the patient's permission, take photographs that can be entered into the electronic health record (EHR). If strangulation has occurred, describe any loss of consciousness or near syncope, describe any bruising or swelling around the neck, and describe any hoarseness or vocal changes. If sexual assault has occurred, a rape kit should be done if possible.

Over the course of assessing the patient, which may take more than one visit, document screening for other associated medical conditions, such as depression, PTSD, suicidal ideation, substance abuse, or alcohol dependence.

In the assessment and plan, document that IPV was discussed, safety issues addressed, and resources were made available for the patient. This documentation protects the provider by documenting appropriate responses to IPV and informs other providers who may provide care in the future.

The EHR has made some important improvements in documentation, but, with sensitive issues such as IPV, some caution is needed. Written summaries of the visit are often printed out to give the patient. These summaries may include the problem list. IPV needs to be on the problem list so other members of the care team are alerted; however, it is important for it not to appear on the summary for the patient because it may be acquired by the perpetrator. Similarly, many patients now have open access to their full health records, including visit notes, via computer. Care must be exercised to make sure that confidential information cannot be accessed by the abuser.

LEGAL ISSUES

Laws and mandates around IPV vary from state to state and sometimes from county to county. Knowledge of local laws applicable to the health care setting is essential. Patients should have access to information on how to obtain protection orders. Mandatory arrest is the standard policy in certain regions, requiring police to arrest the primary perpetrator if called for a domestic disturbance. The perpetrator is often kept in jail for 24 hours, allowing the victim time to get assistance from domestic violence advocates. In some states prosecutors can prosecute perpetrators of severe IPV without the victim being present in court, which allows victims to be able to escape a significant abuser and not be retraumatized in court. Medical documentation can be used establish the seriousness of the assault in court.

Mandatory reporting laws are also variable from state to state. Mandatory reporting for elder and child abuse is fairly uniform across the United States. Most states require a police report for any injury by a gun or knife regardless of the perpetrator. Some locales include felony assaults, such as broken bones or injuries requiring hospital admission, as mandated for reporting. A few states require all IPV cases to be reported regardless of the preference of the primary victim. If in doubt about the requirements, a call to Adult Protective Services or the local prosecutor's office is advised.

SELF-DETERMINATION

Just as a medical provider would not start a medication for hypertension and then not schedule a follow-up visit, the diagnosis of IPV requires ongoing monitoring and support. IPV is a complex issue and 1 approach does not fit all patients. Patient-centered care is paramount, providing support and education but ultimately allowing patients to determine the pace and process for change. The resources the patient needs will also change over the course of time. A patient may initially need more safety planning, but later may need help with PTSD symptoms.

Many providers express frustration when a patient does not leave a violent relationship but it is important to understand some of the barriers victims face:

- Fear of death, for themselves or their families
- Fear of reprisal
- Fear of loss of child custody
- Fear of deportation
- Protection of the perpetrator from arrest or deportation
- Religious prohibitions
- Cultural isolation and language barriers
- Lack of job skills
- Poor self-esteem
- Depression

Leaving the relationship is not the only path to safety for patients; other options may exist and providers should be open to these possibilities. Providing a safe, respectful, compassionate place where a patient can reveal IPV is an important first step. Providing education and support in a nonjudgmental and caring manner empowers patients to make healthy changes and end the violence in their lives.

REFERENCES

1. CDC. Available at: http://www.cdc.gov/violenceprevention/intimatepartnerviolence/index.html. Accessed February 20, 2015.
2. WHO. Available at: http://www.who.int/violence_injury_prevention/violence/world_report/factsheets/en/ipvfacts.pdf. Accessed February 20, 2015.
3. Johnson MP, Ferraro K. Research on domestic violence in the 1990s: making distinctions. J Marriage Fam 2000;62:948–63.
4. Miller J. A specification of the types of intimate partner violence experienced by women in the general population. Violence Against Women 2006;12: 1105–31.
5. Stith S, McCollum E, Amanor-Boadu Y, et al. Systemic perspectives on intimate partner violence treatment. J Marital Fam Ther 2012;38(1):220–40.
6. Whitaker K, Haileyesus T, Swahn M. Differences in frequency of violence and reported injury between relationships with reciprocal and nonreciprocal intimate partner violence. Am J Public Health 2007;97(5):941–7.
7. Breiding MJ, Chen J, Black MC. Intimate partner violence in the United States – 2010. Atlanta (GA): National Center for Injury Prevention and Control, Centers for Disease Control and Prevention; 2014.
8. Kann L, Kinchen S, Shanklin SL, et al. Youth risk behavior surveillance – United States, 2013. MMWR Surveill Summ 2014;66(Suppl 4):1–172.
9. Miller E, Decker M, Raj A, et al. Intimate partner violence and health care-seeking patterns among female users of urban adolescent clinics. Matern Child Health J 2010;14:910–7.
10. Silverman J, Raj A, Mucci L, et al. Dating violence against adolescent girls and associated substance use, unhealthy weight control, sexual risk behavior, pregnancy, and suicide. JAMA 2001;286(5):572–9.

11. Walters ML, Chen J, Breiding MJ. The National Intimate Partner and Sexual Violence Survey (NISVS): 2010 findings on victimization by sexual orientation. Atlanta (GA): National Center for Injury Prevention and Control, Centers for Disease Control and Prevention; 2013.
12. Finneran C, Stephenson R. Intimate partner violence among men who have sex with men: a systematic review. Trauma Violence Abuse 2012;14(2):168–85.
13. Ard K, Makadon H. Addressing intimate partner violence in lesbian, gay, bisexual, and transgender patients. J Gen Intern Med 2011;26(8):930–3.
14. Sprague S, Goslings JC, Hogentoren C, et al. Prevalence of intimate partner violence across medical and surgical health care settings: a systematic review. Violence Against Women 2014;20(1):118–36.
15. Bhandari M, Sprague S, Dosanjh S, et al, The PRAISE Investigators. The prevalence of intimate partner violence across orthopaedic fracture clinics in Ontario. J Bone Joint Surg Am 2011;93(2):132–41.
16. Ernst A, Nick T, Weiss S, et al. Domestic violence in an inner-city ED. Ann Emerg Med 1997;30:190–7.
17. Kramer A, Lorenzon D, Mueller G. Prevalence of intimate partner violence and health implications for women using emergency departments and primary care clinics. Womens Health Issues 2004;14:19–29.
18. El-Bassel N, Gilbert L, Wu E, et al. Intimate partner violence prevalence and HIV risks among women receiving care in emergency departments: implications for IPV and HIV screening. Emerg Med J 2007;24:255–9.
19. Abbot J, Johnson R, Koziol-McLain J, et al. Incidence and prevalence in an emergency department population. JAMA 1995;273:1763–7.
20. Dearwater S, Coben J, Campbell J, et al. Prevalence of intimate partner abuse in women treated at community hospital emergency departments. JAMA 1998; 280(5):433–8.
21. Weinsheimer R, Schermer C, Malcoe L, et al. Severe intimate partner violence and alcohol use among female trauma patients. J Trauma 2005;58:22–9.
22. Gazmararian J, Lazorick S, Spitz A, et al. Prevalence of violence against pregnant women. JAMA 1996;275:1915–20.
23. Covington D, Dalton V, Diehl S, et al. Improving detection of violence among pregnant adolescents. J Adolesc Health 1997;21:18–24.
24. Rickert VI, Wiemann C, Harrykissoon S, et al. The relationship among demographics reproductive characteristics, and intimate partner violence. Obstet Gynecol 2002;187:1002–7.
25. Coker A, Davis K, Arias I, et al. Physical and mental health effects of intimate partner violence for men and women. Am J Prev Med 2002;23(4):260–8.
26. Campbell J, Jones A, Dienemann J, et al. Intimate partner violence and physical health consequences. Arch Intern Med 2002;162:1157–63.
27. Wuest J, Merritt-Gray M, Ford-Gilboe M, et al. Chronic pain in women survivors of intimate partner violence. J Pain 2008;9(11):1049–57.
28. Campbell J. Health consequences of intimate partner violence. Lancet 2002;359: 1331–6.
29. McCauley J, Kern D, Kolodner K, et al. The "Battering Syndrome": prevalence and clinical characteristics of domestic violence in primary care internal medicine practices. Ann Intern Med 1995;123(10):737–46.
30. Breiding M, Black M, Ryan G. Chronic disease and health risk behaviors associated with intimate partner violence. Ann Epidemiol 2008;18:538–44.
31. Drossman D, Talley N, Leserman J, et al. Sexual and physical abuse and gastrointestinal illness. Ann Intern Med 1995;123:782–94.

32. Drossman D, Leserman J, Nachman G, et al. Sexual and physical abuse in women with functional or organic gastrointestinal disorders. Ann Intern Med 1990;113:828–33.
33. Bonomi A, Anderson M, Reid R, et al. Medical and psychosocial diagnoses in women with a history of intimate partner violence. Arch Intern Med 2009; 169(18):1692–7.
34. Holmes S, Krantz D, Rogers H, et al. Mental stress and coronary artery disease: a multidisciplinary guide. Prog Cardiovasc Dis 2006;49(2):106–22.
35. McCloskey L, Williams C, Lichter E, et al. Abused women disclose partner interference with health care: an unrecognized form of battering. J Gen Intern Med 2007;22:1067–72.
36. Coker AL, Smith PH, Bethea L, et al. Physical health consequences of physical and psychological intimate partner violence. Arch Fam Med 2000;9(5):451–7.
37. Bauer H, Gibson P, Hernandez M, et al. Intimate partner violence and high-risk sexual behaviors among female patients with sexually transmitted diseases. Sex Transm Dis 2002;29(7):411–6.
38. Wu E, El-Bassel N, Witte S, et al. Intimate partner violence and HIV risk among urban minority women in primary health care settings. AIDS Behav 2003;7(3): 291–301.
39. Sareen J, Pagura J, Grant B. Is intimate partner violence associated with HIV infection among women in the United States? Gen Hosp Psychiatry 2009;31: 274–8.
40. Devries K, Child J, Bacchus L, et al. Intimate partner violence victimization and alcohol consumption in women: a systematic review and meta-analysis. Addiction 2013;109:379–91.
41. El-Bassel N, Gilbert L, Frye V, et al. Physical and sexual intimate partner violence among women in methadone maintenance treatment. Psychol Addict Behav 2004;18(2):180–3.
42. Waller M, Iritani B, Christ S, et al. Relationships among alcohol outlet density, alcohol use, and intimate partner violence victimization among young women in the United States. J Interpers Violence 2012;27(10):2062–86.
43. Nowotny K, Graves J. Substance use and intimate partner violence victimization among white, African American, and Latina women. J Interpers Violence 2013; 28(17):3301–18.
44. Devries K, Mak J, Bacchus L, et al. Intimate partner violence and incident depressive symptoms and suicide attempts: a systematic review of longitudinal studies. PLoS Med 2013;10(5):e1001439.
45. Dutton M, Green B, Kaltman S, et al. Intimate partner violence, PTSD, and adverse health outcomes. J Interpers Violence 2006;21(7):955–68.
46. Pico-Alfonso M, Garcia-Linares I, Celda-Navarro N, et al. The impact of physical, psychological, and sexual intimate male partner violence on women's mental health: depressive symptoms, posttraumatic stress disorder, state anxiety, and suicide. J Womens Health 2006;15(5):599–611.
47. Gill J, Szanton S, Page G. Biological underpinnings of health alterations in women with PTSD: a sex disparity. Biol Res Nurs 2005;7(1):44–54.
48. Gielan A, McDonnel K, O'Campo P, et al. Suicide risk and mental health indicators: do they differ by abuse and HIV status. Womens Health Issues 2005;14:89–95.
49. Cerulli C, Stephens B, Bossarte R. Examining the intersection between suicidal behaviors and intimate partner violence among sample of males receiving services form the Veterans Health Administration. Am J Mens Health 2014;8(5): 440–3.

50. Olson L, Huyler F, Lynch AW, et al. Guns, alcohol, and intimate partner violence: the epidemiology of female suicide in New Mexico. Crisis 1999;20(3):121–6.
51. Parks SE, Johnson LL, McDaniel DD, et al, Centers for Disease control and Prevention. Surveillance for violent deaths - National Violent Death Reporting System, 16 states, 2010. MMWR Surveill Summ 2014;63(1):1–33.
52. Pallitto C, Campbell J, O'Campo P. Is intimate partner violence associated with unintended pregnancy? Trauma Violence Abuse 2005;6(3):217–35.
53. Goodwin M, Gazmararian J, Johnson C, et al, the PRAMS Working Group. Pregnancy intendedness and physical abuse around the time of pregnancy: findings from the pregnancy risk assessment monitoring system, 1996-1997. Matern Child Health J 2000;4(2):85–92.
54. Miller E, Decker M, McCauley H, et al. Pregnancy Coercion, Intimate Partner Violence, and Unintended Pregnancy 2010;81(4):316–22.
55. Hathaway J, Willis G, Zimmer B, et al. Impact of partner abuse on women's reproductive lives. J Am Med Womens Assoc 2005;60(1):42–5.
56. Bailey B. Partner violence during pregnancy: prevalence, effects, screening, and management. Int J Womens Health 2010;2:183–97.
57. Dietz P, Gazmararian J, Goodwin M, et al. Delayed entry into prenatal care: effect of physical violence. Obstet Gynecol 1997;90(2):221–4.
58. Janssen P, Holt V, Sugg N, et al. Intimate partner violence and adverse pregnancy outcomes: a population-based study. Am J Obstet Gynecol 2003;188: 1341–7.
59. Coker A, Sanderson M, Dong B. Partner violence during pregnancy and risk of adverse pregnancy outcomes. Paediatr Perinat Epidemiol 2004;18:260–9.
60. Watson L, Taft A. Intimate partner violence and the association with very preterm birth. Birth 2013;40(1):17–23.
61. Sarkar N. The impact of intimate partner violence on women's reproductive health and pregnancy outcomes. J Obstet Gynaecol 2008;28(3):266–71.
62. Murphy C, Shei B, Myhr T, et al. Abuse: a risk factor for low birth weight? A systematic review and meta-analysis. CMAJ 2001;164(11):1567–72.
63. Decker M, Miller E, McCauley H, et al. Recent partner violence and sexual and drug-related STI/HIV risk among adolescent and young adult women attending family planning clinics. Sex Transm Infect 2014;90:145–9.
64. Exner-Cortens D, Echenrode J, Rothman E. Longitudinal associations between teen dating violence victimization and adverse health outcomes. Pediatrics 2013;131:71–8.
65. Wu V, Huff H, Bhandari M. Pattern of physical injury associated with intimate partner violence in women presenting to the emergency department: a systematic review and meta-analysis. Trauma Violence Abuse 2010;11(2):71–82.
66. Muelleman R, Lenaghan P, Pakieser R. Battered women: injury locations and types. Ann Emerg Med 1996;28:486–92.
67. Catalano S. Intimate partner violence: attributes of victimization, 1993-2011. Available at: http://www.bjs.gov/index.cfm?ty=pbdetail&iid=4801. Accessed September 5, 2014.
68. Kothari C, Rhodes K. Missed opportunities: emergency department visits by police-identified victims of intimate partner violence. Ann Emerg Med 2006; 47(2):190–9.
69. Catalano S. Female victims of violence. Available at: http://www.bjs.gov/index.cfm?ty=pbdetail&iid=2020. Accessed September 5, 2014.
70. Bossarte R, Simon TR, Barker L. Characteristics of homicide followed by suicide incidents in multiple states, 2003-04. Inj Prev 2006;12(Suppl 2):ii33–8.

71. Krulewitch C. Epidemiology of intimate partner homicide-suicide events among women of childbearing age in Maryland, 1994-2003. Am J Forensic Med Pathol 2009;30(4):362–5.
72. Smith S, Fowler K, Niolon P. Intimate partner homicide and corollary victims in 16 states: national violent death reporting system, 2003-2009. Am J Public Health 2014;104:461–6.
73. De Boinville M. ASPE Policy brief: screening for domestic violence in health care settings. Available at: http://aspe.hhs.gov/hsp/13/dv/pb_screeningDomestic.pdf. Accessed February 20, 2015.
74. Moyer V, on behalf of the USPSTF. Screening for intimate partner violence and abuse of elderly and vulnerable adults: U.S. Preventive Services Task Force Recommendation Statement. Ann Intern Med 2013;158:478–86.
75. O'Doherty L, Taft A, Hegarty K, et al. Screening women for intimate partner violence in healthcare settings: abridged Cochrane Systematic Review and meta-analysis. BMJ 2014;348:g2913.
76. Rabin R, Jennings J, Campbell J, et al. Intimate partner violence screening tools. Am J Prev Med 2009;36(5):439–45.
77. Sherin K, Sinacore J, Li X, et al. HITS: a short domestic violence screening tool for use in a family practice setting. Fam Med 1998;30(7):508–12.
78. Shakil A, Smith D, Sinacore J, et al. Validation of the HITS domestic violence screening tool for males. Fam Med 2005;37(3):193–8.
79. Ernst A, Weiss S, Cham E, et al. Detecting ongoing intimate partner violence in the emergency department using a simple 4-question screen: the OVAT. Violence Vict 2004;19(3):375–84.
80. Feldhaus KM, Koziol-McLain J, Amsbury HL, et al. Accuracy of 3 brief screening questions for detecting partner violence in the emergency department. JAMA 1997;277(17):1357–61.
81. McFarlane J, Parker B, Soeken K, et al. Assessing for abuse during pregnancy. Severity and frequency of injuries and associated entry into prenatal care. JAMA 1992;267(23):3176–8.
82. Brown JB, Lent B, Brett PJ, et al. Development of the woman abuse screening tool for use in family practice. Fam Med 1996;28(6):422–8.
83. Nelson H, Bougatsos C, Blazina I. Screening women for intimate partner violence: a systematic review to update the U.S. Preventive Services Task Force recommendations. Ann Intern Med 2012;156:796–808.
84. Campbell J, Webster D, Glass N. The danger assessment: validation of a lethality risk assessment instrument for intimate partner femicide. J Interpers Violence 2009;24(4):653–74.
85. Snider C, Webster D, O'Sullivan C, et al. Intimate partner violence: development of a brief risk assessment for the emergency department. Acad Emerg Med 2009;16:1208–16.
86. The National Consensus Guidelines on Identifying and Responding to Domestic Violence Victimization in Health Care Settings. Available at: http://www.futureswithoutviolence.org/userfiles/file/Consensus.pdf. Accessed February 20, 2015.

Care of Women Veterans

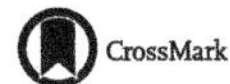

Ximena A. Levander, MD*, Maryann K. Overland, MD

KEYWORDS

- Women veterans • Military cultural competency
- Functional gastrointestinal disorders • Chronic pain syndromes
- Post-traumatic stress disorder • Military sexual trauma • Veteran homelessness

KEY POINTS

- Over the coming decades, as more women join and then complete their service in the US military, women veterans are expected to become an ever-increasing proportion of the total veteran population.
- Health care providers must be aware of the various unique aspects of military culture and understand how the experiences women veterans face during their military service impact their medical, psychiatric, and psychosocial wellbeing.
- Women veterans have been shown to be at higher risk for certain conditions that providers should be aware of and be able to recognize.
- There are extensive national and local resources available to support and to provide comprehensive care to women veterans.
- In order to open the conversation about the potential impacts of military service on patient health, providers must ask all patients about whether they served in the military, especially as some veterans may not initially volunteer this information.

INTRODUCTION

Ms V is a 28-year-old woman coming in to the clinic to establish with a new primary care provider. She complains of neck, lower back, and bilateral hip and knee pain, all of which have limited her ability to do many of the activities and work-related responsibilities she would like to do. She also has issues related to diffuse abdominal discomfort and intermittent constipation and diarrhea. Later on in the appointment, she relays that she had previously been in the Army Reserves. How does this change how one would think about her conditions? Would this information change how one would evaluate and treat her?

Women have a long tradition of service with the US military, having participated in every war since the American Revolution. Early in their military history, women had to

Department of Medicine, VA Puget Sound Health Care System, University of Washington, 1959 Northeast Pacific Street, Seattle, WA 98195-6421, USA
* Corresponding author. 1959 Northeast Pacific Street, Box 356421, Seattle, WA 98195-6421.
E-mail addresses: Ximena@u.washington.edu; ximena@uw.edu

Med Clin N Am 99 (2015) 651–662
http://dx.doi.org/10.1016/j.mcna.2015.01.013 medical.theclinics.com
0025-7125/15/$ – see front matter

disguise themselves as men in order to serve, and it was not until 1901 with the formation of the Army Nurse Corps that women officially became part of the US armed forces.[1]

The percent of women in the military was held stagnant until 1973, when the Congressional legislative cap on women's military participation was lifted.[2] From 1950 to 1980, women comprised just 2% of uniformed personnel, while in 2011 women comprised 14% of active duty and 18% of National Guard and Reserves forces.[3]

Operation Enduring Freedom/Operation Iraqi Freedom/Operation New Dawn (OEF/OIF/OND), collectively known as the Global War on Terrorism (GWOT), resulted in a dramatic increase in the rate of enlistment of women. Upon completion of their service duties, these women have become a part of the US veteran population. Of the over 1 million GWOT veterans who have become eligible and have utilized Veterans (VA) health care, just over 12% are women.[4]

It is estimated that the women veteran population will double over the next decade, with women comprising over 10% of the veterans population by 2020 and almost 18% by 2040.[3,5] This is in the setting of the overall total number of Veterans decreasing over the next few decades from just over 22 million veterans down to an estimated 15 million veterans by 2040.[5]

With the creation of the Women Veterans Task Force of the Department of Veterans Affairs in 2012, the VA has recognized that women veterans represent a unique patient population with specific medical, psychiatric and psychosocial care needs, and that the VA system will need to change in order to optimally deliver health care to this evolving population.[3]

Women veterans are different from male veterans in several ways[3,6]:

- On average women veterans are younger, with an average age of 48, compared with male veterans, who average 62 years of age.
- Women veterans seeking care at the VA are more likely to have a service-connected (SC) disability rating (55% compared with 41% of male veterans). An SC disability is defined as the onset of symptoms or diagnosis during military service regardless of specific cause of symptoms or diagnosis.
- Women veterans with an SC disability rating were more likely than male veterans to have a disability rating greater than 50% (26% compared to 19% of male veterans).
- Women veterans tend to use outpatient services more heavily than male veterans, and this is more likely to be the case in women veterans with concomitant medical and mental health conditions.

Although women veterans have many differences compared with male veterans, due to the changing nature of warfare during the GWOT, women are being subjected to more hostile military environments.[3] Women veterans are sustaining injuries and developing deployment-related medical conditions, such as those outlined in subsequent sections, in a similar fashion to their male counterparts (**Table 1**).

Women veterans are also distinct from civilian, active duty, and national guard/reserve women. Although women veterans have several factors considered to be protective for overall health and wellness, such as increased education and incomes when compared with civilian women, surveys have shown women veterans are more likely to smoke, be sedentary, be overweight/obese, and suffer from depressive disorders.[7]

All health care providers should recognize the complex needs of women veterans, as this population often receives much of its care outside the VA system. It is estimated that 24% of women veterans use the VA Health Care System, and only 5.1% use the VA exclusively.[8] Studies indicate that significant numbers of women

Table 1
Conditions diagnosed in Global War on Terrorism veterans at Veterans Affairs health care system

Disease Categories (ICD-9 Diagnostic Codes)	Number	Percent
Diseases of musculoskeletal system connective tissue disorders (710–739)	634,569	60.0
Mental disorders (290–319)	593,583	56.1
Symptoms, signs, and ill-defined conditions (780–799)	590,446	55.8
Diseases of the nervous system/sense organs (320–389)	515,586	48.7
Diseases of the digestive system (520–579)	392,351	37.1
Diseases of the endocrine/nutritional/metabolic systems (240–279)	384,065	36.3
Injury/poisonings (800–999)	331,258	31.3
Diseases of respiratory systems (460–519)	299,072	28.3
Diseases of the skin (680–709)	250,069	23.6
Diseases of the circulatory system (390–459)	246,506	23.3
Diseases of the genitourinary system (580–629)	181,137	17.1
Infectious and parasitic diseases (001–139)	178,940	16.9
Benign neoplasms (210–239)	84,998	8.0
Diseases of blood and blood-forming organs (280–289)	48,672	4.6
Malignant neoplasms (140–209)	16,491	1.6

Adapted from Analysis of VA Health Care Utilization among Operation Enduring Freedom, Operation Iraqi Freedom, and Operation New Dawn Veterans, from 1st Qtr FY 2002 through 2nd Qtr FY 2014. Washington, DC: Epidemiology Program, Post-Deployment Health Group, Office of Public Health, Veterans Health Administration, Department of Veterans Affairs; 2014.Available at: http://www.publichealth.va.gov/docs/epidemiology/healthcare-utilization-report-fy2014-qtr2.pdf. Accessed August, 2014.

who initially receive some care within the VA will eventually seek care from other providers (**Box 1**).[9]

This article will outline the distinct medical, psychiatric and psychosocial needs of women veterans within the context of their military background and shared cultural values to give all providers, not just those within the VA system, the ability to care for this growing population deserving of optimal patient care.

MILITARY CULTURAL COMPETENCY

Ms. V relays that she was deployed to Afghanistan twice as part of her military service with the Army Reserves during Operation Enduring Freedom. She worked as part of a delivery envoy and she often found herself on edge because of concerns about improvised explosive devices. She reports repeated exposures to smoke and fumes from large roadside burn pits. Since completing her 2 tours of duty, she has had difficulty reintegrating back with her friends and family and prefers to spend time alone or with 1 friend from the military who lives nearby. What more would one want to know about her military service? How could her military service be impacting her presentation in the clinic today? Could her past experiences impact how she interacts with the health care system now and in the future?

Integral to providing care for women veterans like Ms. V and their wide array of medical, psychological, and psychosocial care needs is recognizing their varied experiences and understanding how their military service has impacted their overall health. Unfortunately, many providers working with women veterans may be unaware of the long history of women serving in the US military and on the potential impacts their service can have

Box 1
Reasons women may choose care outside VA system

- Long distance to travel to nearest VA
- Health care insurance with adequate coverage attained outside the VA
- Lack of awareness of VA benefits or eligibility
- Concerns about health care quality
- Concerns about personal privacy
- Concerns about the environment in which care will be received
- Fragmentation in health care delivery
- Gaps in health care needs
- Lack of access to mental health care services
- Lack of access to women-specific specialty services such as obstetric care
- Underrepresentation in research studies and funding
- Underutilization of VA resources
- Need for child care for appointments
- Homelessness
- Unemployment or underemployment
- History of MST or PTSD
- Domestic violence

Adapted from Strategies for serving our women veterans. Department of Veterans Affairs Women Veterans Task Force. Draft for Public Comment; 2012. Available at: http://www.va.gov/opa/publications/draft_2012_women-Veterans_strategicplan.pdf. Accessed May 14, 2014; and Hamilton AB, Frayne SM, Cordasco KM, et al. Factors related to attrition from VA health-care use: findings from the national survey of women veterans. J Gen Intern Med 2013;28 Suppl 2:S510–6.

on their health and wellness.[10] This may be partially due to military personnel getting health care not only from military physicians, but also frequently from civilian providers.[11]

As a cultural group, those who currently and previously served in the military share a common set of unifying core values and beliefs (**Fig. 1**). Similar to religious, ethnic, or other cultural groups, they also share a unifying language, set of rules, and codes of conduct.

At the same time, although there is a shared set of core values and beliefs, those who served in the military underwent tremendously varied experiences during their active duty. Providers should be aware of how different situations such as exposures, combat, prolonged tours, to name a few, may impact a patient's current medical state, as well as their degree of interaction with the medical system.

"Are you currently serving or have you ever served in the military?" This question is often not a standard one asked on outpatient clinic, emergency department, or hospital intake forms. However, asking that 1 question can begin a dialogue that can bring enhanced patient insight and risk factor assessment.[12] Asking about military service can also improve therapeutic alliances between patients and their health care providers and the overall healthcare system.[12]

A comprehensive military history can be extensive, especially in the setting of a recent return from deployment. However, a basic military history (**Box 2**) can include

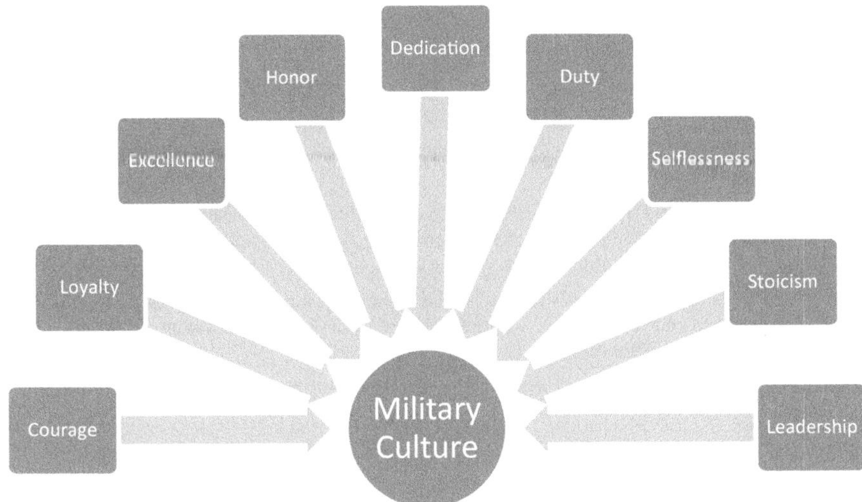

Fig. 1. Military—shared core values and beliefs.

a few questions that can provide health care workers with a starting point and framework in understanding the impact military service has had on their patients and, if indicated, in facilitating appropriate referrals to needed specialty services or to learn more through available resources (**Box 3**).

Taking a military history is a skill that health care providers can develop with practice and by simply learning more about military culture and history. Providers must also be aware of their own attitudes about the military, as these biases could impede the patient–provider care alliance.[11] Providers can also play a pivotal role in the destigmatization of conditions such as depression, post-traumatic stress disorder, anxiety, and substance abuse, which can lead to earlier mental health intervention and treatment.[11]

FUNCTIONAL GASTROINTESTINAL DISORDERS

Functional gastrointestinal disorders, including irritable bowel syndrome (IBS) and functional dyspepsia, are a result of dysfunction of brain–gut interactions. Stressful life events can exacerbate IBS and dyspepsia symptoms. Psychological distress,

Box 2
Basic military history taking

- When and where did you serve?
- What did you do while in the service?
- How has military service affected you?
- What were the challenges and rewards associated with your service?
- Did you experience any combat during your military service?
- How have things been going for you since being out of the military?
- What are your plans having completed military service?
- Acknowledgments of service

Box 3
Resources for providers on military culture and women veterans

Center for Women Veterans. US Department of Veterans Affairs. Available at: http://www.va.gov/womenvet/cwv/index.asp. Accessed September, 2014.

D'Amico F, Weinstein L. Gender camouflage: women and the US military. New York: New York University Press; 1999.

Department of Defense Deployment Health Clinical Center—For clinicians providing post-deployment care to service members, veterans and their families. Available at: www.pdhealth.mil/main.asp. Accessed September, 2014.

Goldenberg M, Hamaoka D, Santiago P, et al. Basic training: a primer on military life and culture for health care providers and trainees. MedEdPORTAL; 2012. Available at: www.mededportal.org/publication/9270. Accessed September, 2014.

Holm J. Women in the military: an unfinished revolution. revised edition. Novato (CA): Presidio Press; 1992.

Iskra DM. Women in the United States armed forces: a guide to the issues. Santa Barbara (CA): Praeger; 2010.

Women Veterans Health Care. US Department of Veterans Affairs. Available at: http://www.womenshealth.va.gov/. Accessed September, 2014.

trauma, depression, anxiety, and post-traumatic stress disorder (PTSD) are all more prevalent in patients with functional gastrointestinal disorders than those with organic gastrointestinal disorders.[13]

Women veterans have higher rates of functional gastrointestinal disorders than civilian women. In 1 study, 38% of women veterans reported IBS, and 21% reported dyspepsia.[13] Among those with IBS and dyspepsia, there were higher reports of anxiety, depression, and PTSD.[13] The associations were strongest for anxiety, with a greater severity of anxiety being associated with an up to 16-fold increase in IBS and a more than 40-fold increase in dyspepsia.[13]

Another study found the excess odds of IBS symptoms are fourfold greater in women with PTSD than in women without dyspepsia, and the odds of dyspepsia are fivefold greater in women with PTSD than in women without PTSD.[14] Of those women with IBS, 56% had been forced to have sex against their will versus 42% of women without IBS.[14] Thirty-six percent of patients with IBS reported other situations with attempted force or unwanted sexual contact versus 21% of patients without IBS.[14] Women veterans with IBS were significantly more likely to have PTSD (22.1% vs 10.7%) and depression (44.2% vs 29.5%) than those without IBS.[14]

These studies support a possible biologic link between experiences of trauma and functional gastrointestinal disorders, which is likely related to the relationship between the enteric nervous system and neuroendocrine systems.[14]

FUNCTIONAL AND OTHER PAIN DISORDERS

The prevalence of functional pain disorders, including noncyclic breast pain (mastalgia), menstrual symptoms, chronic pelvic pain, and fibromyalgia is higher in women with PTSD and a history of sexual trauma than in populations without a psychiatric history. Additionally, women veterans have higher rates of chronic musculoskeletal pain than male veterans who experience similar training and deployment exposures.

One study of mastalgia among women veterans reported a 55% prevalence of this finding in women veterans in the past year. Those with frequent mastalgia (greater than once weekly) were more likely to screen positive for PTSD, depression, panic disorder, and alcohol misuse disorders. Those with mastalgia also reported higher rates of fibromyalgia and irritable bowel syndrome.[15]

Another study found that 71% of women Veterans reporting menstrual symptoms (premenstrual syndrome, menorrhagia, irregular menstruation, and dysmenorrhea) had experienced sexual assault while in the military. They also had significantly lower overall health status than women without menstrual symptoms, even after controlling for sociodemographic and psychosocial characteristics. In fact, the difference in overall health status and impact on daily functioning between women Veterans with menstrual symptoms and those without was similar to differences seen with other chronic illnesses, including chronic pulmonary disease, arthritis, and angina.[16]

Chronic pelvic pain is defined as "noncyclic pain of at least 6 months duration, severe enough to require medical care or cause disability, and occurring in locations such as the pelvis, anterior abdominal wall at or below the umbilicus, lower back, or buttocks."[17] Among women treated at a referral-based pelvic pain clinic, half reported a history of physical or sexual abuse. Thirty-one percent screened positive for PTSD, with higher rates among those reporting at least 2 lifetime traumas. Those with PTSD and chronic pelvic pain had significantly lower healthy physical functioning and functioning without pain, more medical symptoms, a higher number of surgeries for their pelvic pain, and a higher number of days in bed because of illness. Those reporting at least 2 traumas had physical functioning similar to patients with other serious medical conditions such as diabetes, rheumatoid arthritis, and chronic liver disease.[18]

Fibromyalgia is also frequently diagnosed in women Veterans, and it has been linked to PTSD. In 1 study of consecutive fibromyalgia syndrome (FMS) patients with age-matched controls, 45.3% of those with FMS met criteria for PTSD as opposed to 3% of population controls. In two-thirds of the patients, trauma preceded FMS symptoms, whereas 30% reported PTSD/trauma after the onset of their chronic widespread pain. In 4% of the sample, PTSD and FMS symptoms occurred in the same year. Based on this study, FMS and PTSD are both risk factors for one another and are commonly comorbid conditions associated with traumatic experiences.[19]

In addition to functional pain disorders, women veterans are more likely than their male counterparts to develop chronic musculoskeletal pain after their military service. Women experience a high rate of injuries during basic training and deployment, and are particularly prone to stress fractures. The odds of having back pain, joint disorders, and other musculoskeletal disorders are higher in women than male veterans, and increase yearly for at least 7 years after return from deployment.[20] Women with chronic musculoskeletal pain report higher pain intensity, greater pain-related interference with function, and more disability days than men.[21]

Because of the links between functional and other pain syndromes and a history of trauma in women veterans, women with unexplained pain syndromes should be screened for psychiatric disorders, alcohol misuse, and trauma.

POST-TRAUMATIC STRESS DISORDER AND MILITARY SEXUAL TRAUMA

Women veterans are not only increasing in their total numbers, but they are also advancing and expanding in the positions they hold while on active duty. Although women were not utilized as combat troops officially until US approval in 2013, the distinction between combat and noncombat roles has become less clear in war zones without a front line such as those in Iraq and Afghanistan. Women have held positions with significant exposure to combat, including military police, convoy transportation, intelligence, pilots, medics, and mechanics.[22] Fifteen percent of women veterans in 1 sample reported exposure to combat while deployed to Afghanistan.[22]

Although the risk of combat-related trauma is high among women veterans of the GWOT, the risk of trauma at the hands of one of their military colleagues is even higher. Experiences of sexual assault and harassment during military service are associated with mental health problems including PTSD, depression, anxiety disorders, and substance abuse disorders.[22] There is also a strong correlation with the development of general physical health problems and financial and occupational hardships. Sexual assault and harassment incurred during military service appear to cause more lasting and significant trauma as these experiences are more strongly associated with subsequent mental health problems when compared with sexual trauma that occurred before or occurs after military service.[22]

Military sexual trauma (MST) is defined by the Department of Veterans Affairs as "sexual harassment that is threatening in character or physical assault of a sexual nature that occurred while the victim was in the military, regardless of geographic location of the trauma, gender of the victim, or the relationship to the perpetrator." The reported prevalence of MST is most commonly noted around 20% to 40% for women and 1% to 2% for men.[23]

MST is more predictive of developing PTSD than other types of military trauma or civilian sexual trauma. Indeed, 40% to 60% of women survivors of MST go on to develop PTSD. This incidence is 40% higher than those who suffered other kinds of military or civilian trauma.[24]

Risk factors for MST include entering the military at a younger age, being of the enlisted (as opposed to officer) rank, and having a lower level of educational attainment.[23,25,26] In addition, veterans with a history of childhood sexual abuse and those who enlisted to escape their home environment have higher rates of sexual assault as adults.[27,28] Recent military conflicts also have seen women and men in more isolated and vulnerable positions compared with previous conflicts and wars, and the subsequent rates of reported MST are higher.[22]

Social support among military personnel has been identified as a protective factor against military-related stressors. Higher perceptions of peer social support are associated with improved psychological wellbeing; unit cohesion reduces the risk of PTSD in the face of military trauma. However, deployed women are less likely to perceive positive social support from fellow service members, and thus their traumatic military exposures are often compounded by this lack of social support from their team.[22]

Undergoing traumatic events, especially MST, has been linked to the development of other mental health conditions. Among women Veterans with MST, 60% screen positive for depression, and 27% report eating disorders. They have a rate of alcohol abuse disorders twice as high and a rate of PTSD 5 times as high as their counterparts without a history of MST.[29,30]

The consequences of MST are not purely mental health, but also physical. Women with MST report an increased number of physical symptoms and more chronic health problems than women without MST. They have increased cardiovascular risk factors, including obesity, smoking, and sedentary lifestyles.[31]

The complete evaluation, management, and treatment of PTSD and MST are beyond the scope of this article. However, it is critical that all providers be aware of these conditions in their women veteran patients, especially in those with other often coexisting disorders, including depression, chronic pain, and substance abuse or medically unexplained conditions for screening purposes (**Table 2**), and referrals should be made as appropriate.[32]

Women veterans with the diagnosis of PTSD or MST who are interested are eligible for treatment through the VA in their area.[32] There are also numerous resources available to providers and patients for further information about PTSD and MST (**Box 4**).

Table 2
Mental health screening tools

Depression Screening	
Patients are asked to respond with "not at all," "several days," "more than half the days," or "nearly every day."	During the past 2 wk, how often have you been bothered by little interest or pleasure in doing things?
A positive screen is ≥3 points out of a possible 6	During the past 2 wk, how often have you been bothered by feeling down, depressed or hopeless?
PTSD Screening	
A positive screen is a positive answer to 3 of 4 questions.	Have nightmares about it?
In your life, have you ever had any experience that was so frightening, horrible, or upsetting that in the past month it has caused you to...	Try hard not to think about it, go out of your way to avoid situations that remind you of it? Be constantly on guard, watchful, or easily startled? Be numb or detached from others, activities, or your surroundings?
Military Sexual Trauma Screening	
A "yes" answer to either question is considered a positive screen.	When you were in the military, did you ever receive uninvited or unwanted sexual attention (ie, touching, cornering, pressure for sexual favors, or verbal remarks)? Did someone ever use force or threat of force to have sexual contact with you against your will?

Box 4
Post-traumatic stress disorder and military sexual trauma resources

Department of Defense Deployment Health Clinical Center resources for evaluation and treatment of PTSD. Available at: www.pdhealth.mil/clinicians/ptsd.asp#it3. Accessed September, 2014.

Veterans Affairs National Center for PTSD. Available at: www.ptsd.va.gov/index.asp. Accessed September, 2014.

US Department of Veterans Affairs/Department of Defense. Essentials for posttraumatic stress disorder: provider tool; 2013. Available at: http://www.healthquality.va.gov/guidelines/MH/ptsd/DCoEPTSDTool2ProviderTool23May2013v1HiResPrint.pdf. Accessed September, 2014.

US Department of Veterans Affairs/Department of Defense. Clinical practice guideline for management of post-traumatic stress disorder and acute stress reaction; 2010. Available at: http://www.healthquality.va.gov/guidelines/MH/ptsd/cpg_PTSD-FULL-201011612.pdf. Accessed September, 2014.

US Department of Veterans Affairs. Military sexual trauma center. Available at: http://www.mentalhealth.va.gov/msthome.asp. Accessed September, 2014.

Veterans Crisis Line 1-800-273-8255 press 1. Available at: http://www.Veteranscrisisline.net/. (Live chat available online).

US Department of Veterans Affairs. PTSD Coach mobile application. Available at: www.ptsd.va.gov/public/pages/PTSDcoach.asp. Accessed September, 2014.

Box 5
Veterans' homelessness resources

US Department of Veterans Affairs. Homeless veterans—housing assistance for veterans. Available at: http://www.va.gov/homeless/housing.asp. Accessed September, 2014.

Department of Housing and Urban Development—VA Supportive Housing (HUD-VASH). HUD-VASH Resource Guide for Permanent Housing and Clinical Care. Available at: http://www.va.gov/HOMELESS/docs/Center/144_HUD-VASH_Book_WEB_High_Res_final.pdf. Accessed September, 2014.

Veterans Affairs National Call Center for Homeless Veterans at 1-877-4AID-VET (1-877-424-3838). Free telephone and online chat available. Neither VA registration nor enrollment in VA healthcare is required.

HOMELESSNESS

Women veterans are 3 to 4 times more likely than civilian women to be homeless.[33] Risk factors for homelessness among women veterans include history of military sexual trauma, unemployment, disability, worse overall health status, anxiety disorder, and PTSD. Protective factors include being married and being a college graduate.

Homeless women are more likely to access mental health services and receive at least some of their care at that VA than housed women.[34] Despite efforts on the part of the VA to end homelessness among veterans, many of these programs are designed to accommodate male veterans and do not adequately address the privacy or other concerns of women veterans.[34] More recently, the VA has been specifically identifying women veterans and their families in an effort to reserve transitional housing for this at-risk group.

A study based on focus groups of homeless women veterans described several inter-related pathways to homelessness among women veterans.[35] These included

1. Premilitary adversity
2. Military trauma or substance abuse
3. Postmilitary interpersonal violence and abuse
4. Termination of intimate relationships
5. Postmilitary mental illness, substance abuse, and medical issues
6. Unemployment

Acknowledging these pathways can help health care providers identify women who are at risk for homelessness. Likewise, health care providers who care for homeless women should be prepared to screen for veteran status, and refer veterans for available veteran-specific services as appropriate (**Box 5**).

SUMMARY

Women veterans present to health care providers with a broad spectrum of medical, psychiatric, and psychosocial conditions, many of which may be directly or indirectly correlated with their previous military service. Research efforts at the VA to better characterize the relationship between military-related exposures and disease progression are ongoing. However, these efforts have escalated in the women veteran population to include over 60 studies specifically addressing women's health.[36] There is much that still needs to be studied about the health of women veterans and this type of research, focused on topics specific to women, will continue to provide further answers and guidance on caring for this patient population with unique health needs.

REFERENCES

1. America's women veterans: military service history and VA benefit utilization statistics. Department of Veterans Affairs National Center for Veterans Analysis and Statistics; 2011. Available at: http://www.va.gov/vetdata/docs/SpecialReports/Final_Womens Report_3_2_12 v 7.pdf. Accessed September, 2014.
2. Atkins D. Health services research on women veterans: a critical partner on the road to patient-centered care. J Gen Intern Med 2013;28(Suppl 2):S498–9.
3. Strategies for serving our women veterans. Department of Veterans Affairs Women Veterans Task Force; 2012. Available at: http://www.va.gov/opa/publications/draft_2012_women-Veterans_strategicplan.pdf. Accessed August, 2014.
4. Analysis of VA Health Care Utilization among Operation Enduring Freedom. Operation Iraqi Freedom, and Operation New Dawn veterans, from 1st qtr fy 2002 through 2nd qtr FY 2014. Washington, DC: Epidemiology Program, Post-Deployment Health Group, Office of Public Health, Veterans Health Administration, Department of Veterans Affairs; 2014. Available at: http://www.publichealth.va.gov/docs/epidemiology/healthcare-utilization-report-fy2014-qtr2.pdf. Accessed August, 2014.
5. Veteran population projections: FY2010 to FY2040. Office of the Actuary, Department of Veterans Affairs; 2013. Available at: http://www.va.gov/vetdata/docs/QuickFacts/Population_slideshow.pdf. Accessed August, 2014.
6. Frayne SM, Yu W, Yano EM, et al. Gender and use of care: planning for tomorrow's Veterans Health Administration. J Womens Health 2007;16(8):1188–99.
7. Lehavot K, Hoerster KD, Nelson KM, et al. Health Indicators for military, veteran, and civilian women. Am J Prev Med 2012;42(5):473–80.
8. Women veteran profile. United States Department of Veterans Affairs Prepared by the National Center for Veterans Analysis and Statistics; 2013. Available at: http://www.va.gov/vetdata/docs/SpecialReports/Women_Veteran_Profile5.pdf. Accessed August, 2014.
9. Hamilton AB, Frayne SM, Cordasco KM, et al. Factors related to attrition from VA healthcare use: findings from the national survey of women veterans. J Gen Intern Med 2013;28(Suppl 2):S510–6.
10. Murdoch M, Bradley A, Mather SH, et al. Women and war: what physicians should know. J Gen Intern Med 2006;21:S5–10.
11. Gleeson TD, Hemmer PA. Providing care to military personnel and their families: how we can all contribute. Acad Med 2014;89:1201–3.
12. Convoy S, Westphal RJ. The importance of developing military cultural competence. J Emerg Nurs 2013;39:591–4.
13. Savas LS, White DL, Wieman M, et al. Irritable bowel syndrome and dyspepsia among women veterans: prevalence and association with psychological distress. Aliment Pharmacol Ther 2009;29(1):115–25.
14. White DL, Savas LS, Daci K, et al. Trauma history and risk of the irritable bowel syndrome in women veterans. Aliment Pharmacol Ther 2010;32(4):551–61.
15. Johnson K, Bradley K, Bush K, et al. Frequency of mastalgia among women veterans: association with psychiatric conditions and unexplained pain syndromes. J Gen Intern Med 2006;21:S70–5.
16. Barnard K, Frayne S, Skinner K, et al. Health status among women with menstrual symptoms. J Womens Health 2003;12(9):911–9.
17. ACOG Committee on Practice Bulletins—Gynecology. ACOG Practice Bulletin No. 51. Chronic pelvic pain. Obstet Gynecol 2004;103:589–605.

18. Melzer-Brody S, Leserman J, Zolnoun D, et al. Trauma and posttraumatic stress disorder in women with chronic pelvic pain. Obstet Gynecol 2007; 109(4):902–8.
19. Häuser W, Galek A, Erbslöh-Möller B, et al. Posttraumatic stress disorder in fibromyalgia syndrome: prevalence, temporal relationship between posttraumatic stress and fibromyalgia symptoms, and impact on clinical outcome. Pain 2013; 154(8):1216–23.
20. Haskell S, Ning Y, Krebs E, et al. Prevalence of painful musculoskeletal conditions in female and male veterans in 7 years after return from deployment in Operation Enduring Freedom/Operation Iraqi Freedom. Clin J Pain 2012;28(2):163–7.
21. Stubbs D, Krebs E, Bair M, et al. Sex differences in pain and pain-related disability among primary care patients with chronic musculoskeletal pain. Pain Med 2010;11:232–9.
22. Street AE, Vogt D, Dutra L. A new generation of women veterans: stressors faced by women deployed to Iraq and Afghanistan. Clin Psychol Rev 2009; 29:685–94.
23. Suris A, Lind L. Military sexual trauma: a review of prevalence and associated health consequences in veterans. Trauma Violence Abuse 2008;9:250–69.
24. Yaeger D, Himmelfarb N, Cammack A, et al. DSM-IV diagnosed posttraumatic stress disorder in women veterans with and without military sexual trauma. J Gen Intern Med 2006;21:S65–9.
25. Sadler AG, Booth BM, Cook BL, et al. Factors associated with women's risk of rape in the military environment. Am J Ind Med 2003;43:262–73.
26. Coyle BS, Wolan DL, Van Horn AS. The prevalence of physical and sexual abuse in women veterans seeking care at a Veterans Affairs medical center. Mil Med 1996;161:588–93.
27. Sadler A, Booth B, Mengeling M, et al. Life span and repeated violence against women during military service: Effects on health status and outpatient utilization. J Womens Health 2004;13:799–811.
28. Merrill L, Newell C, Thomsen C, et al. Childhood abuse and sexual revictimization in a female Navy recruit sample. J Trauma Stress 1999;12(2):211–25.
29. Skinner K, Kressin N, Frayne S, et al. The prevalence of military sexual assault among female Veterans' Administration outpatients. J Interpers Violence 2000; 15(3):291–310.
30. Suris A, Lind L, Kashner TM, et al. Sexual assault in women veterans: an examination of PTSD risk, health care utilization, and cost of care. Psychosom Med 2004;66:749–56.
31. Frayne S, Skinner K, Sullivan L, et al. Sexual assault while in the military: violence as a predictor of cardiac risk? Violence Vict 2003;18:219–25.
32. Sessums LL, Jackson JL. In the clinic. Care of returning military personnel. Ann Intern Med 2013;159:ITC1–15.
33. Gamache G, Rosenheck R, Tessler R. Overrepresentation of women veterans among homeless women. Am J Public Health 2003;93(7):1132–6.
34. Washington D, Yano E, McGuire J, et al. Risk factors for homelessness among women veterans. J Health Care Poor Underserved 2010;21:81–91.
35. Hamilton A, Poza I, Washington D. "Homelessness and trauma go hand-in-hand": pathways to homelessness among women veterans. Womens Health Issues 2011;21:S203–9.
36. Women's health research at VA: fact sheet. Department of Veterans Affairs; 2012. Available at: http://www.research.va.gov/media_roundtable/wh-factsheet.pdf. Accessed August, 2014.

Preconception Care and Reproductive Planning in Primary Care

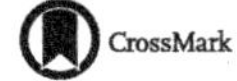

Lisa S. Callegari, MD, MPH[a,b,*], Erica W. Ma, BA[b],
Eleanor Bimla Schwarz, MD, MS[c]

KEYWORDS

- Preconception care • Reproductive life plan • Reproductive planning
- Reproductive-aged women • Primary care

KEY POINTS

- Primary care for women of childbearing age should include routine assessment of a woman's reproductive goals and pregnancy intentions ("reproductive planning").
- Women who could potentially become pregnant should be assessed for preconception risks and educated about the importance of maternal health in ensuring healthy pregnancies.
- Women may be motivated to address modifiable health risks by learning about the way their health will affect a future pregnancy.
- For women not intending pregnancy in the short term, preconception care should include counseling on effective contraception.
- Women with chronic medical conditions should be counseled about highly effective reversible methods such as intrauterine devices and contraceptive implants, which have few medical contraindications.

It's not a question of whether you provide preconception care, rather it's a question of what kind of preconception care you are providing.
—Joseph Stanford and Debra Hobbins

The authors report no conflicts of interest.
L.S. Callegari was supported by a VA Health Services Research and Development Postdoctoral Fellowship (TPM 61-041).
The findings and conclusions in this report are those of the authors and do not represent the views of the Department of Veterans Affairs or the United States Government.
[a] Department of Obstetrics & Gynecology, University of Washington, 1959 NE Pacific St, Seattle, WA 98195, USA; [b] Health Services Research and Development (HSR&D), Department of Veterans Affairs, VA Puget Sound Health Care System, 1660 S. Columbian Way S-152, Seattle, WA 98108, USA; [c] Department of Medicine, University of California, Davis, 4150 V Street, Suite 3100, Sacramento, CA 95817, USA
* Corresponding author. Health Services Research and Development (HSR&D), Department of Veterans Affairs, VA Puget Sound Health Care System, University of Washington, 1660 S. Columbian Way S-152, Seattle, WA 98108.
E-mail address: lcallega@uw.edu

Med Clin N Am 99 (2015) 663–682
http://dx.doi.org/10.1016/j.mcna.2015.01.014
0025-7125/15/$ – see front matter Published by Elsevier Inc.
medical.theclinics.com

INTRODUCTION

The United States has one of the highest rates of maternal mortality in the developed world,[1] with a growing proportion of maternal deaths attributable to chronic medical conditions.[2] In addition, the United States ranks behind most other industrialized nations in infant mortality, primarily because of congenital anomalies and preterm birth.[3] As prenatal care is often initiated too late to meaningfully impact pregnancy outcomes, a growing body of evidence highlights the prepregnancy or preconception period as critical to addressing high rates of maternal and fetal mortality.[4] Preconception care has been defined broadly as a set of interventions to identify and modify biomedical, behavioral, environmental, and social risks to the health of a woman or her baby before pregnancy occurs.[4] Primary care physicians (PCPs) care for large numbers of reproductive-aged women before, between, and after their pregnancies and thus are ideally positioned to help women identify and modify preconception health risks.[5]

Despite national campaigns by organizations such as the Centers for Disease Control and Prevention (CDC),[4,5] many PCPs lack training and knowledge of preconception care. Few PCPs routinely ask women about their pregnancy intentions or discuss how their health status or medications can impact pregnancy.[6,7] For example, one national study found that contraceptive counseling was provided in less than 20% of health care visits that documented use of a potential teratogen by a woman of childbearing age.[8] Furthermore, many women remain unaware of the importance of their prepregnancy health to both maternal and fetal pregnancy health outcomes, and few seek preconception counseling from providers.[9–11]

Given that more than 50% of pregnancies in the United States are unplanned,[12] PCPs should proactively conduct a preconception risk assessment as part of routine primary care for women of childbearing age.[4,13] The substantial overlap between the goals of comprehensive primary care and preconception care suggests that high-quality preconception care need not be viewed as a new set of interventions for PCPs, but rather as a different lens through which to view standard preventive care. This review focuses primarily on aspects of conditions commonly managed by PCPs that may benefit from targeted preconception intervention.

REPRODUCTIVE PLANNING

The first step in identifying a reproductive-aged woman's need for preconception risk screening and counseling is to assess her pregnancy desires and plans. CDC[4] and the American Congress of Obstetricians and Gynecologists (ACOG),[14] recommend that providers routinely ask women about their reproductive goals and encourage women to create a "reproductive life plan." More recent data indicate that longer term planning may be difficult for many women, therefore asking women about reproductive goals in a shorter time frame, such as 1 year, may be more widely acceptable to women.[15,16] The "Before, Between, and Beyond" provider toolkit recently released by the National Preconception Health and Health Care Initiative recommends the question, "Are you hoping to become pregnant in the next year?" to initiate reproductive planning conversations in routine primary care.[17]

Additional questions to help women think about their reproductive goals and related health needs are listed in **Table 1**. For women who desire pregnancy in the next year, preconception risk assessment and counseling are indicated. For women who do not desire pregnancy in the next year, information about effective contraception is essential, including information about highly effective reversible contraceptives that

Table 1
Reproductive planning questions

Questions to Ask if Desires Pregnancy in the Future	Questions to Ask if Never Desires Pregnancy in the Future
How many children would you like to have?	What family planning method will you use to avoid pregnancy?
How long would you like to wait until you (or your partner) become pregnant?	How sure are you that you will be able to use this method without any problems?
What family planning method do you plan to use until you (or your partner) are ready to become pregnant? How sure are you that you will be able to use this method without any problems?	People's plans change. Is it possible you or your partner could ever decide to become pregnant?

Adapted from National Preconception Health and Health Care Initiative. Before, between and beyond toolkit. Available at: http://beforeandbeyond.org/toolkit/reproductive-life-plan-assessment/. Accessed September 27, 2014.

are safe for virtually all women (eg, intrauterine or subdermal contraceptives). Because women's pregnancy intentions often change over time, a key feature of reproductive planning is the integration of contraceptive and preconception counseling. For example, a woman who desires pregnancy at a later time can benefit from counseling on both effective contraception and preconception risk modification to optimize future pregnancy health. Many women not intending pregnancy in the short term will nonetheless experience unintended pregnancy[12]; PCPs should therefore proactively address a woman's contraceptive plans and preconception health risks whenever possible at each visit. At a minimum, these are important components of annual well-woman visits for this population.[17]

Provision of information on the impact of maternal age on fertility and birth outcomes is an important component of reproductive planning for some women. A large amount of literature describes age-related pregnancy risks and demonstrates a continual increase in risks over the age of 35, rather than a threshold effect.[18] In one meta-analysis, increasing age was significantly associated with miscarriage (adjusted odds ratio [aOR] 2.0 and 2.4 for ages 35–39 years and age 40 years and older, respectively), chromosomal abnormalities (aOR 4.0 and 9.9), congenital anomalies (aOR 1.4 and 1.7), gestational diabetes (aOR 1.8 and 2.4), placenta previa (aOR 1.8 and 2.8), and cesarean delivery (aOR 1.6 and 2.0).[18] Women aged 40 or older also experienced increased risk for abruption (aOR 2.3), preterm delivery (aOR 1.4), low birth weight (aOR 1.6), and perinatal mortality (aOR 2.2).[18] Another important aspect of reproductive planning is the provision of information about recommended interpregnancy intervals (IPIs, defined as the time from delivery to subsequent conception). Data indicate that an IPI shorter than 6 months results in increased risk of preterm birth, low birth weight, and small for gestational age and that an IPI between 18 and 59 months appears to be safest.[19] For women over the age of 35, however, a shorter IPI may be appropriate to balance risks of age-related fertility declines and pregnancy risk.

Reproductive planning conversations are perceived as valuable and important to women from a variety of backgrounds.[16,20,21] Studies suggest that women appreciate having their PCP initiate conversations about reproductive planning that are nonjudgmental (ie, there are no right or wrong answers) and delivered in a caring and supportive manner.[16,20] Women who are not interested in a pregnancy in the next year may find messages related to "being prepared for the unexpected"[16] or "investing in themselves" for a healthy future[22] more relevant than information about "planning for pregnancy." Additional information on reproductive life plans and reproductive planning is available on the Before, Between, and Beyond Web site.[17]

OPTIMIZATION OF CHRONIC CONDITIONS

Diabetes

The prevalence of pregestational diabetes among women in their childbearing years is rising, fueled by the obesity epidemic.[23] One study of nearly 200,000 pregnancies identified an increase in diagnosed pregestational diabetes from 0.81% in 1999 to 1.82% in 2005.[23] Elevated serum glycemic levels are a powerful teratogen,[24] and thus, prepregnancy optimization of glycemic control is critically important to ensure healthy pregnancy outcomes. Women in poor glycemic control during organogenesis (approximately 4–10 weeks of gestation) are at substantially increased risk of spontaneous abortion and of congenital anomalies, including cardiac structural defects, neural tube defects (NTDs), and sacral agenesis.[25–27] The overall risk of one or more congenital anomalies is 6% to 7% among women with pregestational diabetes, more than twice the baseline prevalence,[24] and increases with glycosylated hemoglobin (HgA1c) levels.[28] Later in pregnancy, prepregnancy diabetes is associated with fetal risks including fetal macrosomia (birth weight more than the 90th percentile for gestational age), preterm birth, stillborn, and neonatal death. Maternal risks include worsening of diabetic retinopathy and nephropathy, hypertension, and preeclampsia. Children born to women with diabetes mellitus may be at increased risk of developing diabetes, and hyperglycemia during pregnancy may result in metabolic effects on the fetus that predispose to later life obesity and metabolic syndrome.[29] Data indicate that women who can lower their HgA1c levels to the normal range can reduce their risks to close to that of a nondiabetic woman.[30]

Counseling and education in both inpatient and outpatient settings can improve maternal and fetal outcomes among women with diabetes.[26,31–33] One meta-analysis of 8 retrospective and 8 prospective studies of preconception counseling interventions for type 1 and type 2 diabetic women found reductions in both major congenital anomalies (those involving death such as abortion or intrauterine fetal death, surgical correction, or medical therapy) and minor congenital anomalies as well as in first-trimester HgA1c levels.[34] A second meta-analysis found similar reductions in fetal anomalies and first-trimester HgA1c levels as well as a reduction in rates of preterm delivery.[31]

The American Diabetes Association (ADA) recommends a target HgA1c of less than 7% before conception.[35] Both ADA[36] and the ACOG[37] advise that insulin therapy be the mainstay for glycemic control in pregnancy, although a growing body of literature supports the safety of using metformin during pregnancy.[38] Women with preexisting diabetes who are planning pregnancy should have a comprehensive eye examination, documentation of baseline renal function, thyroid function screening (type 1 diabetes), and baseline cardiovascular risk screening (eg, electrocardiogram). Review of medications should also be performed to address safety in pregnancy (see "Review of medications" section).[36] Angiotensin-converting enzyme (ACE) inhibitors have been associated with congenital anomalies, intrauterine growth restriction, and fetal/neonatal demise. Data are more limited for angiotensin receptor blockers (ARBs) but suggest similar risks to ACE inhibitors; therefore, both classes are contraindicated in pregnancy.[39]

ACOG recommends a minimum of 0.4 to 0.8 mg/d of folic acid for women with pregestational diabetes, with higher doses (4 mg/d) if additional risk factors for NTDs are present.[37] The Society of Obstetricians and Gynaecologists of Canada recommends a higher dose of 5 mg/d of folic acid for women with insulin-dependent pregestational diabetes.[40] Because folic acid is water-soluble and easily excreted, the risks of high doses are minimal, although evidence suggesting benefit of these doses remains limited.[41] The ADA recommends 0.6 mg/d for women with pregestational diabetes.[36]

Women with pregestational diabetes who do not desire pregnancy should be counseled about effective contraception and encouraged to use highly effective reversible options such as the intrauterine device (IUD) or contraceptive implant. The US Medical Eligibility Criteria (US MEC) for contraceptive use published by the CDC provides specific recommendations regarding safety of contraceptives in women with diabetes in a user-friendly format with summary charts (**Box 1**).[42]

Summary of recommendations

- Women should be educated about the risks of diabetes in pregnancy and advised that normalizing blood glucose before pregnancy will reduce their risks to the level of a nondiabetic woman. ADA recommends target HgA1c of less than 7%.
- All women with preexisting diabetes who are planning pregnancy should be screened for end-organ damage, including retinopathy, nephropathy, and cardiovascular disease.
- Medications should be reviewed to address potential teratogenic risks.
- Women who have elevated HgA1c levels should be counseled about the benefits of short-term use of effective contraception to enable optimization of glycemic control before conception.

Hypertension

Approximately 8% of women of reproductive age have hypertension, according to data from the National Health and Nutrition Examination Survey.[43] Women who have chronic hypertension, whether controlled on antihypertensive drug treatment or not, are more likely to experience fetal and maternal complications, including fetal growth restriction, stillbirth, iatrogenic preterm birth, maternal pulmonary edema and stroke, superimposed preeclampsia, and cesarean delivery.[30,44] Women with moderate or severe renal disease before pregnancy are at risk for developing worsened renal function during pregnancy.[30]

For women with severe hypertension or end-organ damage, continued medical therapy during the preconception period and pregnancy is recommended. Women planning a pregnancy should be transitioned to a regimen that is safe in pregnancy. β_1-selective β-blockers such as atenolol have been associated with growth restriction, and diuretics may prevent physiologic expansion of blood volume in pregnancy; therefore, these drugs are generally not recommended. ACE inhibitors and ARBs are generally contraindicated in pregnancy. ACOG suggests labetalol (a β-blocker with both α-adrenergic and β-adrenergic blocking activity), nifedipine, or methyldopa

Box 1
Additional resources

Before, between, and beyond provider toolkit. Available at: www.beforeandbeyond.org

Reprotox information on medication safety. Available at: www.reprotox.org

CDC Preconception Care. Available at: http://www.cdc.gov/preconception/index.html

March of Dimes. Available at: http://www.marchofdimes.org/pregnancy/get-ready-for-pregnancy.aspx

US Medical Eligibility Criteria for Contraceptive Use. Available at: http://www.cdc.gov/reproductivehealth/unintendedpregnancy/usmec.htm

as first-line options in women who are pregnant or planning pregnancy to achieve a target blood pressure range of 120/80 to 160/105 mm Hg.[45]

Medical therapy in women with mild hypertension may be discontinued with close follow-up if women are planning pregnancy. According to both ACOG and the National High Blood Pressure Education Program Working Group on Blood Pressure in Pregnancy, women with blood pressures less than 160 mm Hg systolic or 105 mm Hg diastolic who have no evidence of end-organ damage do not require treatment during pregnancy.[45,46] The American Heart Association agrees that milder hypertension in pregnancy does not require treatment, but defines systolic pressures greater than 150 mm Hg and diastolic pressures greater than 100 mm Hg as warranting treatment to reduce stroke risk.[47]

Women with hypertension who do not desire pregnancy should be encouraged to use highly effective contraceptive methods such as the IUD and contraceptive implants, which have few medical contraindications. The US MEC for contraceptive use provides specific recommendations on the use of contraceptives among women with hypertension (see **Box 1**).[42]

Summary of recommendations

- Women with chronic hypertension should be counseled about associated pregnancy risks and possible need to change medications when planning a pregnancy.
- Women with mild hypertension can be transitioned off of medication with careful monitoring before pregnancy to ensure pressures remain under SBP less than 150 to 160 mm Hg and DBP less than 100 to 110 mm Hg.
- Women with hypertension of several years' duration should be evaluated for end-organ damage, such as ventricular hypertrophy, retinopathy, and renal disease before pregnancy.
- Medications such as ACE inhibitors and ARBs should be discontinued before attempting pregnancy, with transition to agents with established safety in pregnancy, such as labetalol, nifedipine, or methyldopa.
- For hypertensive women who wish to avoid pregnancy, highly effective reversible methods, such as IUDs and contraceptive implants, are preferred.

Obesity

One-third of reproductive-aged women in the United States are obese,[48] defined as a body mass index (BMI) 30 kg/m^2 or more. Compared with women with a normal BMI (<25 kg/m^2), obese women are at increased risk of a wide range of adverse pregnancy outcomes, including gestational diabetes mellitus (GDM), pregnancy-related hypertensive disorders such as preeclampsia, iatrogenic preterm delivery, dysfunctional labor, postterm pregnancy, large for gestational age (LGA) infant, shoulder dystocia, fetal and infant death, congenital anomalies, cesarean delivery, and postpartum complications.[49–52] Associated congenital anomalies include NTDs, cardiovascular defects, cleft palate and lip, anorectal atresia, and limb abnormalities.[52] Newborns born to obese mothers are more likely to develop childhood obesity, type 2 diabetes, and cardiovascular disease later in life.[53,54] Obese women also are at increased risk of subfertility and miscarriage.[54]

Weight loss before pregnancy is thus one of the most important preconception lifestyle changes a woman can make. Women should be educated about the pregnancy risks associated with obesity and encouraged to engage in a weight-reduction program before attempting to conceive.[55] Once pregnancy occurs, significant weight loss is no longer a recommended goal, although obese women are encouraged to avoid excess gestational weight gain.[56] Effective contraception before, between, and after pregnancies to allow women to achieve their weight loss goals is critical.[57] Because the use of depot medroxyprogesterone acetate injections causes undesired weight gain for some women, alternative methods such as the IUD and implant should be considered. Additional information on the safety and efficacy of contraceptives in women with obesity is available in the US MEC for contraceptive use.[42]

Few data exist on whether lifestyle or dietary interventions are effective in helping women to lose weight before conception.[33] Several trials have examined interventions aimed at postpartum weight loss, with mixed results.[58–60] Data from observational cohort studies suggest that decreases in prepregnancy weight between pregnancies are associated with reduced risk in many pregnancy complications, including gestational diabetes, LGA infant, preeclampsia, cesarean delivery, and failed vaginal birth after cesarean.[61–66] The amount of weight loss needed to reduce pregnancy risks is not clear; some studies found risk reductions with change from obese to normal BMI,[61,62] while others found risk reductions with loss of 1 to 2 BMI units (from 2.7 to 5.4 kg for a woman of average height).[63–66]

Women can be counseled that modest to moderate weight loss (5%–15%) can improve health outcomes.[67] The 2013 Obesity Guidelines for Managing Overweight and Obesity in Adults provide guidelines for providers, which can also be applied to women planning pregnancy.[68] These guidelines recommend that overweight individuals engage in comprehensive lifestyle programs for 6 months or more that support low-calorie diets and physical activity with the use of behavioral therapies, including self-monitoring of weight and food, environmental control, contingency planning, and stress management. Programs should be "intensive" and preferably delivered face-to-face or by telephone by a trained interventionist.[68]

Women who have undergone bariatric surgery should be advised to wait 12 to 18 months following surgery to attempt conception, to both allow for optimal postsurgery weight loss and avoid potential adverse effects of nutritional deficiencies.[69] Procedures that may result in malabsorption (such as Roux-en-Y gastric bypass), and to a lesser extent restrictive procedures (such as gastric banding), can cause deficiencies in iron, folate, vitamin B12, calcium, and vitamin D, which can lead to adverse pregnancy outcomes.[70] Nutritional supplementation and monitoring in the preconception period are therefore critical.[69] Specific regimens should be tailored to the individual patient and the type of bariatric procedure performed,[71] with consultation from the bariatric surgeon. Women should be counseled to use effective contraception after surgery, preferable a highly effective reversible method (eg, IUD or implant). Those who undergo malabsorptive procedures should be advised not to use oral contraceptives, because absorption and thus efficacy may be decreased.[42]

Summary of recommendations

1. Women should be educated about obesity-related pregnancy risks and encouraged to pursue weight loss before conception.
2. Women can be encouraged to set achievable goals and counseled that modest reductions in weight can improve both pregnancy and their long-term health outcomes.
3. Women should be counseled to use effective contraception, such as IUDs and implants, to enable them to achieve their weight loss goals before conception.

Depressive and Anxiety Disorders

Depression is a highly prevalent condition among women in the United States.[72] Depression in pregnancy is common, with an estimated period prevalence of perinatal depression ranging from 11% to 32% from conception to 3 months postpartum.[73] A growing body of evidence suggests that depressive symptoms during pregnancy are associated with poor birth outcomes, including low birth weight, preterm delivery, and postpartum depression.[74–76] Anxiety disorders and symptoms are similarly common among women during pregnancy and the postpartum period[77] and have been linked to adverse perinatal outcomes, including low birth weight and preterm birth.[78]

Psychotropic medications prescribed to women with depression and anxiety may also result in adverse pregnancy outcomes. Studies assessing risks, however, have been observational and of variable quality. Observational studies often cannot adequately control for confounding and can be biased by numerous factors, such as the fact that women with more severe illness are more likely to receive medication. Although certain pregnancy risks may be elevated with psychotropic medications, meta-analysis aggregating the available data suggests that the risks seem to be small and of questionable clinical significance.[79]

The selective serotonin reuptake inhibitors (SSRIs) have been associated with low birth weight, small for gestational age (<10th percentile birth weight), preterm birth, and neonatal effects (increased irritability and persistent pulmonary hypertension of the newborn).[74] SSRIs in general have not been shown to be teratogenic with the exception of paroxetine, which has been linked to a small increased risk of congenital cardiac defects.[80] The risk of congenital anomalies with serotonin-norepinephrine reuptake inhibitors such as venlafaxine seems to be low, although these may increase the risk of preeclampsia.[81] Data are limited on other antidepressants, such as bupropion and tricyclic antidepressants; however, teratogenicity risks seem to be low.[74] Although psychotropic medications are all excreted in low levels in breast milk, levels appear to be lowest with sertraline and paroxetine.[82] Sertraline may therefore be a reasonable first-line SSRI among women initiating therapy given safety data in both pregnancy and breastfeeding.

Although most studies focus on associations between antepartum symptoms and outcomes,[76] one study using national data found that preconception depressive symptoms as well as antepartum symptoms were independently associated with postpartum depression risks.[83] Experts recommend that depression and anxiety be addressed in the preconception period to permit time to review treatment options and to work toward euthymia before conception.[74,76] A joint review from the American Psychiatric Association and ACOG suggests that women with mild or no symptoms for 6 or more months may attempt to taper and discontinue medications before pregnancy, with close follow-up. Patients with serious mental illness, including severe depressive disorders, bipolar disorder, psychosis, and prior history of suicidal ideation or attempts, should generally remain on psychotropics to avoid worsened disease states.[74]

Summary of recommendations

1. Women of reproductive age should be screened for common mental illness such as depression and anxiety.
2. Women with mental illness should be counseled about the risks of untreated conditions and the importance of addressing symptoms before conception.
3. Ideally, women should wait for a period of euthymia (eg, 6–12 months) before attempting conception.
4. Women with mild or no symptoms for 6 or more months may attempt to taper and discontinue medications before pregnancy, with close follow-up.
5. Patients with serious mental illness, including severe depressive disorders, bipolar illness, and psychosis, should generally remain on their medications before and during pregnancy.

Other Medical Conditions

Multiple other medical conditions treated by PCPs, often in conjunction with specialists, can impact maternal and fetal birth outcomes. Women with chronic conditions should be counseled about the potential impact of their condition on pregnancy, and care should be coordinated with specialists to optimize prepregnancy disease control and to choose medication regimens balancing maternal and fetal risks and benefits. **Table 2** provides an overview of selected disease risks and recommendations.

Table 2
Additional selected chronic conditions and preconception recommendations

Disease	Adverse Effects	Recommendations
Asthma	Preterm birth, low birth weight, preeclampsia, stillbirth, and neonatal death	Counsel regarding importance of asthma control before pregnancy. Inhaled and systemic steroids appear to be low risk, with benefits generally outweighing the pregnancy risks[30]
Cardiovascular disease	Maternal morbidity and mortality. Fetal congenital heart disease is increased among women with congenital heart disease	Counsel about the importance of preconception consultation with maternal-fetal medicine specialist and cardiologist before conception[30]
Seizure disorders	Increased frequency of seizures during pregnancy, congenital anomalies (independent of medication-related anomalies), miscarriage, low birth weight, developmental disabilities Anticonvulsants are known teratogens (see **Table 3**)	Optimize medication before pregnancy with specialist input. Valproate should be avoided when possible, given its teratogenicity. Monotherapy is preferred with lowest dose needed for seizure prevention. Folic acid supplementation of 4 mg/d is recommended[30]
Systemic lupus erythematosus	Hypertension, preeclampsia, preterm birth, growth restriction, stillborn, and neonatal lupus	A period of quiescence of 6 mo or more is recommended before pregnancy[30]
Thrombophilia	Increased risk of thromboembolic events and preeclampsia during pregnancy and postpartum. Warfarin is teratogenic (see **Table 3**)	Management of anticoagulation in the preconception period should be addressed with specialist input and generally involves transition to low-molecular-weight heparin or heparin[30]
Thyroid disorders	Hypothyroidism: Preterm birth, preeclampsia, placental abruption, postpartum hemorrhage, low birth weight, stillborn, and impaired neuropsychological development among children Hyperthyroidism: Preeclampsia, maternal heart failure and thyroid crisis, placental abruption, low birth weight, preterm birth, and stillbirth	Universal prepregnancy screening is not recommended, but women with symptoms of thyroid imbalance should be screened. Women with known thyroid disorders should be counseled about the importance of achieving euthyroidism before attempting pregnancy[30]

Table 3
Common medications with known or suspected teratogenic effects

Medication	Adverse Effects	Recommendations
ACE inhibitors and ARBs	First-trimester exposure: Cardiovascular and central nervous system defects Second- and third-trimester exposure: Impaired fetal/neonatal renal function leading to oligohydramnios and resulting pulmonary hypoplasia, limb contractures, and skeletal deformations. Hypocalvaria, retinopathy, and prolonged neonatal hypotension	Consider alternative antihypertensives, such as nifedipine, labetalol, or methydopa[45]
Antibiotics	Tetracycline: Bone and teeth staining Trimethoprim: Theoretic risk of NTDs due to lowered folic acid levels	Consider alternatives such as penicillins or cephalosporins
Antidepressants (SSRIs)	First-trimester exposure: Paroxetine may increase risk of some congenital malformations, predominantly congenital heart disease (results not consistent) Third-trimester exposure: Postnatal neurobehavioral effects (long-term effects not known)	Discuss risks and benefits, because risks are low. Consider sertraline as first-line option given good safety profile and low levels secreted in breast milk[74]
Antiepileptics	Valproate: NTDs, facial dysmorphology, autism, atrial septal defect, cleft palate, hypospadias, polydactyly, and craniosynostosis Phenytoin: Risk of fetal hydantoin syndrome, consisting of facial dysmorphology, cleft palate, ventricular septal defect, and growth and mental retardation Carbamazepine: Facial dysmorphology, NTDs, cardiovascular defects, and urinary tract defects	Consult specialist for optimization of medication, including monotherapy and avoidance of valproate[30]
Folic acid antagonists (methotrexate)	Risk of spontaneous abortion, malformations, including microcephaly, meningomyelocele, hydrocephalus, cleft palate, and mental retardation	Women who plan to conceive should discontinue methotrexate and use contraception for at least 3 mo (ideally 6 mo) before conception, with folic acid supplementation[85]

(*continued on next page*)

Table 3
(continued)

Medication	Adverse Effects	Recommendations
Immunosuppressants	Mycophenolate: Miscarriage, abnormalities of the ear, distal limbs, heart, esophagus, kidney, and cleft lip/palate Cyclophosphamide: Inconsistent effect in humans, but may cause malformations	Effective contraception necessary during and for 6 wk to 3 mo after cessation of immunosuppressants[85]
Isotretinoin	Risk of spontaneous abortion and multiple anomalies, including anomalies of the face (facial dysmorphia, cleft palate), central nervous system, and cardiovascular system	Recommend effective contraception and cessation at least 1 mo before attempting conception[86]
Lithium	Low risk of cardiac anomalies, including Ebstein anomaly	Use lowest amount necessary to achieve therapeutic level and consider prenatal cardiac anomaly screening[87]
Nonsteroidal anti-inflammatory drugs (ibuprofen, aspirin)	First trimester: Data on effects not consistent Third trimester: Premature closure of the ductus arteriosus	Avoid use in pregnancy. Alternatives include acetaminophen[85]
Statins (HMG-CoA reductase inhibitors statins)	Decreased cholesterol synthesis may affect fetal development. Animal studies indicate teratogenicity; data in humans are limited	Avoid during pregnancy given paucity of data[88]
Warfarin	Bone and cartilage deformities, mental retardation, and vision problems	Refer to specialist for conversion to heparin or low-molecular-weight heparin[89]

REVIEW OF MEDICATIONS

One in 6 women of reproductive age receive a prescription for a potentially teratogenic medication each year in the United States.[8] Given high unintended pregnancy rates in the United States,[12] education about the potential teratogenic risks of mediations is critical for all women of reproductive age who could become pregnant. Medications with clearly documented teratogenic effects should be avoided in women who desire pregnancy or could become pregnant. For many women, however, medications with some potential teratogenicity also have important benefits, such as psychotropic medications and antiepileptic medications. The benefits of medications with low absolute risk of teratogenicity may outweigh the risks in certain circumstances. Conversations should therefore be individualized and address the risks and benefits of medications to an individual woman. Dietary supplements should also be reviewed with patients to assess for safety in pregnancy, and nonessential supplements without clear safety data should be stopped before attempting conception. **Table 3** includes a list of commonly prescribed medications. Consultation with online resources or experts regarding the risks of medications is recommended (see **Box 1**).

Table 4
Recommendations for additional preconception risk factors

Risk Factor	Adverse Effects	Recommendations
Inadequate folic acid consumption	NTDs and other congenital anomalies	Folic acid supplements: 0.4 mg/d for low-risk women and 4 mg/d for women at high risk for NTDs (previous affected child, on anticonvulsants).[90] Some experts recommend 4–5 mg/d for women at intermediate risk, including insulin-dependent diabetes and obesity[40]
Alcohol use	A continuum of adverse outcomes, including birth defects and developmental disabilities, with fetal alcohol syndrome as the most severe (microcephaly, mental retardation, growth retardation, facial dysmorphogenesis, abnormal ears, small palpebral fissures)	Women should be screened for risky drinking. Brief interventions, including education and motivational interviewing, have been shown to be effective in reducing alcohol-exposed pregnancies in randomized controlled trials[33]
Drug use	Marijuana: Data inconclusive, possible childhood neurodevelopmental effects Cocaine: Low birth weight, prematurity, perinatal death, placental abruption Heroin and other narcotics: Spontaneous abortion, placental insufficiency, preterm birth, intrauterine death	Substance use should be obtained in a screening history. Women should be educated and referred to treatment programs that support abstinence and rehabilitation[91]
Tobacco use	Spontaneous abortion, preterm birth, low birth weight, placental previa, placental abruption, and stillbirth	Women should be screened for tobacco use. Provide brief intervention for smoking cessation (eg, the 5 As) and counseling about pharmacotherapies. Few interventions have been studied in the preconception period, although randomized trials of counseling interventions during pregnancy have demonstrated efficacy.[33,92]

Sexually transmitted diseases	HIV, Hepatitis B, and Hepatitis C: Vertical transmission Syphilis: Spontaneous abortion, fetal hydrops, growth restriction, and congenital syphilis Chlamydia/gonorrhea: Pelvic inflammatory disease and resulting impaired fertility. Neonatal eye infections and pneumonia	Screen according to CDC guidelines, which include annual HIV screening for women engaging in unsafe sex and HIV screening for all women not at increased risk of unsafe sex at least once. Women engaging in unsafe sex and all sexually active women <25 should be screened for chlamydia and gonorrhea annually. Women with risk factors should be vaccinated against hepatitis B per CDC recommendations[93]
Other infection exposures	Toxoplasmosis, cytomegalovirus (CMV), rubella, and varicella: Congenital anomalies. Varicella can cause severe pneumonia in pregnant women Listeria: Spontaneous abortion, preterm labor, neonatal sepsis, meningitis, and fetal death	*No vaccine available—toxoplasmosis, CMV, listeria* Toxoplasmosis: Avoid cat litter, undercooked and raw meats. CMV: Practice frequent hand washing, especially when in contact with children. Listeria: Avoid cold cuts, unpasteurized milk and soft cheeses, and unwashed raw produce. *Vaccine available—rubella and varicella* Women should be screened if immunization status unknown and vaccinated before pregnancy. Avoid pregnancy for 1 mo after vaccination, as both are live vaccines[94]
Environmental exposures	Lead: Spontaneous abortion, birth defects, and impaired fetal growth and neurodevelopment. Mercury: Impaired neurodevelopment including lower IQ and poor language and motor development	Test serum lead levels in woman with exposure history; consult with environmental health specialist as needed. Lead: Avoid potential sources (paint, construction, ceramics). Mercury: Eat low mercury fish (2 servings/wk). Avoid swordfish, shark, king mackerel, and tile fish[95]
Intimate partner violence and reproductive coercion	Intimate partner violence: Maternal depression, poor pregnancy weight gain, substance abuse, infection, low birth rate, preterm birth, perinatal death Reproductive coercion, including birth control sabotage and pregnancy coercion: Increased risk of unintended pregnancy	Screen all women for intimate partner violence and reproductive coercion. Refer women who screen positive to local or state services dedicated to women with IPV[96]

Table 5
Pregnancy history and genetics

Risk Factor	Screening Question	Recommendations
Pregnancy history[97]	In your past pregnancy(s), have you had: a. Recurrent miscarriage b. Low birth weight c. Preterm delivery d. GDM e. Baby with NTD (eg, spina bifida) f. Baby with other birth defects g. Stillbirth	Refer to obstetrician/gynecologist For history of GDM, ensure patient has been screened for type 2 diabetes For women with a history of a NTD, prescribe folic acid 4 mg/d
Genetic disease[98]	Do you have a personal or family history of a. β-thalassemia or α-thalassemia b. Cystic fibrosis c. Sickle cell disease d. Tay-Sachs disease e. Mental retardation or Fragile X syndrome	Refer to obstetrician/gynecologist or genetic counselor

SCREEN FOR ADDITIONAL PRECONCEPTION RISK FACTORS

Many routine preventive health interventions provided by PCPs are important for preventing maternal and fetal complications in addition to promoting overall health. Examples include tobacco use screening and cessation interventions and screening for sexually transmitted diseases and intimate partner violence (IPV). Several preventive interventions are specifically relevant to women contemplating a pregnancy, such as counseling about folic acid supplementation and confirming rubella immunization. **Table 4** presents an overview of recommended interventions with potential impact on maternal and fetal health.

SCREEN FOR PRIOR POOR PREGNANCY OUTCOMES AND GENETIC DISEASE

Women's prior pregnancy history and family history can impact the health of future pregnancies. Although a detailed reproductive and genetic history is outside the scope of many PCPs, brief screening questions can identify women who would benefit from referral to a specialist for preconception evaluation and risk modification. **Table 5** provides a brief list of selected screening questions.

SUMMARY

Few women present to primary care visits requesting preconception care; however, an estimated 10% of US women of reproductive age become pregnant each year.[84] PCPs who care for women have a critical role to play in helping women to identify preconception risks, both modifiable and nonmodifiable, and to make informed decisions about planning pregnancy and contraception. Screening women for their pregnancy intentions and initiating conversations with women about their pregnancy goals are critical first steps in providing preconception counseling and care. Emphasizing the overlap between a woman's own health goals and preconception goals can help empower women to invest jointly in their own long-term health and the health of their future families.

REFERENCES

1. Kassebaum NJ, Bertozzi-Villa A, Coggeshall MS, et al. Global, regional, and national levels and causes of maternal mortality during 1990-2013: a systematic analysis for the Global Burden of Disease Study 2013. Lancet 2014;384(9947): 980–1004.
2. Berg CJ, Callaghan WM, Henderson Z, et al. Pregnancy-related mortality in the United States, 1998 to 2005. Obstet Gynecol 2011;117(5):1230.
3. MacDorman MF, Hoyert DL, Mathews TJ. Recent declines in infant mortality in the United States, 2005-2011. NCHS Data Brief 2013;(120):1–8.
4. Johnson K, Posner SF, Biermann J, et al. Recommendations to improve preconception health and health care–United States. A report of the CDC/ATSDR Preconception Care Work Group and the Select Panel on Preconception Care. MMWR Recomm Rep 2006;55(RR-6):1–23.
5. Floyd RL, Johnson KA, Owens JR, et al. A national action plan for promoting preconception health and health care in the United States (2012-2014). J Womens Health (Larchmt) 2013;22(10):797–802.
6. Williams JL, Abelman SM, Fassett EM, et al. Health care provider knowledge and practices regarding folic acid, United States, 2002-2003. Matern Child Health J 2006;10(Suppl 5):S67–72.
7. Chuang CH, Hwang SW, McCall-Hosenfeld JS, et al. Primary care physicians' perceptions of barriers to preventive reproductive health care in rural communities. Perspect Sex Reprod Health 2012;44(2):78–83.
8. Schwarz EB, Maselli J, Norton M, et al. Prescription of teratogenic medications in United States ambulatory practices. Am J Med 2005;118(11):1240–9.
9. Dunlop AL, Logue KM, Thorne C, et al. Change in women's knowledge of general and personal preconception health risks following targeted brief counseling in publicly funded primary care settings. Am J Health Promot 2013;27(Suppl 3): S50–7.
10. Frey KA, Files JA. Preconception healthcare: what women know and believe. Matern Child Health J 2006;10(Suppl 5):S73–7.
11. Schwarz EB, Sobota M, Gonzales R, et al. Computerized counseling for folate knowledge and use: a randomized controlled trial. Am J Prev Med 2008;35(6): 568–71.
12. Finer LB, Zolna MR. Shifts in intended and unintended pregnancies in the United States, 2001-2008. Am J Public Health 2014;104(Suppl 1):S43–8.
13. Dunlop AL, Jack B, Frey K. National recommendations for preconception care: the essential role of the family physician. J Am Board Fam Med 2007;20(1):81–4.
14. American College of Obstetricians and Gynecologists. ACOG Committee Opinion number 313, September 2005. The importance of preconception care in the continuum of women's health care. Obstet Gynecol 2005;106(3):665–6.
15. Borrero S, Nikolajski C, Steinberg JR, et al. "It just happens": A qualitative study exploring low-income women's perspectives on pregnancy intention and planning. Contraception 2015;91(2):150–6.
16. Callegari LS, Nelson K, Borrero S, et al. Integrating reproductive planning into VA primary care: a qualitative study of acceptability to women Veterans. Arlington (VA): Abstract presentation at the VA Health Services Research & Development (HSR&D). National Meeting on Partnerships for Research & Care of Women Veterans. July 2014.
17. Before, between and beyond toolkit. Available at: http://beforeandbeyond.org/toolkit/reproductive-life-plan-assessment/. Accessed September 27, 2014.

18. Cleary-Goldman J, Malone FD, Vidaver J, et al. Impact of maternal age on obstetric outcome. Obstet Gynecol 2005;105(5 Pt 1):983–90.
19. Conde-Agudelo A, Rosas-Bermudez A, Kafury-Goeta AC. Birth spacing and risk of adverse perinatal outcomes: a meta-analysis. JAMA 2006;295(15):1809–23.
20. Bello JK, Adkins K, Stulberg DB, et al. Perceptions of a reproductive health self-assessment tool (RH-SAT) in an urban community health center. Patient Educ Couns 2013;93(3):655–63.
21. Dunlop AL, Logue KM, Miranda MC, et al. Integrating reproductive planning with primary health care: an exploration among low-income, minority women and men. Sex Reprod Healthc 2010;1(2):37–43.
22. Squiers L, Mitchell EW, Levis DM, et al. Consumers' perceptions of preconception health. Am J Health Promot 2013;27(Suppl 3):S10–9.
23. Lawrence JM, Contreras R, Chen W, et al. Trends in the prevalence of preexisting diabetes and gestational diabetes mellitus among a racially/ethnically diverse population of pregnant women, 1999-2005. Diabetes Care 2008;31(5):899–904.
24. Greene MF. Spontaneous abortions and major malformations in women with diabetes mellitus. Semin Reprod Endocrinol 1999;17(2):127–36.
25. Kitzmiller JL, Buchanan TA, Kjos S, et al. Pre-conception care of diabetes, congenital malformations, and spontaneous abortions. Diabetes Care 1996; 19(5):514–41.
26. Ray JG, Vermeulen MJ, Shapiro JL, et al. Maternal and neonatal outcomes in pregestational and gestational diabetes mellitus, and the influence of maternal obesity and weight gain: the DEPOSIT study. Diabetes Endocrine Pregnancy Outcome Study in Toronto. QJM 2001;94(7):347–56.
27. Verheijen EC, Critchley JA, Whitelaw DC, et al. Outcomes of pregnancies in women with pre-existing type 1 or type 2 diabetes, in an ethnically mixed population. BJOG 2005;112(11):1500–3.
28. Jensen DM, Korsholm L, Ovesen P, et al. Peri-conceptional A1C and risk of serious adverse pregnancy outcome in 933 women with type 1 diabetes. Diabetes Care 2009;32(6):1046–8.
29. Clausen TD, Mathiesen ER, Hansen T, et al. Overweight and the metabolic syndrome in adult offspring of women with diet-treated gestational diabetes mellitus or type 1 diabetes. J Clin Endocrinol Metab 2009;94(7):2464–70.
30. Dunlop AL, Jack BW, Bottalico JN, et al. The clinical content of preconception care: women with chronic medical conditions. Am J Obstet Gynecol 2008; 199(6 Suppl 2):S310–27.
31. Wahabi HA, Alzeidan RA, Bawazeer GA, et al. Preconception care for diabetic women for improving maternal and fetal outcomes: a systematic review and meta-analysis. BMC Pregnancy Childbirth 2010;10:63.
32. Tieu J, Middleton P, Crowther CA. Preconception care for diabetic women for improving maternal and infant health. Cochrane Database Syst Rev 2010;(12):CD007776.
33. Shannon GD, Alberg C, Nacul L, et al. Preconception healthcare and congenital disorders: systematic review of the effectiveness of preconception care programs in the prevention of congenital disorders. Matern Child Health J 2014; 18:1354–79.
34. Ray JG, O'Brien TE, Chan WS. Preconception care and the risk of congenital anomalies in the offspring of women with diabetes mellitus: a meta-analysis. QJM 2001;94(8):435–44.
35. American Diabetes Association. Standards of medical care in diabetes–2014. Diabetes Care 2014;37(Suppl 1):S14–80.

36. Kitzmiller JL, Block JM, Brown FM, et al. Managing preexisting diabetes for pregnancy: summary of evidence and consensus recommendations for care. Diabetes Care 2008;31(5):1060–79.
37. ACOG Practice Bulletin. Clinical Management Guidelines for Obstetrician-Gynecologists. Number 60, March 2005. Pregestational diabetes mellitus. Obstet Gynecol 2005;105(3):675–85.
38. Cassina M, Dona M, Di Gianantonio E, et al. First-trimester exposure to metformin and risk of birth defects: a systematic review and meta-analysis. Hum Reprod Update 2014;20(5):656–69.
39. Bullo M, Tschumi S, Bucher BS, et al. Pregnancy outcome following exposure to angiotensin-converting enzyme inhibitors or angiotensin receptor antagonists: a systematic review. Hypertension 2012;60(2):444–50.
40. Wilson RD, Johnson JA, Wyatt P, et al. Pre-conceptional vitamin/folic acid supplementation 2007: the use of folic acid in combination with a multivitamin supplement for the prevention of neural tube defects and other congenital anomalies. J Obstet Gynaecol Can 2007;29(12):1003–26.
41. Parker SE, Yazdy MM, Tinker SC, et al. The impact of folic acid intake on the association among diabetes mellitus, obesity, and spina bifida. Am J Obstet Gynecol 2013;209(3):239.e1–8.
42. Curtis KM, Jamieson DJ, Peterson HB, et al. Adaptation of the World Health Organization's medical eligibility criteria for contraceptive use for use in the United States. Contraception 2010;82(1):3–9.
43. Bateman BT, Shaw KM, Kuklina EV, et al. Hypertension in women of reproductive age in the United States: NHANES 1999-2008. PLoS One 2012;7(4):e36171.
44. Bramham K, Parnell B, Nelson-Piercy C, et al. Chronic hypertension and pregnancy outcomes: systematic review and meta-analysis. BMJ 2014;348:g2301.
45. American College of Obstetricians and Gynecologists, Task Force on Hypertension in Pregnancy. Hypertension in pregnancy. Report of the American College of Obstetricians and Gynecologists' task force on hypertension in pregnancy. Obstet Gynecol 2013;122(5):1122–31.
46. Report of the National High Blood Pressure Education Program Working Group on High Blood Pressure in Pregnancy. Am J Obstet Gynecol 2000;183(1):S1–22.
47. Bushnell C, McCullough LD, Awad IA, et al. Guidelines for the prevention of stroke in women: a statement for healthcare professionals from the American Heart Association/American Stroke Association. Stroke 2014;45(5):1545–88.
48. Flegal KM, Carroll MD, Kit BK, et al. Prevalence of obesity and trends in the distribution of body mass index among US adults, 1999-2010. JAMA 2012;307(5):491–7.
49. Robinson HE, O'Connell CM, Joseph KS, et al. Maternal outcomes in pregnancies complicated by obesity. Obstet Gynecol 2005;106(6):1357–64.
50. McDonald SD, Han Z, Mulla S, et al. Overweight and obesity in mothers and risk of preterm birth and low birth weight infants: systematic review and meta-analyses. BMJ 2010;341:c3428.
51. Wuntakal R, Hollingworth T. The implications of obesity on pregnancy. Obstet Gynaecol Reprod Med 2009;19(12):344–9.
52. Stothard KJ, Tennant PW, Bell R, et al. Maternal overweight and obesity and the risk of congenital anomalies: a systematic review and meta-analysis. JAMA 2009;301(6):636–50.
53. Gaillard R, Durmus B, Hofman A, et al. Risk factors and outcomes of maternal obesity and excessive weight gain during pregnancy. Obesity (Silver Spring) 2013;21(5):1046–55.

54. Jungheim ES, Moley KH. Current knowledge of obesity's effects in the pre- and periconceptional periods and avenues for future research. Am J Obstet Gynecol 2010;203(6):525–30.
55. American College of Obstetricians and Gynecologists. ACOG Committee opinion no. 549: obesity in pregnancy. Obstet Gynecol 2013;121(1):213–7.
56. Viswanathan M, Siega-Riz AM, Moos MK, et al. Outcomes of maternal weight gain. Evid Rep Technol Assess (Full Rep) 2008;(168):1–223.
57. Moos MK, Dunlop AL, Jack BW, et al. Healthier women, healthier reproductive outcomes: recommendations for the routine care of all women of reproductive age. Am J Obstet Gynecol 2008;199(6 Suppl 2):S280–9.
58. Ostbye T, Krause KM, Lovelady CA, et al. Active Mothers Postpartum: a randomized controlled weight-loss intervention trial. Am J Prev Med 2009;37(3):173–80.
59. Hoedjes M, Berks D, Vogel I, et al. Effect of postpartum lifestyle interventions on weight loss, smoking cessation, and prevention of smoking relapse: a systematic review. Obstet Gynecol Surv 2010;65(10):631–52.
60. Amorim AR, Linne YM, Lourenco PM. Diet or exercise, or both, for weight reduction in women after childbirth. Cochrane Database Syst Rev 2007;(3): CD005627. Available at: http://onlinelibrary.wiley.com/doi/10.1002/14651858.CD005627.pub2/abstract.
61. Getahun D, Kaminsky LM, Elsasser DA, et al. Changes in prepregnancy body mass index between pregnancies and risk of primary cesarean delivery. Am J Obstet Gynecol 2007;197(4):376.e1–7.
62. Whiteman VE, McIntosh C, Rao K, et al. Interpregnancy BMI change and risk of primary caesarean delivery. J Obstet Gynaecol 2011;31(7):589–93.
63. Villamor E, Cnattingius S. Interpregnancy weight change and risk of adverse pregnancy outcomes: a population-based study. Lancet 2006;368(9542):1164–70.
64. Jain AP, Gavard JA, Rice JJ, et al. The impact of interpregnancy weight change on birthweight in obese women. Am J Obstet Gynecol 2013;208:205.e1–7.
65. Callegari LS, Sterling LA, Zelek ST, et al. Interpregnancy body mass index change and success of term vaginal birth after cesarean delivery. Am J Obstet Gynecol 2014;210(4):330.e1–7.
66. Ehrlich SF, Hedderson MM, Feng J, et al. Change in body mass index between pregnancies and the risk of gestational diabetes in a second pregnancy. Obstet Gynecol 2011;117(6):1323–30.
67. Kushner RF, Ryan DH. Assessment and lifestyle management of patients with obesity: clinical recommendations from systematic reviews. JAMA 2014;312(9): 943–52.
68. Ryan D, Heaner M. Guidelines (2013) for managing overweight and obesity in adults. Preface to the full report. Obesity (Silver Spring) 2014;22(Suppl 2):S1–3.
69. Beard JH, Bell RL, Duffy AJ. Reproductive considerations and pregnancy after bariatric surgery: current evidence and recommendations. Obes Surg 2008; 18(8):1023–7.
70. Poitou Bernert C, Ciangura C, Coupaye M, et al. Nutritional deficiency after gastric bypass: diagnosis, prevention and treatment. Diabetes Metab 2007;33(1):13–24.
71. Guelinckx I, Devlieger R, Vansant G. Reproductive outcome after bariatric surgery: a critical review. Hum Reprod Update 2009;15(2):189–201.
72. Weissman MM, Olfson M. Depression in women: implications for health care research. Science 1995;269(5225):799–801.
73. Gaynes BN, Gavin N, Meltzer-Brody S, et al. Perinatal depression: prevalence, screening accuracy, and screening outcomes. Evid Rep Technol Assess (Full Rep) 2005;(119):1–8.

74. Yonkers KA, Wisner KL, Stewart DE, et al. The management of depression during pregnancy: a report from the American Psychiatric Association and the American College of Obstetricians and Gynecologists. Obstet Gynecol 2009;114(3):703–13.
75. Grote NK, Bridge JA, Gavin AR, et al. A meta-analysis of depression during pregnancy and the risk of preterm birth, low birth weight, and intrauterine growth restriction. Arch Gen Psychiatry 2010;67(10):1012–24.
76. Frieder A, Dunlop AL, Culpepper L, et al. The clinical content of preconception care: women with psychiatric conditions. Am J Obstet Gynecol 2008;199(6 Suppl 2):S328–32.
77. Ross LE, McLean LM. Anxiety disorders during pregnancy and the postpartum period: a systematic review. J Clin Psychiatry 2006;67(8):1285–98.
78. Ding XX, Wu YL, Xu SJ, et al. Maternal anxiety during pregnancy and adverse birth outcomes: a systematic review and meta-analysis of prospective cohort studies. J Affect Disord 2014;159:103–10.
79. Ross LE, Grigoriadis S, Mamisashvili L, et al. Selected pregnancy and delivery outcomes after exposure to antidepressant medication: a systematic review and meta-analysis. JAMA Psychiatry 2013;70(4):436–43.
80. Greene MF. Teratogenicity of SSRIs–serious concern or much ado about little? N Engl J Med 2007;356(26):2732–3.
81. Palmsten K, Setoguchi S, Margulis AV, et al. Elevated risk of preeclampsia in pregnant women with depression: depression or antidepressants? Am J Epidemiol 2012;175(10):988–97.
82. Fortinguerra F, Clavenna A, Bonati M. Psychotropic drug use during breastfeeding: a review of the evidence. Pediatrics 2009;124(4):e547–56.
83. Witt WP, Wisk LE, Cheng ER, et al. Poor prepregnancy and antepartum mental health predicts postpartum mental health problems among US women: a nationally representative population-based study. Womens Health Issues 2011;21(4): 304–13.
84. Curtin SC, Abma JC, Ventura SJ, et al. Pregnancy rates for U.S. women continue to drop. NCHS Data Brief 2013;(136):1–8.
85. Ostensen M, Khamashta M, Lockshin M, et al. Anti-inflammatory and immunosuppressive drugs and reproduction. Arthritis Res Ther 2006;8(3):209.
86. Cragan JD, Friedman JM, Holmes LB, et al. Ensuring the safe and effective use of medications during pregnancy: planning and prevention through preconception care. Matern Child Health J 2006;10(Suppl 5):S129–35.
87. Burt VK, Bernstein C, Rosenstein WS, et al. Bipolar disorder and pregnancy: maintaining psychiatric stability in the real world of obstetric and psychiatric complications. Am J Psychiatry 2010;167(8):892–7.
88. Godfrey LM, Erramouspe J, Cleveland KW. Teratogenic risk of statins in pregnancy. Ann Pharmacother 2012;46(10):1419–24.
89. Dunlop AL, Gardiner PM, Shellhaas CS, et al. The clinical content of preconception care: the use of medications and supplements among women of reproductive age. Am J Obstet Gynecol 2008;199(6 Suppl 2):S367–72.
90. Cheschier N. ACOG practice bulletin. Neural tube defects. Number 44, July 2003. (Replaces committee opinion number 252, March 2001). Int J Gynaecol Obstet 2003;83(1):123–33.
91. Floyd RL, Jack BW, Cefalo R, et al. The clinical content of preconception care: alcohol, tobacco, and illicit drug exposures. Int J Gynaecol Obstet 2008;199(6 Suppl 2):S333–9.
92. Temel S, van Voorst SF, Jack BW, et al. Evidence-based preconceptional lifestyle interventions. Epidemiol Rev 2014;36(1):19–30.

93. Workowski KA, Berman S. Sexually transmitted diseases treatment guidelines, 2010. MMWR Recomm Rep 2010;59(RR-12):1–110.
94. Coonrod DV, Jack BW, Stubblefield PG, et al. The clinical content of preconception care: infectious diseases in preconception care. Am J Obstet Gynecol 2008; 199(6 Suppl 2):S296–309.
95. Sathyanarayana S, Focareta J, Dailey T, et al. Environmental exposures: how to counsel preconception and prenatal patients in the clinical setting. Am J Obstet Gynecol 2012;207(6):463–70.
96. ACOG Committee Opinion No. 518: intimate partner violence. Obstet Gynecol 2012;119(2 Pt 1):412–7.
97. Stubblefield PG, Coonrod DV, Reddy UM, et al. The clinical content of preconception care: reproductive history. Am J Obstet Gynecol 2008;199(6 Suppl 2): S373–83.
98. Solomon BD, Jack BW, Feero WG. The clinical content of preconception care: genetics and genomics. Am J Obstet Gynecol 2008;199(6 Suppl 2):S340–4.

Index

Note: Page numbers of article titles are in **boldface** type.

Med Clin N Am 99 (2015) 683–690
http://dx.doi.org/10.1016/S0025-7125(15)00057-7 medical.theclinics.com

G

H

I

O

W